# PROGRESS IN BRAIN RESEARCH

## VOLUME 33

## COMPUTERS AND BRAINS

# PROGRESS IN BRAIN RESEARCH

# PROGRESS IN BRAIN RESEARCH

## VOLUME 33

# COMPUTERS AND BRAINS

EDITED BY

## J. P. SCHADÉ

AND

## J. SMITH

*Central Institute for Brain Research,*
*IJdijk 28, Amsterdam (The Netherlands)*

## ELSEVIER PUBLISHING COMPANY

AMSTERDAM / LONDON / NEW YORK

1970

ELSEVIER PUBLISHING COMPANY
335 JAN VAN GALENSTRAAT,
P.O. BOX 211, AMSTERDAM, THE NETHERLANDS

ELSEVIER PUBLISHING CO. LTD.
BARKING, ESSEX, ENGLAND

AMERICAN ELSEVIER PUBLISHING COMPANY, INC.
52 VANDERBILT AVENUE, NEW YORK, N.Y. 10017

LIBRARY OF CONGRESS CATALOG CARD NUMBER 70-110965

ISBN 0-444-40855-x

PRINTED IN THE NETHERLANDS

# List of Contributors

W. R. ADEY, Departments of Anatomy and Physiology, Space Biology Laboratory, Brain Research Institute, University of California, Los Angeles, U.S.A.

J. L. BLOM, Netherlands Central Institute for Brain Research and Mathematical Center, Amsterdam, The Netherlands.

E. J. COLON, Central Institute for Brain Research, Amsterdam, The Netherlands.

F. A. DODGE, JR., IBM Thomas J. Watson Research Center, Yorktown Heights, New York, U.S.A.

H. FALLON, IBM Systems Development Division, Yorktown Heights, N.Y., U.S.A.

D. GARFINKEL, Johnson Research Foundation, University of Pennsylvania, Philadelphia, Penna. 19104 U.S.A.

G. GOERTZEL IBM Advanced Systems Development Division, Yorktown Heights, N.Y., U.S.A.

H. HAUG, Department of Anatomy, University of Hamburg, Germany.

R. E. JENSEN, International Medical Support Center, IBM Svenska A.b., Stockholm, Sweden.

E. A. KOLDENHOF, IBM-Netherlands, Amsterdam, The Netherlands.

G. E. MARLER, IBM, Advanced Systems Development Division, Yorktown Heights, N.Y., U.S.A.

A. R. MØLLER, Department of Physiology, Karolinska Institutet, Stockholm, Sweden.

J. OOSTERHOFF, Netherlands Central Institute for Brain Research and Mathematical Center, Amsterdam, The Netherlands.

J. P. C. PEPERKAMP, Central Institute for Brain Research, IJdijk 28, Amsterdam, The Netherlands.

H. PETSCHE, Neurological Institute of the University, Vienna, Austria.

R. W. PULVER, IBM Advanced Systems Development Division, Yorktown Heights, N.Y., U.S.A.

J. P. SCHADÉ, Central Institute for Brain Research, IJdijk 28, Amsterdam, The Netherlands.

G. J. SMIT, Central Institute for Brain Research, IJdijk 28, Amsterdam, The Netherlands.

J. SMITH, Central Institute for Brain Research, IJdijk 28, Amsterdam, The Netherlands.

J. C. DE VALOIS, Central Institute for Brain Research, IJdijk 28, Amsterdam, The Netherlands.

R. WIGGERS, Netherlands Central Institute for Brain Research and Mathematical Center, Amsterdam, The Netherlands.

H. VAN WILGENBURG, Central Institute for Brain Research, IJdijk 28, Amsterdam, The Netherlands.

*Other volumes in this series:*

PROGRESS IN BRAIN RESEARCH

Volume 17: *Cybernetics of the Nervous System*
Edited by Norbert Wiener† and J. P. Schadé

Volume 18: *Sleep Mechanisms*
Edited by K. Akert, Ch. Bally and J. P. Schadé

Volume 19: *Experimental Epilepsy*
by A. Kreindler

Volume 20: *Pharmacology and Physiology of the Reticular Formation*
Edited by A. V. Valdman

Volume 21A: *Correlative Neurosciences. Part A: Fundamental Mechanisms*
Edited by T. Tokizane and J. P. Schadé

Volume 21B: *Correlative Neurosciences. Part B: Clinical Studies*
Edited by T. Tokizane and J. P. Schadé

Volume 22: *Brain Reflexes*
Edited by E. A. Asratyan

Volume 23: *Sensory Mechanisms*
Edited by Y. Zotterman

Volume 24: *Carbon Monoxide Poisoning*
Edited bij H. Bour and I. McA. Ledingham

Volume 25: *The Cerebellum*
Edited by C. A. Fox and R. S. Snider

Volume 26: *Developmental Neurology*
Edited by C. G. Bernhard

Volume 27: *Structure and Function of the Limbic System*
Edited by W. Ross Adey and T. Tokizane

Volume 28: *Anticholinergic Drugs*
Edited by P. B. Bradley and M. Fink

Volume 29: *Brain Barrier Systems*
Edited by A. Lajtha and D. H. Ford

Volume 30: *Cerebral Circulation*
Edited by W. Luyendijk

Volume 31: *Mechanisms of Synaptic Transmission*
Edited by K. Akert and P. G. Waser

Volume 32: *Pituitary, Adrenal and the Brain*
Edited by D. de Wied and J. A. W. M. Weijnen

# Preface

The understanding of processing and storage of information in the nervous system depends upon a thorough insight into the structure and function of the neurons. Since the brain processes both properties of digital and analogue computers, a comparison between the function and structure of brains and computers may shed more light on how the human mind functions.

This was the theme of a workshop, sponsored by the Netherlands Government, the NATO Advanced Study Institute Programme, and I.B.M.

The participants originated from various disciplines, and one of the main goals of the organizing committee was to stimulate a cross fertilization between the computer sciences and the brain sciences.

Concise reviews by leading scientists on recent developments in the computer and brain sciences, as well as specialized reports on the computer analysis of specific neurobiological problems are gathered together in this volume.

J. P. Schadé

# Contents

# Brain–Computer Relationships

R. E. JENSEN

*International Medical Support Center, IBM Svenska A.b., Stockholm (Sweden)*

A knowledge of the structure, the function, and the behavior of computers is important for an understanding of how they can best be utilized in various applications of the fields of biology and medicine.

There is much discussion about the behavior of computers and their capabilities. On one hand, they are considered only as calculators or adding machines which can do arithmetic calculations very rapidly; on the other hand, they sometimes are thought of as having magical powers, of giving some information which is above and beyond that which we can otherwise get, like the oracle on the mountain. Obviously the true meaning in utilization of computers lies somewhere in between these extremes. This is the area which needs to be defined in more specific detail.

Within the field of neurophysiology, it is very tempting to discuss this definition of computers in terms of physiology, anatomy, and perhaps psychology. However, this would lead to philosophical discussions and enter into such areas as whether computers think, which is not the purpose of this paper. Nevertheless, drawing certain parallels between the operation of the central nervous system and the operation of computers will perhaps give a better understanding of just how they differ, and how best computers can be used as an aid to extending man's intellectual capabilities. The major thing that needs to be done for better understanding is to improve the man–machine interaction in order to make more intelligent use of computers. It is much the same as the problem of making intelligent use of human beings. In the study of the central nervous system, investigators are trying to learn more about the underlying mechanisms of the nervous system in order to better understand human behavior. In the computer area engineers and mathematicians have designed certain machines to make certain calculations, so one knows the mechanisms quite well. Now one must search for ways to better use these techniques that have already been developed. At the same time, there is a parallel between finding new mechanisms in the central nervous system and applying these techniques to the evolution of the computer.

In history, mankind first had mechanical devices to aid in overcoming natural obstacles of labor, for example, the wheel, and now many examples of machinery. Later there were devices for extension of the senses which were and are particularly useful in the investigative and scientific areas, for example, the microscope. Many other instruments have allowed us to extend our sensory perception to gather greater amounts of detailed information. The advent of the computer is an extension of this process, now providing additional aid to our brain power and intellectual ability. The computer is useful particularly in taking care of the routine sort of intellectual processes, so that man is allowed to devote more time to the things which can be done most effectively by human brainpower. The computer can be used to control machinery and correlate the sensory instrument data, as well as to store information for later recall.

Based on this general introduction, one must now consider the taxonomy of computers because there are many different kinds, which are commonly thrown together in a general classification called "computers".

Like the general trend through mechanics and electronics of our other aids for labor and senses, computers also started out as primarily mechanical devices. Many of the calculators and adding machines that are used are mechanical. The big steps in the evolution of computing devices has been the use of electronics. However, we still speak of computers as machines.

There are a number of diverse categories that are included in the class of computers or computing machines. The first computers were called calculators, reflecting their primary arithmetical role. More recently, the concept of information machines has developed, which is a broader category emphasizing that information other than numbers can be handled. An extension of this is work concerned with machines with so-called artificial intelligence. One can see the trend here between a machine that only adds and subtracts to one that may be doing more in the area of aiding our intellectual processes, that is, enabling us to understand problems. Another major category of computers is simulators, sometimes called automata or automation machines where there is control of other devices by means of a computing type element.

Most of these devices generally go under the heading "computer", which means by definition essentially the calculator part. Modern computers may more accurately be called computer systems because they combine a number of functions in their operation using various computer elements, storage, input and output devices, some mechanical and some electronic.

Among these various type of computers one can define two types of methods which are used for the processing of data. There are analogue computers and digital computers. A particular system may include various analogue elements, digital elements or the combination in terms of a hybrid computer system. The brain can be said to operate as the analogue of a hybrid system.

What is the major difference between computers that are called analogue and those called digital? The term "analogue", means essentially an analogue or a model of a particular process. Many computers do exactly that. They can be very small or very large depending on the complexity of the model. More basically, analogue computers are those that take measurements for continuous analyses of data. In the electronic computer they use measurements of voltage as their active means of processing data. In the "digital" computer (the term coming from counting on the fingers) the technique is to count, which is a discrete type of operation rather than a continuous one. Both of these techniques (analogue and digital) have their role in the processing of data. In some cases the analogue techniques are faster and allow one an easier continuous manipulation of the data. In other cases, the digital computer, which has a much higher precision, is the one of choice. And finally more and more there is the tendency to combine the analogue and digital processes in a single system in order to make use of the advantage of both. The growing use of analogue to digital and digital to analogue converters in the biomedical area is an example of this trend. One can see the parallels with the central nervous system of both analogue field effects and the digital all-or-none impulses which combine together in the data processing sense. These are also the two basic mechanisms which allow the various types of computers to operate and give the required results.

The major question still not answered as yet is why modern computers are becoming more than adding machines or more than simple models of the process that we want to study. One might again look at the evolution of computers, which has been particularly rapid over the past twenty years, to see at what transition points the operation of computers have become more meaningful in the sense of assisting us in making decisions. The mechanical computers were developed, even in the 1600's, and particularly in the 1800's various analytical machines and devices with gears and wheels could be used to calculate very complex mathematical expressions. They were not in the same class as the machines that we have now, but in a sense did much the same thing in terms of adding. It was not really until we came along with the electronic techniques that we were able to make an enormous jump in the capabilities of the computing machine.

The first major step in computer evolution was electronics and then the further developments in electronics, particularly the transistor techniques for making the small core memories and most recently solid state circuits. These technological developments in the electronics area, coming over the past 10 or 15 years, have been major evolutionary steps leading already to the three generations of computers.

In addition to the evolution of hardware another path, which is probably even more significant, is development of the concept of a stored program in the computer which is modifiable by the user or the computer. The computer needs the right programs and rules so that it can carry out the particular operations that need to be accomplished. In the digital computer these instructions are stored in the same form as the data, and because of this they can be modified in the same way as the data by still other instructions. One now has not only a system which remembers its instructions but also can change those instructions depending upon the input data as well as the answers to various questions that may come into the system. This also points out the fact that the memory capability of computers is one of their very essential parts and computers get more and more useful, in general, as the size of their memory for instructions and data increases. Early computers had very small memories compared with present systems.

Another evolutionary factor which has come along in the last ten years is the languages for the user to communicate with computers. Earlier computers had to be communicated with in the basic language of the computer which not only involved the operator's learning the details of operation of computers but also involved the time and complexity of actually setting down large amounts of instructions. This would be rather like setting up a series of electronic pulses in order to get a particular reaction from a person instead of telling him in a general language what to do. Over the past ten years more and more effort has been devoted to building up a library of stored programs or instruction sets in the computer and then telling the system, using more concise language, which instruction set to use in this library.

Further evolution rests very much on this communication problem between man and the computer which is one of the most important in the use of computers. The problem is to tell the computer how to give the required answer in the shortest possible time.

As a result of having a stored program in memory a computer can aid in decisions as well as doing addition, subtraction and other mathematical manipulations. Digital computers have the ability to test a result and to do something different on the basis of the result of the test. There is therefore the ability to make a decision based upon the result of any mathematical operation. With adding machines and calculators certain sets of data are put in, the result is given back and then a decision is made by the user on whether to analyze another set of data. The capability of modern data processing is that this already can be in the computer as part of the program. Based upon the results of calculations it proceeds automatically to the next step. The program itself selects the various alternatives.

The above examples show the major ways computers and the techniques in using them are evolving. By understanding these trends, computers can be more efficiently used now as well as planned for in the future with regard to their impact on medical science.

In order to better understand how computers have evolved to carry out these basic functions one may go into more detail as far as the morphology, the anatomy, or the "hardware" structure of the system to give a better feeling of what the modern digital computer actually consists of. Then, one can relate the physiology or functioning of this hardware and finally consider how best to communicate with this computer to solve particular problems.

Again there are certain parallels between the operation of the central nervous system and computers which help one to understand what sort of problems are very difficult for computers and perhaps easy for people, and also those which are very difficult for people, but easy for computers. This is of specific importance in utilizing computers in the most efficient and optimal fashion. By understanding the structural and functional mechanisms of computers, one can do this. The surface has barely been scratched in utilizing modern computers the way they can and should be used, the way that they have the capability of being used. Certainly the hardware, the technology itself, is way beyond what has been utilized so far as being able to tell it what to do in the right instructions and programs. Indeed the technology is still rapidly developing with newer techniques of operating on the data and making its utilization easier.

The structure and function of the digital computer will be discussed here because it is the one that has particularly the characteristics mentioned above, *i.e.*, the ability to make decisions.

The heart of the computer is called the central processing unit or CPU. The central processing unit essentially just moves data in, adds it together and puts information back out into the same or another area in the computer memory according to instructions. Consequently the central processor works intimately with the core storage memory of the computer.

This memory storage is also called the high speed memory, because there are other ways of storing information for computer processing which the CPU can use at slower speeds. The basic units of the core memory of the computer which gives it its name are iron cores which are little rings. One might think of the analogue of their being the "neurons" of the computer.

The size of these cores is approximately the size of the head of a pin, consequently large number of such units can be packaged in a small volume. This has been one of the main factors in miniaturization of computer systems. The way the memory cores function is by being polarized either in one direction or in another direction, depending upon the impulse of the pair of intersecting wires which are threaded through a core ring. A string or set of these cores, representing a computer word will then store a pattern of polarization or on-off state which can represent a number or instruction. Another wire can read the sequential state of these rings to bring the information out of storage.

In the typical large computer, there are millions of these small core units. The cost of a digital computer is directly related to the number of memory units. A small computer typically has a core storage that is 4000 or 8000 computer words while large ones have 500 000 and more. Each word is made up of 8 or 16 core units. Each unit holds a bit as related to the word or byte.

The major factors determining the capability of the computer are the core memory capacity and the speed with which the central processing unit moves information in and out of storage.

In addition to these particular high speed core memory units which can be used in fractions of micro-seconds, there are slower types of information banks in most computer systems which can hold even more information, for example a hundred million or more different words. These include disks, drums, and tape drives. These so-called peripheral storage units can be used in milliseconds or seconds by the CPU to transfer data and instructions into the high speed memory when the program and activities demand.

In addition to the central processing unit and the memory storage units, a system which makes up a modern computer must have means to get information into the computer and back out, that is input and output communication with the user and outside world. This is information communicated to or from the computer in terms of pulses being present or not present. An early method of input which is still a primary means of entering information into the core storage was to set up a series of pulses by means of holes in a punch card representing a number or letter. Everyone is familiar with punch cards. There are many ways to communicate with or enter information into the computer, but this one is basic and illustrates the principle of all methods.

The basic type of computer output is the typewriter, either in its common form or as a high speed printing mechanism. Here the computer is programmed to output a series of pulses which will convert into graphs, numbers and words readable by the user on the printed page.

There is more and more use of terminals to communicate with the system. They are used either remotely or locally to enter the data and the programs. The ease of terminal operation is illustrated by the fact that terminals may appear the same to the user whether he is communicating to another person or to a computer. A variety of functions and displays are now included on terminals.

One must also consider input or entry of analogue types of information as well as digital. Of particular interest are the systems where one can enter analogue information for digital processing and use the decision-making characteristics of the digital computer to come to conclusions about the data. Analogue or graphic output is also commonly used in many scientific areas.

In many respects, the most important function of the computer system is to prepare the results of the processing for the user in the output units. The display unit is the part of the system which communicates most directly with the user.

To summarize the structure of the computer, one should remember that it is a system including a central processor, a memory and appropriate devices for input and output.

The useful functional advantages of computers are in many respects due to their speed. The computer can do millions of operations per second; for example, decisions. It can decide whether a number is larger than another number and can do multiplications, additions, etc., at this rate. It does this generally in a serial fashion, in other words: one calculation or decision after another. Compared with the central nervous system which may comparably operate at about 10 decisions per second, it is obvious that the computer can do certain things much more rapidly than man can.

On the other hand, the brain uses more parallel processing in contrast to the serial sequential operation of the computer. For example, it can rapidly take in perhaps a million pieces of information in one picture. The brain can therefore do rapid parallel processing, but cannot do the rapid serial processing which the computer can do. The computer has difficulty in handling problems like looking at pictures and analyzing patterns of various types, even though it can be very rapid in terms of doing sequential calculations where one needs the answer to one question before going on to the next. On all problems the computer uses a very simple method by always looking at all possible alternatives where the brain may use guesses and approximations. The computer can arrive at more accurate results because of its high speed. However, for some problems where high accuracy is not required it is slow compared to the brain. As an example of how the brain may function differently than the computer for multiplying it generally adds and adds and adds and instead of looking up in its memory bank for a multiplication table as one does when usually doing multiplications, the computer can look things up in tables but it does not do this as efficiently.

An example of how a computer functions and how newer developments in computer use are perhaps affecting its method of operation is given by having a computer play a chess game. The standard way a computer would be programmed for chess is that on every possible move it must examine every other possibility, including moving off the board. This adds up to many combinations on each possible move. It can do this very rapidly, but it is doing it in an obviously very inefficient way compared with the way that the brain attacks this particular pattern problem. There have been a number of developments along the lines of stating the problem to the computer on a basis of looking for the most probable moves that might have the best chance of success in the next set of combinations, and this is a way of perhaps coming closer to the way the brain does it. However, the brain is not as precise as it comes up with probabilistic answers. The computer can be programmed to handle many variables simultaneously, while the brain has difficulty with more than two.

A major problem still remains, that of telling the computer what to do or outlining the rules it should follow to get a specific result from its input data. In a sense this is the same as the problem in writing a course and teaching a student how to carry out a particular operation. It not only involves teaching him by giving him a set of rules, but one has to define what the set of rules should be, and the course structure itself. In many computer applications it is often experienced that after studying the system design concerning the problem of how to tell a computer the way to carry out an operation, one can greatly increase efficiency of the operation even without a computer.

Consequently for man–computer communications, the first step is to set up a very basic set of rules that the computer can follow. This rule set is primarily concerned not so much in the arithmetic function of the computer, but more in the method for making the decisions, comparing certain data and making further decisions. The languages that have been developed for the computer assist the user in this task so that one can say: multiply a number, divide, move information, and most important compare and branch to new instruction. All this is translated into basic computer instructions by other programs. What is really usually desired in order that the computer be used as an information machine rather than a calculator is that if the computer comes up with a particular answer based upon these calculations that it should then move on to another set of instructions. The general method for programming a computer is first to make flow charts of the overall decision process, the same way as setting up a protocol when doing a particular experimental study. Then, this protocol can be translated into the computer operation by the appropriate language instructions.

There are two major ways one can use a program in the scientific area to tell a computer to go through a particular set of operations and give an answer. One of these might be called the inductive technique and the other the deductive. Certainly much scientific research on computers is done by feeding large amounts of data into the computer, and doing very large statistical analyses, and coming out with large amounts of reduced data, the result being certain statistical or deductive correlations.

The second or inductive approach is illustrated by the growing use of computers in an on-line sense, where there is immediate feedback of results or retrieval of information during an experiment. In neurophysiology an example is the measurement of interspike intervals and arriving at certain correlations that would result in the desire to change certain parameters of the experiment. In the program one can set up the computer to bring in analogue information, convert this to a digital form, and ask the computer to look for all changes in data which are characteristics of spikes and therefore detects the time of the spikes or peaks. One can tell the computer to measure and count all the time intervals between spikes. That information can be gained by elementary signal processing and then can be put into another sort of expression for more complex decision computation analysis, and eventual display so that one can have visual or control feedback for the future progress of the experiment.

A clinical example of this sort of on-line data acquisition is the collection of data from severely ill patients. Although more in the cardiovascular area than neurophysiology, it gives an impression of what kind of data can be analyzed by a system. A television screen may be used to display the computer data. The electrocardiogram is taken into the system and by very simple programming for counting the number of heart beats, heart rate is acquired and displayed. Much more complex programs are now being developed and used in this area for intensive care monitoring which include variations in beat patterns, types of arrhythmias, and the timing of other cardiovascular events. Some of the same techniques may be used for neurophysiological signals as well as electrocardiographic. The slower phenomena of respiration, temperatures and blood pressure collected by appropriate instruments can be likewise sent on-line directly to the computer for processing and display of derived results such as heart output and work.

In addition to the instrument analogue data, one always needs a variety of other types of information in a system for biomedical research. This includes manual information, that is the experimental and medical record information that is needed for the complete processing of the data.

It has been the purpose of this paper to define the various types of computers in light of the evolutionary trend of these powerful aids to scientific investigation, to further define their micro- and macro-structure and function and to give examples of how computers can be programmed and used in biomedical research. This information can hopefully make computers easier to use for a variety of life science problems. There are certain parallels between the operation of computers and the brain which may be of interest for computer engineers and biological scientists. The primary task is to distinguish between what computers can and cannot do easily and to use them intelligently for the difficult problems in the life sciences. Likewise, one must look to the future as to what computers may be able to do later on. One can see very definitely the accelerated rate of the increase in capability of computers over the past ten to fifteen years. We can do more than just use computers for automation of old manual techniques of data acquisition and processing. The intelligent use of computers in the basic sciences is still lagging far behind their actual potential capabilities. This is a challenge for all of us.

# Computers of the Brain and Brainmade Computers

J. P. SCHADÉ AND J. SMITH

*Central Institute for Brain Research, Amsterdam (The Netherlands)*

Information-processing systems ordinarily consist of a combination of units including input, processing, storage and output devices. They are devised to handle data at high speeds, with self-checking accuracy.

The most remarkable system, both from the point of view of design and information-handling capacity, is the human brain. In no more than 1400 grammes a complete input and output system is stored and some 30 000 000 000 processing and storage units are interconnected. Although it lacks the speed of electronic machines, the integrative capacities of the human computer far exceed any known electronic computing system. In order to evaluate the superb properties of the nervous system in comparison with ordinary computing systems, it is helpful to examine the digital, analogue and hybrid features of the brain, and thereupon the input, processing, storage and output devices.

*Digital computers* operate with discrete bits of data and can thus be made extremely precise. Their basis is binary arithmetic, the counting operations being performed with only two symbols: 0 and 1. The presence of two basic symbols means that in the machine these can be recognized not merely as counting digits, but as the logic commands YES and NO. They can be grouped in particular sequences to form keys which are able to open particular electronic gates. In this way the computer is endowed with capacities in logic as well as in counting. Speed, accuracy and reliability are its main virtues.

The *electronic analogue computer* is not so versatile as the digital computer; but by virtue of its composition of resistance and capacitance networks, associated with amplifiers, it is able to perform the operation of integration very simply. The charge distribution changes occurring around a collection of these amplifiers and their associated networks enable information to be taken from the array in a continuous voltage form, in contrast to the digital machine, which produces only discrete outputs.

The basic elements of the nervous system perform principally the same operations. The structural and functional unit is called the *neuron*, which consists of a cell body and a number of processes. The cell body and its constituents are the seat of the trophic and genetic functions of the neuron. As a centre for control, steering, and maintenance of the morphological and metabolic integrity of the neuron with its often very long processes, its position and size is more related to these latter functions than to the signal-transmitting properties. The processes, dendrites—the receiving part of the cell—and the axon—the conducting and transmitting part—possess a number of characteristic properties which make them ideally suited for the transmission of signals. The electric properties of an axon are very poor compared with, for instance, those of a cable of copper wire. The membrane of the axon is at least 1 000 000 times leakier to electrical current while the resistance of the interior of the axon is more than 10 000 000 times as great, but it is still adequate for the propagation of electrical energy in our body.

The axon conducts signals by sudden changes in its resting membrane potential, so-called *action potentials*. These potential shifts have a constant amplitude (about 110 millivolt) and a fixed duration of about 1 millisecond. The axon represents the "digital" part of the neuron, its basic operation is binary because the action potential represents the symbol 1, and the interval between two action potentials is divided into parts of 1 millisecond (the duration of an action potential), each representing the symbol 0. Apparently the axon transmits information in a similar way to machine language. A simple add-instruction in programming language of the IBM 1130 system: A 184 may be transmitted by the axon as 10000000000000000000000010111000. The conduction along the axon of this communication would take 32 milliseconds, the symbol 1 standing for an action potential. The transmission *between* neurons is of a different nature. The various phenomena involved in the transition of electric signals from one neuron to another take place at the synapse. The presynaptic fibre ends in an expanded terminal, the synaptic knob, which is closely opposed to a portion of a postsynaptic neuron. The presynaptic axon serves as a transmitter and the postsynaptic neuron as the receiver. The distance of the membranes of these elements is 150–300 Å, more than sufficient to prevent the direct transfer of an electrical signal. To facilitate the communication between neurons, small vesicles containing a chemical substance are located in the presynaptic elements. These substances—neurotransmitters—serve as chemical mediators for the electrical signals. Two opposing phenomena, generally known as *excitatory* and *inhibitory synaptic activity*, provide the basis for the transmission of information between neurons.

Synaptic activity is brought about by a sequence of events: The arrival of action potentials (digital signals) in the presynaptic terminals; the mobilization of synaptic vesicles which move to the presynaptic membrane and their release quanta of transmitter substance in the small space between the neurons (analogue signals); the action of the transmitter substance upon the subsynaptic membrane producing changes in the ionic permeability of the membrane to intracellular and extracellular ions. Dependent on the type of synapse one of two electrical phenomena are generated in the neuron: Excitatory neurotransmitters produce small electrical currents which flow inward under the synapse and outward across the adjacent portions of the postsynaptic membrane. The resulting excitatory potentials are algebraically summated by the initial segment of the axon. If a threshold is reached the axon fires one or more action potentials. Inhibitory neurotransmitters produce opposing electrical currents which flow outward under the synapse and inward across the adjacent portions of the postsynaptic membrane. The resulting inhibitory potentials interfere with the generation of action potentials because the threshold at the initial segment is considerably raised.

It is the receptive pole of the neuron which is the seat of the interplay between the hundreds and thousands of excitatory and inhibitory synapses. One can extrapolate that the receptive pole of a large neuron may make contact with as many as 40 000 to 50 000 presynaptic axonal terminals, a computer unit of immense size and variability. The receptive pole thus represents the analogue element. In following any pathway or circuit in the nervous system we always pass from one system into another; we always meet the transition analogue–digital–analogue, etc. The axon is thus a nerve process stretched between the point of origin of the action potential to the point where this signal fades out and becomes transformed. At the receptive pole of the neuron digital–analogue conversion continuously takes place, whereas at the initial segment analogue–digital conversion occurs.*

The cell body of the neuron is usually located between the D/A and the A/D converters. Since it contains the nucleus (filled with DNA—desoxyribonucleic acid) and a huge amount of RNA—ribonucleic acid—it acts as a master control switch and also as processing and memory device. DNA is instrumental in the formation of complementary RNA molecules, incorporating the same genetic information which travels as messenger-RNA through the nuclear membrane to the cytoplasm where they attach to the endoplasmic reticulum. The latter has in the neuron a rough surface, because the outer membrane is covered with granules containing RNA. This whole complex system is the focal point for steering the outgrowth of processes in the immature nervous system and for control of regeneration and degeneration of neuronal processes both in the immature and mature nervous system. RNA molecules provide a unique basis for the storage and retrieval of long-term and short-term information.

Thus one single neuron possesses the qualities of a *hybrid* computer. Control signals are usually logic signals and the digital part of the machine is always given the job of controlling both its own actions and those of the analogue part. The RNA molecules in the cell body of the neuron provide those control signals. Communication between the digital and analogue parts of a hybrid computer during operation is generally a major problem. The digital machine must be able to vary the information pattern in the analogue in the course of a run according to its own calculations, and the analogue must similarly be able to change the digital calculations when certain conditions are satisfied in its own computing. Therefore, sophisticated D/A and A/D converters are integrated parts of a hybrid computer. In the neuron the synapse acts as D/A converter. It may be regarded as a transistor switch which can open a micro-circuit according to whether it receives a digital 1 or 0 control command. The micro-circuit releases quantal amounts of neurotransmitter. As in the input of an amplifier network these switches act as a relay contact. The binary signals of the presynaptic terminals are supplied to sets of D/A switches (the branched terminals of the presynaptic fibre) each supplying a given voltage to an analogue amplifier (the postsynaptic neuron) the addition given the required voltage.

---

* In a more specialized way all neural signals could be regarded as being analogous (action potentials: discrete analogous, synaptic potentials: continuous analogous).

Each neuron possesses an A/D converter at the initial segment of the axon. In general, in a hybrid system the analogue voltages are first sampled at a predetermined time by a sample/hold unit. This is an amplifier containing in its feedback network a capacitator capable of retaining its charge at any point in time, thus freezing the amplifier output at a constant voltage for examination by the A/D converter. The molecular configuration of the neuronal membranes and the close relationship of these structures to the intraneuronal proteins and nucleic acids provide the submicroscopic substrate for this function. The A/D converter works by successively comparing this input voltage (the resting membrane potential of the neuron is carefully stabilized by enzymatic processes in the membrane itself) with a succession of voltages produced inside it (small excitatory and inhibitory currents and potentials), controlled by D/A switches, which are in turn controlled by binary 1 or 0 signals. These 1 or 0 are arranged to be the output (action potentials generated at the initial segment) in the required binary form.

Let us now turn to the units of the information-processing system: input, processing, storage and output devices. An information-processing system requires devices that can enter data into the system and record data from the system. These functions are performed by input–output units. In electronic computers the input device is a very sophisticated machine that can read or sense coded data that are recorded on a prescribed medium and make this information available to the computer. In man innumerable small input devices—receptors—are located in the periphery and inside the body. Thousands of millions of receptors (for example one eye has 125 000 000 photoreceptors) handle all information which comes from outside or inside. They function in much the same manner: various types of energy (light impulses, sound, touch, etc.) are transformed into electrical signals which are then transmitted as action potentials by the sensory nerves to the brain. Irrespective of the kind of physical stimulus which excites it, the immediate response of any receptor is an electrical change—which is an approximate analogue of the physical stimulus in time and magnitude. The receptors display graded increase of the number of action potentials when the stimulus intensity is increased. In many, the firing frequency is a linear function of the log of the stimulus intensity. Thus the receptors are able to provide continuously graded, frequency-coded information concerning stimulus intensity to the central processing unit.

The various types of receptors are connected to different parts of the central nervous system, where perception and storage of the messages take place. The nervous system seems to work with an outmoded telecommunication method: many parallel lines are used instead of only a few. In the latter case a number of messages are transmitted at the same time and sorted out by the decoding machine at the end. Apparently the nervous system does not take the chance of a failure of the input device. The redundancy of numerous small input devices provides also an extra dimension (localisation and space) to the internal organization of the computer.

At the output devices—effector organs—a reverse transformation occurs. Trains of action potentials are transformed via a number of enzymatic steps into mechanical energy. In this way the tension of muscle fibers changes as part of the contraction of a muscle. The resulting behaviour patterns are the major output of the human nervous system.

Little is known about the exact way in which the neuronal processing and storage units work. The capacity of storage which determines the amount of information that can be held within the system at any time, seems to be infinite. Altogether, 30 000 000 000 units, each containing many millions of RNA storage and protein molecules, provide sufficient storage for all information which is received by the receptors during a whole lifetime. Some brain parts, such as the cerebellum, possess a short-term storage and memory device; all stimuli are faded out in less than 100 milliseconds. Other parts (the cerebral cortex) are able to store information for a period of more than 70 or 80 years. A main asset to this function is the connectivity pattern of the individual units: a neuron possesses from 500 to 500 000 connections with other neurons.

## APPENDIX

### ANNOTATED BIBLIOGRAPHY

AMOSOV, N. M. (1967) *Modeling of Thinking and the Mind*, Spartan Books, New York; MacMillan & Co., London.

A small monograph by a Russian scientist, one of the leading cyberneticists. The following topics are included: Some general assumptions of pre-human living systems and their programs, basic programs of human behaviour, consciousness, thinking, and modeling of mental functions.

ARBID, M. A. (1963) *Brains, Machines, and Mathematics*, McGraw-Hill, New York, 1963.

Mathematics is extensively used to exploit the analogies between the working of brains and the control–computation–communication aspects of machines. The book also gives an outline of the trends in mathematical thought which led up to Godel's work, a proof of his incompleteness theorem, a discussion of its dramatic philosophical consequences for the foundations of mathematics and, finally, a look at its role in the brain–machine controversy.

BRAZIER, M. A. B. (1961) Computer techniques in EEG analysis, *Electroenceph. Clin. Neurophysiol.*, Suppl. **20**.

A survey of the application of the computer to the analysis of spontaneous and evoked potentials of the brain.

CAIANIELLO, E. R. (Ed.) (1968) *Neural Networks*, Springer, Berlin.

This book contains the proceedings of an interdisciplinary workshop on neuronal networks. The following subjects have been discussed:

— On fields of inhibitory influence in a neural network.
— Some ideas on information processing in the cerebellum.
— Neural networks: reverberations, constants of motion, general behavior.
— Probabilistic description of neurons.
— Diffusion models for the stochastic activity of neurons.
— Statistical approach to the study of neuronal networks.
— Statistical mechanics of nervous nets.

DEUTSCH, S. (1967) *Models of the Nervous System*, Wiley, New York.

This book describes simplified engineering models of the nervous system and brain, in order to facilitate the study and analysis of complicated structures under investigation in neurophysiology. The models are examined from a pattern-recognition viewpoint and conjectural models are used where gaps in knowledge exist.

DIXON, W. J. (Ed.) (1965) *BMD Biomedical Computer Programs*, rev. ed., UCLA Medical School, Dept. of Preventive Medicine and Public Health Sciences Computing Facility, Los Angeles.

This book describes in a unified manner the various computer programs which have proved to be useful in many types of medical research projects at UCLA. It contains a number of computer programs for the neurological sciences.

ECCLES, J. C., ITA, M. AND SZENTÁGOTHAI, J. (1967) *The cerebellum as a neuronal machine*, Springer, Berlin.

The thema of the book is to discover the functional meaning of the patterns of neuronal connexion in the cerebellum, both in the cortex and in the various nuclei on its efferent pathways, because all of these structures are organized into very remarkable operational entities. Essentially the cerebellum is constructed of stereotyped and relatively simple neuronal arrangements which can be regarded as neuronal machinery designed to process the input information in some unique and essential manner.

FELLINGER, K. (1968) *Computer in der Medizin. Probleme, Erfahrungen, Projekte*, Hollinek, Wien

Contains documentation on computer applications to psychiatric conditions.

FINLEY, M. (1967) *An experimental Study of the Formation and Development of Hebbian Cell-Assemblies by Means of Neural Network Simulation*, Univ. Michigan, Ann Arbor, Mich.

In this study a description is given of a structural and dynamic characterization of Hebbian cell-assemblies in terms of a particular class of models of neural networks.

KABRISKY, M. (1966) *A proposed Model for Visual Information Processing in the Brain*, Univ. of Illinois Press, Urbana–London.

A description is given of the nervous system of the vertebrate animal analyzed as an information-processing device, with particular emphasis on the human visual system. A generalized two-dimensional cross correlation function is introduced and it is shown that known biological structures could be able to perform such a calculation.

KOZHEVINSKOV, V. A. (1900) *Probability Models in the Study of Bioelectrical Brain Reaction,* Pavlov Institute of Physiology, Academy of Sciences, Leningrad, USSR.

Review of Russian investigations on the mathematical approach to brain function.

LEDLEY, R. S. AND WILSON, J. B. (1965) *Use of Computers in Biology and Medicine,* McGraw-Hill, New York.

The book presents the methods by which the computer is coded, the application of computer methods to biological problems and some of the more important mathematical concepts frequently involved.

LIVANOV, M. N. AND RUSINOV, V. S. (1968) *Mathematical Analysis of the Electrical Activity of the Brain,* Harvard Univ. Press, Cambridge, Mass., U.S.A.

In view of the development of electronic computing techniques, and the penetration of mathematics into all fields of science, various attempts have been made to supplement visual analysis of the electroencephalogram by mathematical methods. The book includes the reports of a small interdisciplinary meeting on these problems.

MACGREGOR, R. J. (1966) *A Digital Computer Model of Spike Elicitation by Postsynaptic Potentials in Single Nerves,* Rand Corp., AD-640268.

A simulation of the information-processing function of nerve cells is presented. The computer model simulates the portion of the neuron at which spike potentials are initiated. Values for parameters were specified on the basis of neuroelectric recordings so that the results obtained might be pertinent to actual nerve cells.

MCLACHLAN, G. AND STEGOG, R. A. (Eds.) (1968) *Computers in the Service of Medicines; Essays on Current Research and Applications;* 2 vols., Oxford Univ. Press.

The first of the two volumes of this book is devoted to the use of computers in arrangements for the improvement of patient care. These reports cover some early practical applications and illustrate the diversity of objectives and of the operational methods employed. In the second volume, the theme has changed to the range of problems met in analysing those medical procedures which must be clarified if the systematic use of computers is to be developed to full advantage.

MINSKY, M. L. (1954) *Theory of Neural-Analog Reinforcement Systems and its Application to the Brain-Model Problem,* Princeton Univ., N.J.

An approach to the problem of how the brain works. A series of "brain models" are developed. The theory of neural nets is examined and the notion of "random net" is introduced.

OCKERMAN, D. L. (1965) *Computer Simulation of Visual Data Processing in the Human Brain,* Air Force Inst. of Technology, Wright-Patterson AFB, AD-619394.

The operation of the visual portion of the human brain has been simulated on the IBM 1620 and IBM 7094. The simulation is designed using the cross-correlation method postulated by Kabrisky. The model stores new patterns, standardizes pattern sizes, rotates the input pattern and recognizes identical or similar patterns. The model is evaluated by inserting twenty test patterns. The model did seem to simulate the human visual recognition system for these input patterns. The model will recognize patterns that are reduced, enlarged, shifted or rotated. After analyzing the satisfactory results recommendations are made for the design of larger and more intricate models. The computer programs and sample results are included.

STACY, R. W. AND WAXMAN, B. D. (Eds.) (1965) *Computers in Biomedical Research*, Vol. 1; by W. R. ADEY, TH. L. BRANNICK, M. A. B. BRAZIER *et al.*; Academic Press, New York.

This book provides information on the present state of biomedical computing and automatic data processing, and furnishes guidelines for those who will enter this field in the near future. Sections are: Computers and mathematics in the life sciences— Computer simulation of life processes—Computer analysis of specific biosystems— Computer uses in neurophysiology—Computers in clinical medicine—Computers in psychology and psychiatry.

TURSKY, B., SHAPIRO, D. AND LEIDERMAN, P. H. (1965) *Automatic Data Processing in Psychophysiology: a System in Operation*, Harvard Univ., AD-613177.

An automatic system for processing physiological data is described. Through the use of this system and proper programming, the complex and varied data-processing problems of psychophysiological research can be handled appropriately and with relative ease. The system has the following advantages: (1) The data are stored in dynamic form for easy retrieval. (2) The flexible sampling arrangement meets the needs of psychophysiological experiments independent of their time course. (3) The output is in a format compatible with high-speed computing facilities.

STARK, L. (1968) *Neurological Control Systems*, Plenum Press, New York.

Concerned with an engineering science approach to four neurological motor feedback systems—the pupil, the lens, eyeball rotation, and hand movement—this book explores new, ethical models to deal with the awake, intact brain rather than classical decerebrate and anesthetized animals. Using digital and analog computers to make mathematical models of neurological systems, the work suggests quantitative formulations for deeper interpretation and understanding.

UTTAL, W. R. (1968) *Real-time Computers: Technique and Application in the Psychological Sciences*. Harper & Row, New York.

The first part of this book is devoted to providing the basics of laboratory computers, with an emphasis on the organization and operation of the hardware. Part II discusses three areas of behavioral science applications, giving examples of computational techniques and citing actual instances of applications.

WALTER, D. O. AND BRAZIER, M. A. B. (1968) Advances in EEG-analysis, *Electroenceph. Clin. Neurophysiol.*, suppl. **27**.

An attempt has been made to answer the following questions: How and when might a research-EEG'er anticipate that some of the recent intensive efforts in statistical or computarized study of the EEG may become useful to his work? Can a clinical EEG'er anticipate any useful assistance from such efforts in seaking better diagnosis of the human EEG's? Therefore this booklet deals mainly with the practical applications of the frequency approach to EEG-analysis.

WIENER, N. AND SCHADÉ, J. P. (1963) *Nerve, Brain and Memory Models, Progress in Brain Research,* Vol. **2**, Elsevier, Amsterdam.

This volume contains the proceedings of the Symposium on Cybernetics of the Nervous System, held at the Royal Netherlands Academy of Sciences, Amsterdam, in April 1962. In this collection of 20 papers an account is given of several important aspects of neurocybernetics, a branch of bionics. The interdisciplinary conference was organized around three main subjects: nerve, brain and memory models.

WIENER, N. AND SCHADÉ, J. P. (1965) *Cybernetics of the Nervous System, Progress in Brain Research,* Vol. **17**, Elsevier, Amsterdam.

This volume contains a series of interdisciplinary papers on cybernetics of the nervous system. Among others, the following subjects are discussed: organismic reliability, artificial intelligence, pattern recognition, information theory in relation to human perception, mathematical models for verbal learning, probability statistical models of brain organization, neuron models and learning mechanisms in the brain.

The book also contains a complete biography and bibliography of Norbert Wiener.

YOUNG, J. Z. (1964) *A Model of the Brain*, Oxford Press, Oxford.

The model is mainly built on data from anatomy and behavioural experiments on octopus. Two of the most important questions are discussed by the author: What can the nervous system do? and: How are its units connected to enable it to carry out its functions?

ZIMMER, H. (1966) *Computers in Psychophysiology*, Thomas, Springfield, Ill.

A book on the utilization of digital computer systems in the psychophysiology laboratory, which contains accounts of representative systems. With one exception the systems included produce data in a format suitable as input to a general purpose computer.

On the following pages a number of tables are listed with data which may be useful for the comparison of structure and function of brains and computers.

For an extensive survey of data of the human brain the reader is referred to:

BLINKOV, S. M. and I. I. GLEESER (1968) *The Human Brain in Figures and Tables*, Plenum Press, New York.

## TABLE 1

BIOPHYSICAL CHARACTERISTICS OF MYELINATED NERVE FIBERS*

(Approximate values)

*Axoplasm*
  resistance 15 M $\Omega$/mm

*Myelin sheath*
  resistance    300 m $\Omega$/mm
  capacitance   1.5 pF/mm

*Node of Ranvier*
  membrane resistance    40 M $\Omega$
  membrane capacitance   1.5 pF

internal $K^+$ concentration   120   m$M$
external $K^+$ concentration     2.5 m$M$
internal $Na^+$ concentration   13.5 m$M$
external $Na^+$ concentration 115   m$M$

$K^+$ permeability constant        1.2  $\times$ $10^3$ cm/sec
$Na^+$ permeability constant      8   $\times$ $10^3$ cm/sec
non-specific permeability constant 0.54 $\times$ $10^3$ cm/sec

* Conductive part of the neuron.

## TABLE 2

PRINCIPAL MOSSY FIBER PATHWAYS IN CEREBELLAR CORTEX*

(According to Eccles)

| Excitatory Pathway | | Inhibitory Pathway | |
|---|---|---|---|
| Divergence number | Convergence number | Divergence number | Convergence number |
| Mossy fibers | | Mossy fibers | |
| ↓   600 | 4 | ↓   600 | 4 |
| Granule cells | | Granule cells | |
| ↓ | | Parallel fibers | |
| Parallel fibers | | ↓ | |
| ↓   300 | 100 000 | Basket cells   ~30 | ~10 000 |
| Purkinje cells | | Basket cell axons | |
| | | ↓ | |
| | | Purkinje cell axons   ~50 | 20 |

* The major divergence and convergence properties of one of the input systems of a neuronal circuit in the cerebellum.

## TABLE 3

NUMBER OF NEURONS IN CORTEX OF ONE CEREBRAL HEMISPHERE IN MAN*

| Author | Number of neurons |
|---|---|
| Meynert, 1872 . . . . . . | 612 000 000 |
| Thompson, 1899 . . . . . | 9 200 000 000 |
| Berger, 1921 . . . . . . . | 5 512 000 000 |
| Von Economo, 1925 . . . | 7 000 000 000 |
| Shariff, 1953 . . . . . . . | 6 900 000 000 |
| Sholl, 1956. . . . . . . . | 5 000 000 000 |
| Haug, 1959 . . . . . . . | 8 200 000 000 |

* Estimate, which exemplifies the size of the most important information-processing part of the brain.

## TABLE 4

RELATIVE SIZE OF THE BODY OF THE NEURON AND ITS DENDRITES IN THE OPTIC AND MOTOR CORTEX OF THE CAT*

(Sholl, 1953)

| Type of cell | Depth of situation (in $\mu$) | Volume of cell (in $\mu^3$) | Surface of cell (in $\mu^2$) | Length of dendrites (in $\mu$) | Number of branches of dendrites |
|---|---|---|---|---|---|
| | | Optic cortex | | | |
| P | 250 | 1030 | 470 | 1736 | 46 |
| P | 420 | 1680 | 660 | 2534 | 49 |
| P | 950 | 3560 | 1700 | 2521 | 47 |
| P | 1260 | 4080 | 1270 | 4962 | 79 |
| P | 840 | 4310 | 1840 | 3970 | 78 |
| P | 1050 | 9160 | 2250 | 2848 | 49 |
| P | 1470 | 19620 | 3870 | 4832 | 78 |
| S | 1050 | 1700 | 690 | 1129 | 26 |
| S | 685 | 3890 | 1100 | 1523 | 34 |
| S | 865 | 4850 | 1390 | 3405 | 71 |
| S | 840 | 9010 | 2250 | 1529 | 30 |
| S | 714 | 14140 | 1700 | 3775 | 38 |
| | | Motor cortex | | | |
| P | 1220 | 540 | 310 | 1596 | 41 |
| P | 392 | 680 | 360 | 2377 | 38 |
| P | 364 | 700 | 390 | 2468 | 44 |
| P | 396 | 1060 | 510 | 2205 | 40 |
| P | 660 | 1280 | 570 | 3286 | 48 |
| P | 1300 | 8620 | 1950 | 4706 | 83 |
| P | 1080 | 11500 | 2520 | 6384 | 75 |
| S | 860 | 890 | 490 | 1300 | 18 |
| S | 893 | 1770 | 1710 | 4895 | 62 |
| S | 473 | 5580 | 1520 | 2096 | 28 |
| S | 730 | 8180 | 1960 | 3043 | 36 |
| S | 690 | 1280 | 570 | 2355 | 44 |

P = pyramidal cell; S = stellate cell.
Depth of situation = distance of body of neuron from surface of pia mater.
* Analysis of the size of the receptive pole of neurons in the cerebral cortex. The neuronal membrane of this receptive pole is densely packed with presynaptic endings of other neurons.

## TABLE 5

### ESTIMATES OF CORTICAL PARAMETERS

Some evolutionary aspects of the cerebral cortex in mammals.

|  | Rat | Rabbit | Cat | Man |
|---|---|---|---|---|
| Brain weight (g) | 2.4 | 10.5 | 29.5 | 1450 |
| Cortex volume (cm³) | 0.2 | 0.9 | 2.9 | 290 |
| Neuron density | | | | |
| ($\times 10^3$/mm³) | 105 | 58 | 41 | 15 |
| Total number in cortex | $2.1 \times 10^7$ | $5.2 \times 10^7$ | $12 \times 10^7$ | $435 \times 10^7$ |
| Length dendrites ($\mu$) | 1650 | 2500 | 3000 | 7000 |
| Dendritic field factor | 29 | 31 | 38 | 58 |
| Cortex capacity factor | $61 \ \times 10^7$ | $161 \ \times 10^7$ | $456 \times 10^7$ | $25000 \times 10^7$ |

## TABLE 6

### NUMBER OF CELLS IN SPINAL GANGLIA AND NUMBER OF FIBRES IN POSTERIOR AND ANTERIOR ROOTS AND IN SPINAL NERVES OF SEVEN SEGMENTS IN MAN*

| Segment | Posterior root | | | Anterior root | |
|---|---|---|---|---|---|
|  | Number of cells in ganglion | Total number of fibers (silver impregnation) | Number of nonmedullated fibers | Total number of fibers (silver impregnation) | Number of nonmedullated fibers |
| $C_{II}$ | 49 000 | 38 000 | 13 000 | 3800 | 450 |
| $C_{VI}$ | 60 000 | 61 000 | 26 000 | 12 500 | 500 |
| $T_{IV}$ | 24 000 | 20 500 | 9500 | 9800 | 2700 |
| $T_{IX}$ | 30 500 | 29 000 | 18 500 | 7200 | 1600 |
| $L_{III}$ | 59 000 | 57 500 | 25 000 | 9600 | 600 |
| $S_{III}$ | 56 000 | 50 000 | 27 500 | 6100 | 1500 |
| $S_V$ | 3400 | 3240 | 1720 | 1410 | 780 |

* Afferent fibers of spinal and cranial nerves serve as input units to the brain and spinal cord. Efferent fibers can be regarded as the major output units. Data are given for a number of spinal segments in man.

## TABLE 7

NUMBER OF FIBERS IN OPTIC NERVE OF ANIMALS IN A COMPARATIVE ANATOMICAL SERIES

Comparative data on the fiber content of one of the major sensory systems.

| Species | Number of fibers |
|---|---|
| Macaque | 1 210 000 |
| Cat | 119 000 |
| Dog | 154 000 |
| | (Varying from |
| | 149 320 to 192 160) |
| Opossum | 82 100 |
| Pig | 681 000 |
| Sheep | 649 000 |
| Bat | 6940 |
| Rabbit | 265 000 |
| Albino rat | 74 800 |
| Gray rat | 80 100 |
| Guinea pig | 126 000 |
| Duckbill | 32 000 |
| Pigeon | 988 000 |
| Duck | 408 000 |
| Chicken | 414 000 |
| Canary | 428 000 |

## TABLE 8

RELATIONSHIP BETWEEN PERIPHERAL, SUBCORTICAL, AND CORTICAL SUBDIVISIONS OF THE GENERAL SENSORY, OPTIC, AND AUDITORY SYSTEMS IN THE RAT

Convergence and divergence characteristics of three sensory systems.

| General sensory system | Optic system | Auditory system |
|---|---|---|
| Number of fibers in posterior roots on one side 80 000–90 000 (Agduhr) | Number of fibers in optic nerve 75 000 (Bruesch and Arey) | Number of fibers in auditory nerve 3000 (Droogleever Fortuyn) |
| Number of cells in ventral nucleus of thalamus 13 500 (Abaturova) | Number of cells in lateral geniculate body 13 000 (Sazonova) | Number of cells in medial geniculate body 12 000 (Abaturova) |
| *Number of cells in cortical zone of system* | | |
| 2 800 000 (Abaturova) | 750 000 (Sazonova) | 850 000 (Sazonova) |
| *Ratio between number of cells in cortex and number in immediate subcortex* | | |
| 205 : 1 | 60 : 1 | 70 : 1 |

# On-line Computation in Behavioral Neurophysiology

W. R. ADEY

*Departments of Anatomy and Physiology, Space Biology Laboratory, Brain Research Institute, University of California, Los Angeles, Calif. (U.S.A.)*

## INTRODUCTION

It is a very real pleasure for me to be here in Amsterdam, and to be associated with this program under the auspices of the Central Institute for Brain Research and the Royal Academy, largely because my first teacher in anatomy, Andrew Arthur Abbie, was himself a pupil of Cornelius Ubbo Ariens Kappers here in the late 1920's. My introduction to brain anatomy and brain physiology was at the hands of a man who was himself primarily a morphologist. I have never regretted this association, for the historic role of the systematic anatomist has been and will continue to be very important, even in these days of computer applications in brain science.

The brain anatomist has been responsible for the development of system concepts in cortico-subcortical organization (Elliot Smith, 1910; Herrick, 1933). He has also been responsible with varying degrees of success for the development of concepts of brain as a tissue, often with more error than accuracy.

When in the late 30's it became feasible to test electrically aspects of anatomical organization of cerebral systems and of cerebral tissue, initial studies were in search of evoked potentials. What could one discern about the system if one struck it sufficiently violently with an electrical hammer? We have moved away from that type of electrical stimulation of brain tissue where some motor end point or an evoked potential was the expected outcome of the experiment. Rather, we are looking at the individual in his conscious, unrestrained and performing state.

My assignment is to discuss such studies briefly, with reference to the application of the computer as a tool in the analysis of the very complex data that come from brain systems. As a point of departure in these studies we may consider a model of cortico-subcortical organization in attentive states and in orienting and in discrimination. It is not proposed to discuss the physiological interpretation in great detail, since this has been reported elsewhere (Adey, 1969a), but we will highlight application of the computer by some considerations of the morphology and basic physiology.

### Gross anatomical and physiological aspects of the brain

Those who have been concerned with the brain in almost any aspect are aware of the many studies that have delineated a central core within it (Moruzzi and Magoun,

1949), to which the term *reticular substance* or *reticular formation* has been applied, and which has been presumed to be activated by virtually every sensory modality; from the eye, the ear, as well as from somatic inputs ascending from the spinal cord. Much controversy has existed about the way in which information actually enters it (Proctor and Knighton, 1957). This will not be discussed here, but arising from this reticular formation and distributed to many areas of the cortex are projections from the reticular system. Whereas the broad streams of consciousness in their most basic aspects may be defined by ascending influences, entering the reticular formation, and thence making their way to more rostral levels, it appears that the focusing of attention relates to corticifugal influences that arise, not from all the cortex, but in more restricted ways. Briefly, it appears that these cortico-reticular projections arise in large measure from certain areas of the temporal lobe, which, for the purpose of this discussion, may be termed the hippocampal and amygdaloid projection systems, and certain areas in the frontal lobe, including medial frontal areas and the cingulate region (Adey, Segundo and Livingston, 1957).

Briefly, it should be emphasized that projections from the temporal lobe of the brain appear to be very much concerned with the modulation of ascending reticular influences to other parts of the cortex. I shall exemplify this concept in studies of alerted behavior, in the so-called *orienting responses* to new stimuli in the environment, and in the course of learned discrimination of visual stimuli.

Moreover, as was first shown in 1939 by Klüver and Bucy, bilateral ablation of the temporal lobe in the primate leads to a disruption of those aspects of attention necessary for recent memory, and thus to defects in learning. It is equally apparent, however, that this is not the region where the memories lie, and that there is some alteration in the functions of other parts of the brain, attributable to this interference with the temporal lobe. These are the systems on which I wish to hinge certain points of this discussion of computer applications. I also wish to consider aspects of the organization of cerebral tissue (Adey, 1969c).

### A TRICOMPARTMENTAL MODEL OF BRAIN TISSUE

Let us first consider a model of brain tissue (Fig. 1) which has three compartments (Adey, 1967). The neural compartment is composed of nerve cells. We should emphasize the very large neuronal dendritic fields that Dr. Schadé has described here as overlapping each other. Perhaps the overlap, from both structural and functional indications, may be one in which dendrodendritic contacts can influence adjacent cells (Rall, Shepherd, Reese and Brightman, 1966). At least we can say that the dendrodendritic systems are sufficiently organized to require close scrutiny from the point of view of possible slow electric processes between one nerve cell and another.

As discussed below, studies in our laboratory and those of others have indicated that a large part of the EEG originates in an intracellular wave process of high amplitude and low frequency (Creutzfeldt, Fuster, Lux, and Nacimiento, 1964; Fujita and Sato, 1964; Elul, 1964, 1968). In most instances this is like the EEG on-going in the same domain of tissue, and is clearly a phenomenon of brain nerve

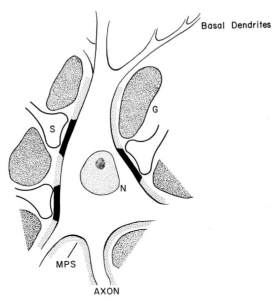

Fig. 1. A tricompartmental model of brain tissue, with a neuron (N) covered on its surface by a hydrated network of macromolecules (shaded) that may also occupy the intercellular space. Darker bands of this material lie in the subsynaptic cleft in conventional electron micrographs (synaptic terminal, S). The third compartment is composed of neuroglial cells (G). (From Adey, 1969c).

cells. It occurs in cortical neurons, in lesser degree in thalamic neurons, but there is not an equivalent wave process in the neurons of the spinal cord. It is emphasized that the wave process may arise in cell regions other than the body, and primarily in the large dendritic tree.

The second component of the tricompartmental arrangement is a neuroglial compartment. Between the neuroglia and the neuron is a substance which is a hydrated net of large molecules, mucopolysaccharides and mucoproteins, specially developed under synapses, and which appears to play a role in the excitability of the cell (Adey, Bystrom, Costin, Kado and Tarby, 1969). It combines preferentially with divalent cations, particularly calcium (Wang and Adey, 1969). Interaction of calcium with surface macromolecular material appears to be a fundamental aspect of excitation in the nerve cell, preceding an exchange of sodium and potassium. This interaction has been observed in all excitable tissue, in muscle, nerve fibre and nerve cell.

From these observations have arisen new models of the excitable membrane, such as that of Schmitt and Davison (1965) in which the lipid double layer is bounded on its external and internal surfaces by mucopolysaccharides or mucoproteins, which might interact with calcium and thus produce a conformation change in the protein. There is a search for electrogenic proteins as a possible basis for excitability, rather than a preoccupation with the traditional role of the lipid double layer.

*References pp. 43–44*

## ACQUISITION OF ELECTROPHYSIOLOGICAL DATA FOR COMPUTATIONAL ANALYSIS

The foregoing discussion has considered brain as a tissue and as a system. We may now consider the types of data that may be collected for computer analysis. What criteria should be applied to them, whether they come from intracellular records or from a domain of tissue as an EEG, to determine their suitability for computation? Highly relevant questions have been asked at this conference about precautions to be taken prior to computation in ensuring that the data are free from artifacts.

There can be no categoric answer, but it is obviously important to know before computation that the data are essentially free of electrical or mechanical artifacts. This is particularly the case in data from the freely moving, performing subject. Such subjects have been the prime interest of our laboratory, where we try to avoid tying a man or an animal to many tons of equipment in a laboratory, and believing incorrectly that thereafter we are carrying out an experiment which can be unhesitatingly correlated with the behavior of the same individual, performing actively in his usual working environment (Walter, Kado, Rhodes and Adey, 1967; Berkhout, Walter and Adey, 1969).

### Electrode connecting cables

In recording the EEG and other electrophysiological data in performing subjects it is of paramount importance that lead connections should not introduce any slow wave artifacts. We routinely use a cable that has a metallic powder deposited between inner and outer plastic sheaths so that electrostatic potentials generated on the cable by bending it are dissipated by the metallic powder (Kado and Adey, 1968). It can be highly deformed without producing any artifacts. It was developed for the missile industry, where missile vibration was for a long time interfering with the quality of strain gauge records. We have used it for more than ten years in experiments with animals and men involving head movements.

### Surface electrode design

There is often a requirement to secure an individual's EEG records while he is performing some quite dexterous and even dangerous task. Our studies have secured EEG records in young men driving on Los Angeles freeways. They normally drive a left hand lane at about 110 km/h, and the EEG is recorded by a helmet making only a sliding contact with the scalp. Nevertheless, records are free of serious artifacts (Kado and Adey, 1968). In this device, the electrodes fit into a light-weight cap. We hope to use this technique in future manned space flights of 28 and 56 days duration. It senses the EEG merely by sitting on the head. Nothing is glued to the scalp and nothing penetrates it. The contact is made by a wetted sponge. The electrode has a little preamplifier built into it. In some instances, a radio transmitter is corporated for transmission of data without connecting wires from the subject.

MULTICHANNEL TELEMETRY SYSTEM FOR EEG

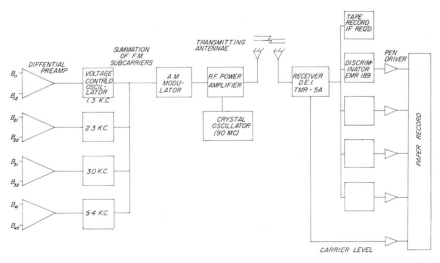

Fig. 2. Multichannel radiotelemetry system for physiological monitoring, characterized by high mechanical, thermal and electrical stability. Voltage controlled oscillators centered on standard (IRIG) audio frequencies are frequency modulated (maximum deviation ± 7.5 per cent) by the physiological signals. These frequency-modulated signals are combined to amplitude modulate a transmitter having quartz crystal frequency control. At the receiver, the subcarriers are separated by appropriate filters, and the physiological signals recovered by FM discriminators. (From Zweizig, Kado, Hanley and Adey, 1967).

These electrodes have evolved in a generic series in our laboratory. They originated in the Soviet Union where it was recognized that a major source of movement artifacts arises from a battery or contact potential, that appears between the metal electrode and whatever fluid surrounds it. In the first Soviet account, metallic tin was in contact with stannous chloride solution. Its contact potential was almost zero. By eliminating the battery, one can move the electrode across the skin and not create an artifact by changing the resistance of the contact. Stannous chloride solution is strongly acid (pH 2). It is quite corrosive on the skin. We have therefore placed a solution of potassium chloride on the external aspect of the electrode, in the form of a wet sponge, and separated it from the stannous chloride solution by a permeable ceramic layer. The ceramic cylinder encloses the stannous chloride solution.

There are several varieties of these electrodes, all constructed on similar principles. Radiotelemetry has become an integral part of these systems.

### Radiotelemetry methods

Our own schemes of telemetry have hinged around designs that have proved relatively insensitive to mechanical vibration and acceleration, and to temperature and battery voltage changes. They use frequency-modulated audio subcarriers centered on standard military (IRIG) frequencies (Zweizig, Kado, Hanley and Adey, 1967). Suitable frequency modulation discriminators are also available commercially for separation of a group of multiplexed subcarriers in the receiver (Fig. 2). The transmitter itself is amplitude modulated by these subcarriers, and its frequency is controlled by a quartz crystal oscillator of high inherent stability. It is noteworthy that one of the first multichannel biotelemetry systems was designed by Dr. Storm van Leeuwen and his colleagues here in Amsterdam some years ago.

We have applied these EEG telemetry techniques to studies in autistic children where head movements and violent body movements are characteristic (Hanley, Zweizig, Kado and Adey, 1968). Although some movement artifacts occur in these records, they remain extremely useful. In fact, children may indulge in such violent activity as jumping from the bed to the floor without producing disastrous blocking of the record.

Much of our interest centers on sleep mechanisms and sleep-walking (Jacobson, Kales, Lehmann and Zweizig, 1965). A contributor here has remarked that one could always tell whether a person is asleep by looking at him. This is dubious even if one is able to look at him. If he happens to be 100 miles up in space, or in some remote location where you cannot look at him, it is important to know whether he is asleep without waking him up. It is equally important to be able to tell what is the stage of sleep. In the clinic, where a child may be sleep-walking, it is an interesting and fundamental physiological problem as to what stage of sleep may be involved. Studies at the UCLA Brain Research Institute have shown that this sleep is not the dream-sleep with rapid eye movements. It is associated with big slow waves (Jacobson, Kales, Lehmann and Zweizig, 1965).

*Combined telephone and radiotelemetry*

More recently in application of the computer to our studies of sleep and wakefulness, and probably for economic reasons in the United States where a hospital bed rarely costs less than $50 per day, it has become desirable to investigate the patient in his own home wherever possible. Children equipped with EEG radiotelemetry packs may play in the vicinity of their homes, while an EEG is being recorded (Fig. 3). A radio receiver in the home is connected to the telephone. Then the data pass directly into our computer facility for immediate on-line analysis (Hanley, Zweizig, Kado, Adey and Rovner, 1969).

We have until this time managed to use ordinary telephone lines with a 3 kHz bandwidth for these studies. Often the records are collected all night long in a "sleep run". We have not asked for special data lines. Recently, in the middle of the night a girl telephone operator apparently heard these peculiar warblings of the audio-subcarriers. She came on the line and said: "Is this line busy?" Dr. Hanley who was in the computer room running the test, very quickly said: "Yes, it is. I am playing my violin to my blind girl friend. Please get off the line, you are interrupting my conversation". The poor girl disappeared and was not heard again. However, I am sure that there is a limit to what you can secure from one dime in terms of EEG data.

DATA FLOW CHART FOR SUBCARRIER TONE
TRANSMISSION BY TELEPHONE

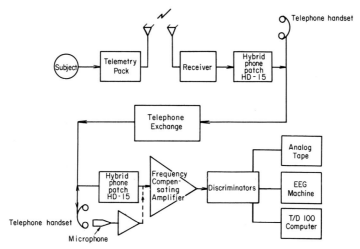

Fig. 3. System for combined radio and telephone telemetry, that allows recording of physiological data from unrestrained patient in his home. (From Hanley, Zweizig, Kado, Adey and Rovner, 1969).

## Coding and editing methods

In presenting data to the computer, and particularly, as I shall explain, in working with shorter and shorter epochs, it is necessary to edit the data, and to provide markers that will allow us to select very short epochs down to about 0.5 sec in duration. We must be able to start the particular epoch to within about 1.0 msec. The question of time coding has therefore become very important.

The codes that we use are of two main varieties: one widely used in the laboratory can be generated as a 3-digit 4-bit member in binary coded decimal (BCD). The numbers can be arranged to appear at regular intervals, or by a manual signal, or by an electrical signal from the experimenter. It can be written at various speeds, but is not suitable for rapid continuous surveillance on the record. However, by looking subsequently at the paper record one can say in hindsight: "I wish to go backwards or forwards so many seconds or so many milliseconds from this code marking point". However, it is often better to use a more rapid code. The second group of codes include so-called IRIG A and B methods that may give a faster coding cycle, but are not usually compatible in their speed with a typical EEG paper record because they are written too fast, and thus cannot be interpreted. The computer can be programmed to recognize any of these codes.

One may also put a step mark or timing pulse on tapes in order to recognize stimulus or behavioral epochs. These should always be applied to the tape in a FM mode, rather than in a direct recording mode if the computer is to handle the signal. Coding pulses recorded in the direct mode may appear ambiguous to the computer by contamination with a variety of electrical and magnetic tape noises.

## CLASSES OF ANALYSES APPLIED TO NEUROPHYSIOLOGICAL DATA

We may turn next to the types of calculations that can be done on-line. This topic could be subtitled, with due respects to our IBM colleagues, "Beware of the industrialist bearing a computer". There are many problems about application of the typical business computer to problems of data handling and data analysis, particularly in an on-line mode. There are two primary problems: one is the mode of access to the computer; the second is the suitability of output methods for rapid, comprehensive on-line display of computed outputs. These problems do not relate to the central processor, which may be quite adequate. But if one is interested in business accounting and punch card entries then one has not usually conceived of the modes of entry that are necessary for high speed handling of massive amounts of physiological data. I will return to this when we discuss specifically the systems in our laboratories.

The first step in preparation of data for handling by the computer involves analog-to-digital conversion. In most cases it is necessary to have quite high precision in the conversion process. We need a word length of the order of 9 bits, or an accuracy of one part in a thousand. If this level of accuracy is not available there is likely to be a loss of precision in calculations on long series of data samples.

Secondly, the data sampling rate must bear a relationship to the bandwidth of the data. This is a very important point. For example, if the EEG is recorded with a bandwidth from D.C. to 50 Hz, then Shannon's sampling theorem points out that at the highest frequencies of that record, the minimum number of samples that would describe it with any accuracy, would be twice the maximum signal frequency, or 100 samples/sec. For safe handling of such a signal the sample rate should be substantially more than twice the maximum signal frequency. If the bandwidth of the data is 0–50 Hz, a reasonable sampling rate would be 200 per second. If this rule is not carefully followed, "aliasing" may occur. For example, with a 60-Hz wave sampled only 40 times/sec, unreal components may appear at 20 Hz in the series of samples. This is particularly liable to happen if, for example, one assumes that an EEG record does not extend to frequencies above 25 Hz. If there is 50 or 60 Hz interference from the AC lines, then one may see components of that line frequency appearing in the EEG pass band. This folding down is referred to as *Nyquist folding*.

When there are many channels of data, as in the typical electroencephalogram a total of 10 channels each sampled at 200/sec will produce 2000 samples/sec. In the usual analog-to-digital converter the channels are sampled in sequence. This sequential examination is called *multiplexing*. A typical modern analog-to-digital converter for electrophysiological studies will incorporate a multiplexing input to handle 10 to 30 channels of data. The total sampling rate is divided between the channels and may allow the investigator to use different rates in different channels depending on the type of data. It is not proposed to deal further with other highly relevant aspects of digital conversion.

Some computational techniques can be used on-line. How much can be done obviously depends upon the size of the central processor and the mode of access to it. One may choose to start simply by averaging, or by correlation analyses. As Dr.

Petsche has pointed out in this meeting, Blackman and Tukey (1959) have warned against correlation analysis as potentially deceptive. *Spectral analysis* was pioneered for EEG investigations by D.O. Walter (1963) in our laboratory. He stressed the value of cross-spectral methods. We shall also consider problems of analyzing short epochs of data.

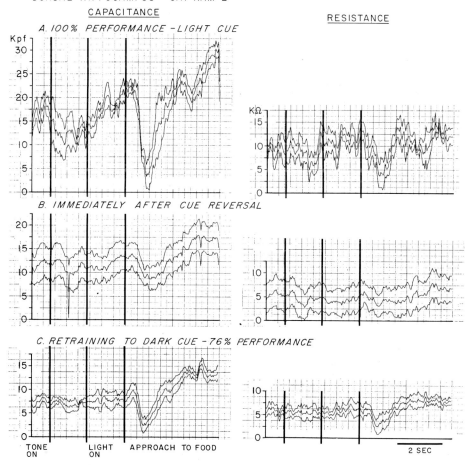

IMPEDANCE IN ALERTING, ORIENTATION AND DISCRIMINATION
COMPUTED MEANS WITH VARIANCE – AVERAGES FOR 5 DAYS
DORSAL HIPPOCAMPUS – CAT KAM 2

Fig. 4. Averages of cerebral electrical impedance in the hippocampus of a performing cat. Each plot covers an 8-sec period, and is computed from data for 5 consecutive days' training, with 30 trials each day. Vertical bars on each plot mark onset of an alerting tone (left), onset of orienting period toward discriminative visual task (middle), and onset of light–dark discrimination task (right). Each plot has 3 graphs, showing the mean, and one standard deviation above and below the mean. For further explanation, see text. (From Adey, Kado, McIlwain and Walter, 1966).

*Averaging of electrophysiological records*

As an example, we may average electrical impedance in the hippocampus of the cat when the animal first alerts, then makes an orienting response, and then a visual discrimination (Adey, Kado, McIlwain and Walter, 1966). Each behavioral change occurs at intervals of 1.5 sec. As shown in Fig. 4, each average is presented as 3 traces. The middle one is the mean, and the other two show one standard deviation above and below the mean. These data were averaged over 5 successive training days, each with 30 trials. At high performance levels a small impedance response occurred during the initial arousal, but very little change followed the orienting stimulus. A large response (of the order of 10 percent of baseline impedance) occurred during the visual discrimination. On reversal of the visual discrimination cues, the impedance response almost disappeared, and the variance increased. With retraining, the variance declined once more and the response during discrimination returned. These data exemplify the power of the computer in detection of consistent time-locked changes.

They also provide important evidence on the tricompartmental model of brain tissue discussed above, and the possible significance of this model to our understanding of learning and information storage in brain tissue. Since the bulk of the measuring current passes through extracellular spaces, rather than through cell membranes, our attention is directed to this space and its content of macromolecules. Our laboratory and others are interested in changes that may occur in mucopolysaccharides and mucoproteins as part of the learning process in brain tissue (Adey, Bystrom, Costin, Kado and Tarby, 1969). It appears that what is happening at the cell surface, rather than in the nucleus, may be the key to the learning process. No longer should we be solely preoccupied with the DNA–RNA mechanisms of the nucleus. Perhaps we should look rather to electrical events at the membrane surface that might produce a mosaic of altered proteins and other macromolecules in structures at the cell surface.

The past experience of the cell would thus alter its excitability, by reason of this modified surface patchwork. Moreover, such an arrangement would probably be a distributed memory through many neurons, and thus accessible to the impedance-measuring technique. Neither the model nor its experimental testing with impedance measurements support the concept of a single engram engulfing the storage capacity of a single neuron.

*Calculations of cross-spectra in multiple EEG records*

Cross-spectral analysis measures the relationship between two simultaneous wave trains, and what is the degree of interrelationship at each frequency in the data epoch, essentially on a wave-by-wave basis (Walter, 1963). This is done by retaining information about phase relations between the two wave trains. Until the arrival of the digital computer we could not say anything about the phase relations of two complex wave trains like this. If they were put through an analog frequency analyzer, information on phase relationships was lost through wide phase shifts in the analog filters. A most useful contribution of applied mathematics to EEG analysis, and to analysis of wave phenomena generally, has been the development of a mathematical expression which in its graphic representation is known as a *digital filter* (Goodman, 1960). It is not something that can be picked up and handled. It is a mathematical expression in the computer. One can specify shoulder and skirt characteristics, as well as the width of what is known as the "flat top". It is possible to construct a set of digital filters if one wishes to examine the spectrum from 0 to 20 Hz, at intervals of 1.0 Hz or less. It is not difficult to program the computer for each computation

## STOCHASTIC MODELS OF EEG

### PROBABILITY BOUNDS ON COMPLEX TRANSFER FUNCTIONS, DORSAL HIPPOCAMPUS TO ENTORHINAL CORTEX

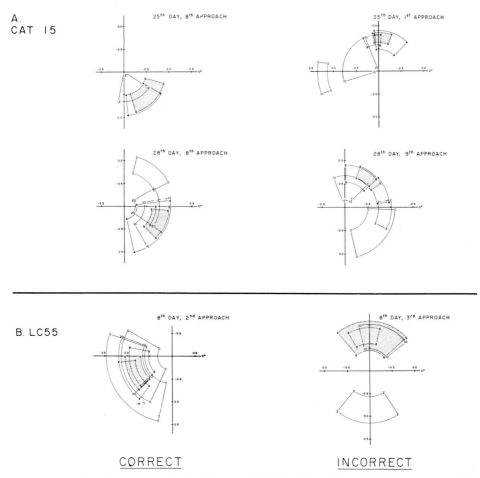

Fig. 5. Polar plots of cross-spectral calculations on EEG data from right and left hippocampi of cats during correct and incorrect visual discriminations in light–dark reward task. Fan-shaped sectors show phase angle relations on circular coordinates, and amplitude transfer functions on radial dimension. Limits of sectors are set at 50% level of probability of significance for that particular epoch. (From Adey and Walter, 1963).

so that filter widths are established for a particular computation on the basis of data bandwidth, duration of the data epoch, and sampling rate.

Digital filters have no phase shift, or a phase shift of 90°, depending on the mode of calculation. Results of cross-spectral analysis can be displayed on a polar plot. Phase angles will then be represented by angular location on a "phase circle". In such a display, the phase representation is not a point. It is a sector, or fan, having certain dimensions (Fig. 5). That is because one can attach a probability function to the relationship between two wave trains at any frequency over that epoch duration. Such a fan for the theta-band in the cat's hippocampal EEG may have its limits set so that a relationship is shown between two EEG wave trains within the angular bounds of the sector for a particular frequency and record length when there is a 50 percent probability or more (Adey and Walter, 1963). Such a display may also show fans for other frequencies.

These fan shaped sectors for different frequencies are often closely grouped in a single sector of the phase circle. This presents us with a remarkable physiological puzzle. How can two parts of the brain, widely separated from each other, be related at very similar phase angles over more than 2 octaves of frequencies, if this relationship depends on a simple pulse coding of impulses between the two regions (Adey, 1969a)? It says a great deal about the complexity of the coding that occurs in the fibre bundles that carry information from one region of the brain to another, something that we scarcely comprehend at this time. It is not enough that we know the interspike intervals in the firing pattern of a particular neuron. That would tell us very little about the fantastically complex behavior of many thousands of neurons. If we could imagine such a pathway as a telephone trunk cable, cut across, and could examine the impulse pattern, we would probably still not see a major component on the firing locked to dominant EEG frequencies (Adey, 1969b). But somehow, in what is carried in that code, a second generation of waves appears at a point several centimeters away from that at which the original generation occurred.

### COMPUTER SYSTEMS FOR NEUROPHYSIOLOGICAL RESEARCH

In our Institute, the main computer is an SDS 9300, originally designed for missile fire control, with a great capacity to interact with the real world in real time, and to accept commands from a variety of inputs (Betyár, 1967). There are many ways of entering commands and data in this computer.

This system is an example of an "interactive processor", which allows the investigators in their laboratories to compute their data in real time, actually during an experiment, with as many as five investigators using the system simultaneously. It involves a series of laboratory consoles (Fig. 6). Each console has 60 keys which allow both "operator" and "operand" modes of command. This means that there are upper and lower cases to the keys, and essentially the user can either command major coding routines and large sub-programs, or he can use this console to program the main computer minutely, step by step. The instructions appear on a display oscilloscope. When the computer executes these commands and performs the com-

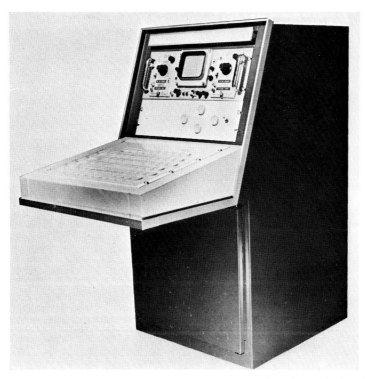

Fig .6. Laboratory console developed at UCLA Brain Research Institute for use in time-shared SLIP (Shared Laboratory Interpretive Processor) system. (From Betyár, 1967).

putation, the output also appears on the oscilloscope, where it may be photographed or plotted graphically, or it may be stored in other ways, as on video tape.

We have looked so far from the central Data Processing Laboratory, with its SDS 9300, back into the laboratory. The SDS 9300 computer also looks outward to a large IBM computer, a 360-91, in the adjacent Health Sciences Computing Facility. The latter can be the central processor by direct tie-lines, or the SDS computer can be used in a "stand-alone" mode, apart from the IBM computer. The SDS 9300 has a 32 000-word, 24-bit memory in magnetic core. It has an 8 000 000-bit disk file. Instructions may be given to the computer on magnetic tape, paper tape, punched cards, or by a typewriter (Fig. 7). Outputs appear on a line printer and on graphic plotters. In a time-shared mode, with five consoles sharing the system at one time, there is a maximum total data transfer rate into the computer of 500 000 bits per second. This is quite fast by comparison with most time-shared systems currently in use. Six tape transports provide storage for intermediate calculations. In a time-shared mode, the system can perform a number of functions simultaneously, such as multichannel high speed A–D conversion, performance of major arithmetic calculations, preparation of output displays on X–Y plotters or on console oscilloscopes, or storage of output on magnetic tape. This flexibility differs in input and output capabilities from that usually available in a typical business computing system. The

*References pp. 43–44*

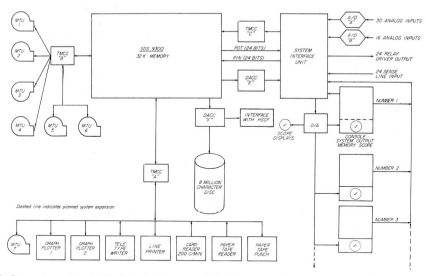

Fig. 7. Computer system in UCLA Brain Research Institute, showing arrangement of magnetic tape storage units (MTU), remote consoles and interface with IBM 360-91 in adjacent Health Sciences Computing Facility (HCSF). (From Betyár, 1967).

A–D converter on the SDS 9300 can handle 32 channels of data at one time, with a maximum overall conversion rate of 100 000 samples/sec.

In recent years the utility of quite modest general purpose computers in comprehensive analyses of physiological data has been substantially augmented by special purpose convolution integral computers that can be attached to a medium-sized digital computer. They were initially designed with emphasis on a very fast multiplying capability, but it was obvious that they could be used to calculate correlation functions and spectral analyses, to average, and to make amplitude or interval histograms. Such devices are thus flexible computers in their own right.

In our applications of this intrument, a TD-100, we can analyze continuously two channels of EEG autospectra, or their cross-spectra. We apply it in continuous spectral analysis of data received in such applications as telephone telemetry. However, when used as a multiplying device as an adjunct to the larger computer, we can have 12 channels of on-line autospectra, continuously calculated, without using the large IBM processor. One can thus convert a relatively limited capability in a medium-sized computer to a much larger capability by adding this type of instrument.

## TYPICAL COMPUTER APPLICATIONS TO NEUROPHYSIOLOGICAL DATA

To the neurophysiologist one of the most challenging applications of the computer is to the problem of the origins of the EEG. It was mentioned by Dr. Petsche at this conference that we do not yet know where the EEG originates. I do not agree completely. It appears that we are much closer to understanding it than we were five years ago, as a result of work by Creutzfeldt (1964) and his colleagues, Fujita and Sato (1964), Jasper and Stefanis (1965) and by Elul (1967, 1968, 1969) in our laboratory. Elul (1964, 1968) recorded intracellularly from unanesthetized cortical neurons of the cat, together with the EEG from the same domain of tissue, with the animal both asleep and awake. It is surprising that many cortical neurons appear to have no fixed resting level of membrane potential. They display big waves that continue ceaselessly, and look very like the EEG. When the cell fires, it does so near the depolarizing peaks of the waves. The amplitude of this intracellular wave is large, up to 20 mV. The EEG by comparison is about 1/100 to 1/200 of this amplitude. This is about what would be expected by a voltage division of this intracellular wave across the membrane resistance.

Moreover, there does not appear to be a fixed firing threshold in the cortical neuron. Depolarization of the cell may occur to the point where it may fire, but firing does not necessarily ensue. One may also observe firing on at least two different thresholds. It is therefore necessary that we either revise our concepts of the window on the cell interior available to us by a microelectrode, or that we must look to the longitudinal organization of the cell and conclude that there are aspects of longitudinal organization from dendrites to soma which will make the susceptibility of the axon hillock (where impulses presumably begin in most cases) differentially susceptible to exciting influences arising in different parts of the dendritic tree. However, we cannot discuss these hypotheses further here.

How much like the EEG is the intracellular wave? The spectra of the gross EEG and the spectra of the intracellular wave do indeed resemble one another. One might then be tempted to say that the EEG is nothing more than the summed activity of many synchronous generators. But the relationship is considerably more complex, because these generators are apparently non-linear, independent and fit a scheme described by Cramer's central limit theorem. My colleague Rafael Elul (1968) has calculated the coherence between the intraneuronal wave and the EEG over epochs as long as 500 sec, with successive analyses at 10-sec intervals, over a spectrum from 0 to 15 Hz (Fig. 8). High coherences typically occurred only with the incidence of a random relationship. Thus, the EEG does not arise simply in summing of synchronous intraneuronal waves.

One may approach this problem of genesis of the EEG from a completely opposite view. From the amplitude distributions of the EEG, one might be able to say something about the contributing generators. If they are randomly related, the generators will show a normal or Gaussian amplitude distribution in their summed activity. In typical examples of the EEG, and contrary to what was said this morning, the distributions tend to be strongly Gaussian (Elul, 1967a; Adey, Elul, Walter and Crandall, 1967; Elul, 1969). On the other hand, intracellular records are virtually never Gaussian in their distribution. What explanation may be offered for the apparent difference between these data and what was discussed this morning? It appears that trends towards a Gaussian distribution depend on the length of the epoch of data analyzed. With short epochs of two seconds, analyzed either at 200 or 7000 samples per second,

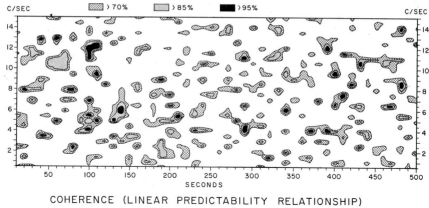

COHERENCE (LINEAR PREDICTABILITY RELATIONSHIP)
BETWEEN NEURONAL WAVES AND EEG

Fig. 8. Estimates of coherence between intracellular wave in cerebral neuron and concurrent EEG in same domain of tissue. High coherence levels in black, low in white. Ordinates are spectral frequencies 0–15 Hz, abscissae cover total period of 500 sec, and successive cross-spectra were calculated on 10 sec epochs. Significant coherence levels do not occur at higher than chance incidence in almost any part of the plot. (From Elul, 1968).

they are Gaussian in most cases. In testing effects of sample length, with EEG durations in excess of 2.0 sec, there is a drop in the probability of a Gaussian distribution. We have compared amplitude distributions with the subject sitting in the dark, sitting quietly anticipating a task in mental arithmetic, and performing the task.

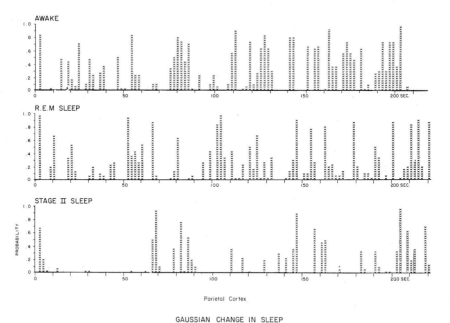

GAUSSIAN CHANGE IN SLEEP

Fig. 9. Probability of Gaussian amplitude distributions in successive 2.0-sec EEG samples in man, when awake, in REM sleep and in Stage II sleep. (From Elul, 1966; Adey, Elul, Walter and Crandall, 1967).

In bifrontal EEG records, task performance increases the tendency to a Gaussian distribution. That is to say, the generators appear less "cooperative".

If one compares Gaussian trends in awake records with those in various stages of sleep (Fig. 9), rapid-eye-movement (REM) sleep associated with dreaming is similar to the awake state, whereas in sleep with a spindling EEG record there is a sharp shift away from a Gaussian distribution, as would be expected from the regularity of waves in each spindle.

We have had the opportunity to study patients with electrodes implanted symmetrically in the hippocampal gyri on both sides. In a patient with an epileptic focus on the right side, the abnormal tissue shows much less tendency to Gaussian amplitude distributions. This could be interpreted as an increased connectivity between the generators in the epileptic tissue.

*Computer applications in behavioral neurophysiology; problems of short data epochs*

One may simply average the EEG when the subject is performing a repetitive task. In such simple daily averages which we made of 40 records from a cat making a visual discrimination, hippocampal theta-trains at 6 Hz contributed strongly to the average (Radulovacki and Adey, 1965). Interspersed with the discrimination trials on the same days were trials in which the animal was orienting by looking towards the task, but was unable to perform it. The averages were totally different during orienting responses. The dominant frequency in the average was much slower, around 4 Hz. By this simple averaging it is possible to clearly separate orienting and discriminating epochs.

LSD produces striking effects in the cat in doses of 25 to 100 $\mu$g/kg. About one hour after injection of the drug, they may paw at invisible objects, or lie stretched out, with claws extended and purring all the time; they may stand rooted to the spot in a catatonic pose; or walk with a peculiar wide-legged gait, tail up, fur erect and suddenly shaking the head as though experiencing some visual illusion (Adey, Bell and Dennis, 1962).

The EEG under LSD is very characteristic in temporal lobe structures. There are episodes of high amplitude slow waves that spread into thalamus, midbrain, and visual cortex. They appear suddenly and last 5 to 10 sec. These acute effects last about 8 hours, but there are other changes that last for many weeks after a single dose of LSD (Fig. 10). There is an augmentation of the theta-trains for about a week after the drug during visual discrimination performances, and gradually, in the second and third weeks there appears much more regular activity in the orienting records than in predrug tests. Augmented orienting behavior is marked in man and animals after LSD.

These studies with averaging techniques have exemplified the power of such simple methods in revealing certain consistent EEG by patterns associated with repetitive performances. In many task performances it would be desirable to analyze quite short epochs that last about a second. It is not possible to deal with these records separately if we wish to perform spectral analyses, with high resolution (*e.g.*, 1.0 Hz

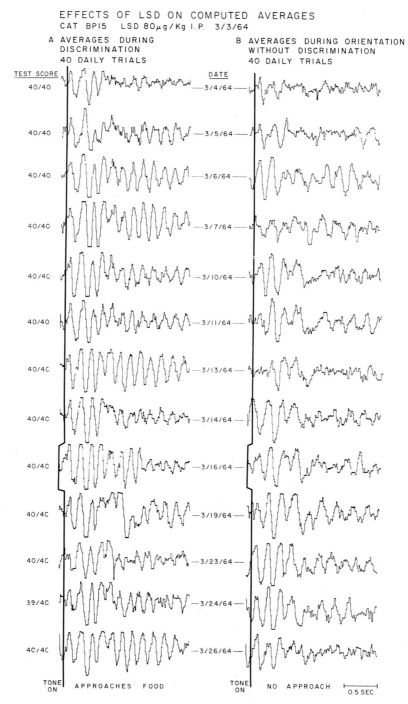

Fig. 10. Daily averages of 2.0-sec EEG epochs of cat hippocampal EEG during light–dark discrimination (left) and randomly interspersed orienting responses (right). These averages were prepared daily following a single dose of LSD (80 μg/kg) prior to the first test day shown here. (From Radulovacki and Adey, 1965).

filter bandwidths). Yet we can perform such a fine analysis on short epochs if we can put them together from repeated trials. We wished to analyze such short epochs about 1.5-sec long, from cats that were successively waiting in the starting box, listening to an alerting tone, running from behind closed doors to make a visual discrimination, and then returning to the starting box (Elazar and Adey, 1967 a and b). We wished to analyze the data with filters only 1.0 Hz wide over the spectrum 0–30 Hz. There are constraints in so doing, determined by the number of degrees of freedom in the data. With very short epochs lasting only about 1.0 sec one must either have very broad filters, 5 to 10 Hz in bandwidth, or one must accept an answer from the computer that is statistically unreliable. That is why our computers have been programmed to first examine the data and ask: "What is the bandwidth of the analysis that you want?" Our response is typically: "0–30 Hz". The computer then asks: "How long is the record and what is the sampling rate?" If we reply that there is less than 5 sec of data and the sampling rate is 200/sec then the computer will say: "These data cannot be analyzed reliably with filters that are less than 2 or 3 Hz wide". Thus one cannot trick a computer into performing an unreliable analysis; at least that is the intention of our instructions.

When such short 1.5-sec epochs are put together to make a total data sample of 10 to 20 sec, the autospectra in the waiting state show a peak in the hippocampus at 4 Hz. When the cat hears the tone, the peak shifts to 5 Hz. When the animal runs

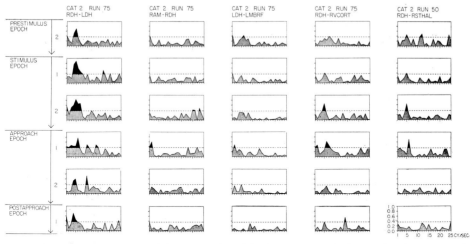

Fig. 11. Estimates of coherence between pairs of brain structures during resting (PRESTIMULUS), alerting (STIMULUS), discriminating (APPROACH) and feeding (POSTAPPROACH) epochs. Each epoch lasted only 1.6 sec, but spectral parameters were estimated from a compilation of 10 repetitions of the test on a single day. Each graph plots coherence on ordinates (0–1.0) and the spectrum (0–25 Hz) on abscissae. Dashed line indicates statistically significant coherence level, and coherence above this level is shown in solid black. Cross-specta were calculated between right and left dorsal hippocampi (RDH–LDH), right amygdala and dorsal hippocampus (RAM–RDH), left dorsal hippocampus and midbrain reticular formation (LDH–LMBRF), right dorsal hippocampus and right visual cortex (RDH–RVCORT), and right dorsal hippocampus and right subthalamus (RDH–RSTHAL). (From Elazar and Adey, 1967b).

to the food it shifts to 6 Hz then reverts to 5 Hz as the animal reaches the food. During eating, the peak drops to 4 Hz. The sequence of dominant frequencies is 4, 5, 6 and 4 Hz. This cannot be reliably detected by looking at the record (Fig. 11).

By the same technique, one can measure coherence between the hippocampus and other regions during this succession of waiting, listening to the tone, and approaching the food. Some remarkable changes appear. A dashed line on each graph is the level above which coherence is significant. The graphs cover from 0–25 Hz and the coherence function is plotted from 0 to 1.0. In the waiting periods there is a broad band of high coherence between right and left hippocampi in the theta band from 4 to 7 Hz. As the animal makes its approach, this peak in coherence narrows to only 1 Hz wide. As the animal completes the approach it tends to broaden out again.

In measurements of coherence between the hippocampus and visual cortex, values are low in the waiting period. As the animal prepares to approach the food goal, a peak of coherence appears between hippocampus and visual cortex at 5 and 6 Hz. During the approach to food with visual discrimination, there is a high peak at 6 to 8 Hz. It declines on attaining the food reward.

Similarly, in coherence measurements between dorsal hippocampus and sub-thalamus, a peak occurs during periods when attention is most sharply focused (Fig. 11). These findings exemplify the brain system model presented at the onset of this discussion. We may postulate pathways on anatomical grounds, and we can evaluate their significance by testing them in the performing subject.

## SUMMARY

In presenting our needs as physiologists to the computer engineer, we should surely point out that if our computations are to be on-line, or as nearly on-line as possible, we will need very high data transfer rates. Moveover, it is inevitable in most physiological experiments that there will be many channels of data. The calculations are usually complex. There must be meaningful display techniques, and as discussed in the next lecture, we will need automatic recognition by the computer of patterns characterizing different classes of EEG records. Historically, the first generation of computers were the calculators that Dr. Jensen discussed at this conference. They were very good at arithmetic, but most difficult to program in a complex series of calculations. The second generation showed much more flexibility in coding and were more successful in analyses and display. Now in the third generation of computers we are moving to the position of allowing the computer to recognize patterns and make decisions about patterns which we cannot perceive with our unaided senses. These will be discussed in the next lecture.

## ACKNOWLEDGMENTS

Studies from our laboratory described here were supported by Grants NB-01883, NB-2503 and MH-03708 from the National Institutes of Health; by Contract AF (49) 638–1387 with the U.S. Air Force Office of Scientific Research; by Contract

NONR 233-91 with the Office of Naval Research; and Contracts NsG 237-62, NsG 502, and NsG 1970 with the National Aeronautics and Space Administration. Our computations in the UCLA Health Sciences Computing Facility were supported by Grant FR-003 from the National Institutes of Health.

## REFERENCES

ADEY, W. R. (1967) Intrinsic organization of cerebral tissue in alerting, orienting and discriminative responses. In: *The Neurosciences*, G. C. QUARTON, T. MELNECHUK, F. O. SCHMITT (Eds.), Rockefeller University Press, New York, pp. 615–633.

ADEY, W. R. (1969a) Spectral analysis of EEG data from animals and man during alerting, orienting and discriminative responses. In: *The Neurophysiology of Attention*, C. EVANS AND T. B. MULHOLLAND (Eds.), Butterworth, London, 1969, pp. 194–229.

ADEY, W. R. (1969b) Spontaneous electrical brain rhythms accompanying learned responses. M.I.T. Neurosciences Research Program. Rockefeller University Press, New York, in press.

ADEY, W. R. (1969c) Neural information processing; windows without and the citadel within. In: *Biocybernetics of the Central Nervous System*, L. D. PROCTOR (Ed.), Little, Brown, Boston, pp. 1–27.

ADEY, W. R., BELL, F. R. AND DENNIS, B. J. (1962) Effects of LSD, psilocybin and psilocin on temporal lobe EEG patterns and learned behavior in the cat. *Neurology*, 12, 591–602.

ADEY, W. R., BYSTROM, B. G., COSTIN, A., KADO, R. T. AND TARBY, T. J. (1969) Divalent cations in cerebral impedance and cell membrane morphology. *Exptl. Neurol.*, 23, 29–50.

ADEY, W. R., ELUL, R., WALTER, R. D. AND CRANDALL, P. H. (1967) The cooperative behavior of neuronal populations during sleep and mental tasks. *Electroenceph. Clin. Neurophysiol.*, 23, 87–88.

ADEY, W. R., KADO, R. T., MCILWAIN, J. T. AND WALTER, D. O. (1966) The role of neuronal elements in regional cerebral impedance changes in alerting, orienting and discriminative responses. *Exptl. Neurol.*, 15, 490–510.

ADEY, W. R., SEGUNDO, J. P. AND LIVINGSTON, R. B. (1957) Corticifugal influences on intrinsic brainstem conduction in cat and monkey. *J. Neurophysiol.*, 20, 1–16.

ADEY, W. R. AND WALTER, D. O. (1963) Application of phase detection and averaging techniques in computer analysis of EEG records in the cat. *Exptl. Neurol.*, 7, 186–209.

BERKHOUT, J., WALTER, D. O. AND ADEY, W. R. (1969) Alterations of the human electroencephalogram induced by stressful verbal activity. *Electroenceph. Clin. Neurophysiol.*, 27, 457–469.

BETYÁR, L. (1967) A user-oriented time-shared online system. *J. Assoc. Computing Machinery*, 10, 413–419.

BLACKMAN, R. B. AND TUKEY, J. W. (1959) *The Measurement of Power Spectra*, Dover, New York.

CREUTZFELDT, O. D., FUSTER, J. M., LUX, H. D. AND NACIMIENTO, A. (1964) Experimenteller Nachweis von Beziehungen zwischen EEG-Wellen und Activität corticaler Nervenzellen. *Naturwissenschaften*, 51, 166–167.

ELAZAR, Z. AND ADEY, W. R. (1967a) Spectral analysis of low frequency components in the hippocampal electroencephalogram during learning. *Electroenceph. Clin. Neurophysiol.*, 23, 225–240.

ELAZAR, Z. AND ADEY, W. R. (1967b) Electroencephalographic correlates of learning in subcortical and cortical structures. *Electroenceph. Clin. Neurophysiol.*, 23, 306–319.

ELLIOT SMITH, G. (1910) Some problems relating to the evolution of the brain. Arris and Gale Lectures. *Lancet*, 1, 147 and 221.

ELUL, R. (1964) Specific site of generation of brain waves. *The Physiologist*, 7, 125.

ELUL, R. (1967a) Amplitude histograms of the EEG as an indicator of the comparative behavior of neuron populations. *Electroenceph. Clin. Neurophysiol.*, 23, 86.

ELUL, R. (1967b) Statistical mechanisms in generation of the EEG. In: *Progress in Biomedical Engineering*, L. J. FOGEL AND F. W. GEORGE (Eds.), Spartan Books, Washington, D.C., pp. 131–150.

ELUL, R. (1968) Brain waves: intracellular recording and statistical analyses help clarify their physiological significance. *Data Acquisition and Processing Biol. Med.*, 5, 93–115.

ELUL, R. (1969) Gaussian behavior of the electroencephalogram: changes during performance of mental task. *Science*, 164, 328–331.

FUJITA, J. AND SATO, T. (1964) Intracellular records from hippocampal pyramidal cells during theta rhythm activity. *J. Neurophysiol.*, 27, 1011–1025.

GOODMAN, N. R. (1960) Measuring amplitude and phase. *J. Franklin Inst.*, **270**, 437–450.

HANLEY, J., ZWEIZIG, R., KADO, R. T. AND ADEY, W. R. (1968) Some applications of biotelemetry. Institute of Electrical and Electronics Engineers, *Proceedings National Telemetry Conference*, pp. 369–373.

HANLEY, J., ZWEIZIG, R., KADO, R. T., ADEY, W. R. AND ROVNER, L. D. (1969) Combined telephone and radiotelemetry. *Electroenceph. Clin. Neurophysiol.*, **26**, 323–324.

HERRICK, C. J. (1933) The functions of the olfactory parts of the cerebral cortex. *Proc. Natl. Acad. Sci. U.S.*, **19**, 7–14.

JACOBSON, A., KALES, A., LEHMANN, D. AND ZWEIZIG, J. R. (1965) Somnambulism: all night electro-encephalographic studies. *Science*, **148**, 975–977.

JASPER, H. H. AND STEFANIS, C. (1965) Intracellular oscillatory rhythms in pyramidal cells of the cat. *Electroenceph. Clin. Neurophysiol.*, **18**, 541–553.

KADO, R. T. AND ADEY, W. R. (1968) Electrode problems in central nervous monitoring in performing subjects. *Ann. N.Y. Acad. Sci.*, **148**, article 1, 263–278.

KLÜVER, H. AND BUCY, P. C. (1939) Preliminary analysis of functions of the temporal lobes in monkeys. *Arch. Neurol. Psychiat.*, **42**, 979–1000.

MORUZZI, G. AND MAGOUN, H. W. (1949) Brain stem reticular formation and activation of the EEG. *Electroenceph. Clin. Neurophysiol.*, **1**, 455–473.

PROCTOR, L. D. AND KNIGHTON, R. (Eds.) (1967) *Reticular Formation of the Brain*, Little, Brown, Boston.

RADULOVACKI, M. AND ADEY, W. R. (1965) The hippocampus and the orienting reflex. *Exptl. Neurol.*, **12**, 68–83.

RALL, W., SHEPHERD, G. M., REESE, T. S. AND BRIGHTMAN, M. W. (1966) Dendrodendritic synaptic pathway for inhibition in the olfactory bulb. *Exptl. Neurol.*, **14**, 44–56.

SCHMITT, F. O. AND DAVISON, P. F. (1965) Brain and nerve proteins: functional correlates. Role of protein in neural function. *Neurosciences Res. Prog. Bull.*, **3** (6), 1–87.

WALTER, D. O. (1963) Spectral analysis for electroencephalograms: mathematical determination of neurophysiological relationships from records of limited duration. *Exptl. Neurol.*, **8**, 155–181.

WALTER, D. O., KADO, R. T., RHODES, J. M. AND ADEY, W. R. (1967) Electroencephalographic baselines in astronaut candidates estimated by computation and pattern recognition techniques. *Aerospace Med.*, **38**, 371–379.

WANG, H. H. AND ADEY, W. R. (1969) Effects of cations and hyaluronidase on cerebral electrical impedance. *Exptl. Neurol.*, **25**, 70–84.

ZWEIZIG, J. R., KADO, R. T., HANLEY, J. AND ADEY, W. R. (1967) The design and use of an FM/AM radio telemetry system for multichannel recording of biological data. *Institute of Electrical and Electronics Engineers, Trans. Biomed. Eng.*, BME-**14**, 230–238.

# Computing Devices of the second and third Generations

W. R. ADEY

*Departments of Anatomy and Physiology, and Space Biology Laboratory, Brain Research Institute,*
*University of California, Los Angeles, Calif. (U.S.A.)*

Previous speakers have emphasized important building blocks that have marked the progress over almost ten years in our use of computers for analytic procedures. There was universal emphasis on the need to have clean neurophysiological data going into the computer, and on adequate amounts of data, and how such factors may determine the nature of analytic methods. About three years ago several groups began to use computers as pattern recognizing devices in the treatment of physiological data (Ramsey, 1969). The two principle fields in these developments are electrocardiography and electroencephalography. Pattern recognition in the electrocardiogram is beyond my special competence, but it has probably received greater public attention than analysis of the EEG. There are major programs to develop pattern recognizing techniques in the EKG for detection of changes with age, and also in management of patients in intensive care.

I wish to discuss use of the computer to assemble data from many computations. These may be computations on data from one individual over a short period, perhaps an hour or two, or it may involve assembling data from many people subjected to the same procedures over a period of months. It became apparent early in these procedures that merely to collect data and put them together in one place defeated the object of the computation, because the size of the computer output on paper was physically much bigger than the EEG records from which they were taken. The piles of paper from the computer exceeded in size the piles of paper from the EEG machine. This was indeed a challenge to both neurophysiologist and computer scientist.

## DEVELOPMENT OF A "LIBRARY" OF NORMAL EEG DATA

In collaboration with Dr. P. Kellaway and Dr. R. Maulsby at the Methodist Hospital, Houston, we undertook to develop a "library" of normal EEG material from young men who wished to be astronauts (Walter, Kado, Rhodes and Adey, 1967). The question of what to do with these data was the first milestone. In a sense we were asked to do something that we should have undertaken voluntarily as physiologists many years ago, namely to study the normal EEG. It was necessary that this base line be established across 200 subjects, and that the data be acquired in ways that would allow its comparison from subject to subject in a highly quantified fashion. We developed an instrument which gave one hour of perceptual and learning tasks to

*References p. 62*

RESPONSES OF ELECTROENCEPHALOGRAM TO DIFFERING SITUATIONS

TOPO-SPECTROGRAPHIC VARIATIONS OF
AVERAGES OVER FIFTY ASTRONAUT CANDIDATES

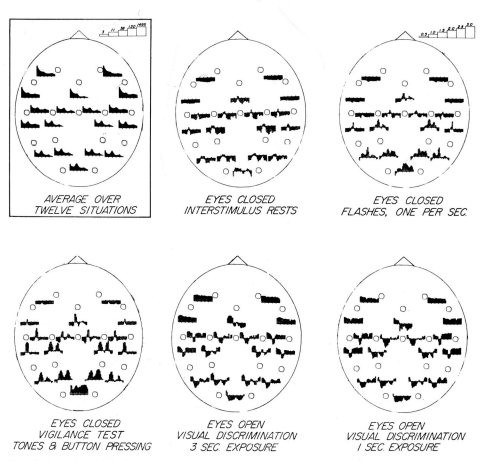

Fig. 1. Examples of data from "normative library" study, showing collective "heads", each prepared for 50 subjects. Electrodes were placed as shown on each subject, according to a modified international 10–20 schema. In handling the data, spectral densities were first separately calculated at each scalp location for each subject in 12 different behavioral situations. The individual spectra were then averaged for each scalp location in 50 subjects, over the 12 behavioral situations (top left). At each scalp location, the graph of spectral density covers frequencies 0–25 Hz. This average over 12 situations was used as a mean for comparison with the 5 separate situations shown, with spectral densities in the separate situations expressed as variance above or below the mean at each frequency. Calibrations: for average over 12 situations in $\mu V^2$/cycle/sec; for individual situations, in standard deviations.
(From Walter, Rhodes, Kado and Adey, 1967.)

each subject from a magnetic tape. Thus, the sequence of tasks was accurately repeated from one subject to another through the magnetic tape control.

This instrument carried as subcarriers magnetic tape signals that delivered physical stimuli in various modalities. It also presented a series of visual tasks on a screen, and auditory tasks from a loudspeaker to test vigilance and recognition of tone sequences. More than 30 parameters from the subjects were recorded on two 16-channel tapes, including 18 channels of EEG. The command signals were also transferred to the data tapes for timing purposes. The subject sat comfortably in a chair with press buttons at his right hand to signal his task responses. There was provision for calibration of the electro-oculogram as a measure of eye movements during the task performance. So many data were accumulated that procedures were necessary to bring them into a common file.

### SPECTRAL PARAMETERS SHARED ACROSS A PERFORMING POPULATION

In first attempts to detect EEG patterns common to this population, data from 50 subjects were put together on a single "head", with a spectral analysis at each point on the head (Fig. 1). The initial spectra were derived as an average over 12 different situations, in which the subjects ranged in behavioral state from sitting quietly with eyes closed, or open, to performing a difficult visual task in 1.0 sec, in circumstances that made success most difficult. The average of the EEG at each point on the head is expressed as a spectrum from 0–25 Hz, and the ordinates show intensity in $\mu V^2/$ cycle/sec. The spectrum thus indicates power density distribution at that point on the head. Succeeding heads on this figure are also for 50 subjects, but set up in a different way. Each situation uses the contour of the initial multi-situational spectrum as its base line. Differences from that base line are expressed in standard deviations above or below the mean. In this collected set of 5 situations, the subjects sat with eyes closed resting; or with eyes closed but with flashes once per second; or with eyes closed during an auditory vigilance test; or performed a visual discrimination of 1 to 6 circles, with 3 sec to make the judgment; or performed the same sort of task but with a smaller difference between the sixth circle and the other 5, and with only a 1-sec exposure, thus making the task quite difficult.

With eyes closed at rest, there was a modest peak above the mean in the $\alpha$-band in the occipital region. The $\alpha$-band was broad, covering frequencies 8 to 12 Hz. The powers at all other frequencies in the occipital region under these conditions were below the mean. In the frontal region none of the powers came up to the mean across the entire spectrum.

Similarly, with eyes closed, but now with flashes at 1/sec, powers in the frontal region remained very low, with the difference that now there was a great exaggeration of all powers in the occipital leads, across the whole spectrum, except at the very low end. This enhancement was partly in the $\alpha$-bands and partly in the $\beta$-bands from 13–25 Hz. Thus, merely by flashing the subject once per sec totally changed the EEG pattern in the posterior half of the head.

In the auditory vigilance task, yet another pattern appeared. The highest powers that we have been able to evoke in the $\alpha$-bands occurred while the subjects were performing this auditory task. Powers remained high at higher frequencies in the occipital region, but still there was no power above the mean in the frontal leads.

Next, they performed a visual discrimination in 3 sec. Immediately the picture in the frontal leads reversed. Very high powers then appeared in frontal leads. At first, it was thought that this might be muscular in orgin, related to activity in the frontal muscles. Very careful checks showed by coherence measurements that this was not likely. Power in the $\alpha$-bands fell substantially below the mean in occipital and other posterior leads, and built up in delta and theta bands at 3–6 Hz. Similarly, theta bands were now quite powerful in temporal leads and in temporovertex placements. Thus, merely changing the behavioral state from paying attention to an auditory stimulus to paying attention to a visual stimulus, with both requiring decision making, changed the pattern completely. Finally, in performing discriminations on visual data presented for only 1.0 sec, the differences were even sharper and qualitatively similar to those in discriminations of 3.0 sec test epochs.

We made similar analyses of EEG records in sleep, covering seven states of drowsiness and sleep in making the initial average. By mere inspections of the collective heads for 30 individuals, it was obvious that they exhibited common features in their EEG at each sleep stage, despite individual differences. It was also clear by simple inspection that individual EEGs bore "signatures" best characterizing them that differed from subject to subject. We thus faced the question: granted that we now have at least a tentative baseline for a population of subjects, what can it tell about the individual subject?

### APPLICATION OF PATTERN RECOGNITION TECHNIQUES TO EEG SPECTRAL PARAMETERS AND TO EVOKED POTENTIALS

As an initial approach to this problem of relating an individual EEG record to a population mean, it appeared potentially useful to test a double color display. For example, the subject's means or group means might be used, and his response in individual situations was then displayed on the trace in another color. This did not help a great deal. It was then decided to try a totally different approach to the broblem by use of stepwise discriminant analysis. In this analysis, a matrix is prepared from parameters calculated in spectral analysis of the EEG. The diagonal of the matrix was examined for the parameters that best distinguished between the situations.

There are various ways in which these discriminant analyses can be displayed. Dr. D. O. Walter first used a simple matrix of successive situations and sought high peaks on the diagonal (Walter, Rhodes and Adey, 1967). The computation is programmed in the following way. The computer is given all numerical data from spectral calculations that include autospectral density, cross-spectral density, coherence, regularity of dominant frequency, and so on. At the first step, a selection is made of the one factor which will best distinguish between a series of 5 or more behavioral situations. Having selected one parameter, the computer selects a second parameter which best distinguishes between them. It is obvious in such a step-by-step analysis that another way to display such a separation would be to indicate the effectiveness of a particular factor in achieving a separation by distance between two points. If plotting it makes a good separation, then the distance between the points will be large, and vice versa. Our display could reflect the differences between two data sets in this way. It is surprising to observe the success of the computer in revealing patterns that the eye cannot see at all, and in making 100% separations in quite a variety of situations, ranging from broad aspects of behavioral states, and correlates with broad classes of task performance, such as those involving auditory or visual discrimination, to finer distinctions between one stress state and another, and into the area of correctness or incorrectness of decision on a predictive basis, where one can tell many seconds beforehand whether a subject will be correct or not.

We may display a simple matrix for EEG parameters in a series of behavioral states including eyes closed, resting; eyes open, resting; eyes closed, performing the auditory discrimination; a visual discrimination in 3 sec; and a visual discrimination in 1 sec. The initial spectral analysis for the 50 subjects took about 1400 hours on an IBM 7094. Most of that time was spent with the computer in a multiplying mode, making 500,000 multiplications per second. The computer output from these calculations was overwhelmingly large. We then faced a new question as to whether a smaller calculation of individual subjects would achieve the goal of this matrix method and of other forms of

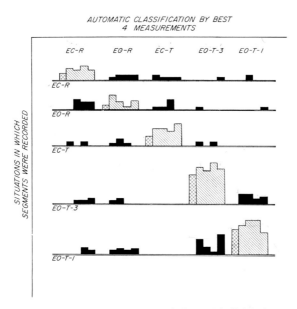

Fig. 2. Discriminant analysis applied to EEG records from 4 individuals separately, and to their records collectively, in situations: eyes closed resting (EC-R); eyes open, resting (EO-R); eyes closed, performing auditory vigilance tasks at 5.0-sec intervals (EC-T); and eyes open, performing identical visual tasks in 1.0 sec (EO-T-I). Matrix display shows on diagonal computed separation of states. Shaded bars of individuals separately; cross-hatched bars are for 4 subjects collectively. The computed separation was over 90 per cent correct for individuals separately. (From Walter, Rhodes and Adey, 1967.)

pattern recognition in allowing recognition by simpler computing devices and with fewer parameters.

An example of discriminant analysis shown in Fig. 2 displays data for 4 subjects. The parameters in each subject came from 4 channels of EEG data, each epoch lasting 10 sec. There were 5 variables per channel. The variables were the spectral density in each filter band, the regularity of the dominant rhythm, the coherence between temporo-vertex leads and temporo-occipital leads, the intensity in the $\beta$-bands and the intensity in the theta-bands, viewed separately in the frontal and temporal leads respectively. These are very simple measures. This final analysis with so few parameters was arrived at after first giving the computer some 80 variables to examine. In a later study we have used as many as 2000 variables. From these studies it appears unnecessary to have either long data epochs or a large number of variables. We shall see that 100% separations of five aspects of behavioral states can be achieved on an automated basis with quite small amounts of data.

In summary, this initial study shows that with four subjects the computer separated the 5 situations. The hatched bar in each case is the summed separation for the 4 people. In every case it is lower than for each as an individual, because it is inherent in group-statistics like this that the efficiency of separation will drop when parameters from different subjects are grouped.

Many of the parameters that were selected by the computer for the individuals were those which the group means from the normative library had indicated would be important. Others were different, and it was concluded that each individual can be characterized by a set of EEG signatures that are peculiarly his own, as well as being in part those which unite him with the group.

We have recently found another interesting method in utilizing discriminant analysis. Gardiner (1969) has recently completed his thesis studies with Dr. D. O. Walter on evoked potentials subjected to discriminant analysis. He recorded evoked potentials on the scalp in music students listening to tones with loudness or pitch differing from a previously tested mean level. The subject was required to report his interpretation in writing after each presentation. Records for evoked potentials relating to these louder or softer, or higher or lower tones were displayed as two evoked potentials that were superimposed and stored separately (Fig. 3). Each is an average of 500 presentations. In applying discriminant analysis to these averaged evoked potentials, the question was asked: what segments of this multiphasic potential make the best distinctions between tones that are louder and tones that are softer? The function that has been graphed below the evoked potential is the measure of the probability that a particular segment of the evoked potential will offer the best discrimination between the one which is louder and the one which is softer. Also shown are the 5.0, 1.0 and 0.1 per cent confidence levels for $F$ for a normal distribution. Discriminant characters in the evoked potential have also been investigated by Donchin (1968).

This probability contour varies very markedly from one part of the potential to another. This interesting probability function is often periodic at about 150 msec, or around 6 or 7 Hz. Although the significance is unknown, it is interesting that there was no evidence of such a rhythmic function in the evoked potentials themselves. One also

MEDIUM BACKGROUND NOISE

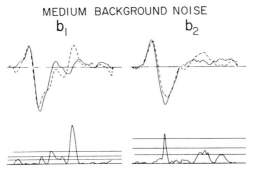

Fig. 3. Discriminant analysis applied to averaged evoked potentials recorded in vertex-mastoid leads of man, with each average based on 500 or more stimulus presentations (see text). $b_1$ and $b_2$: two data sets analyzed from music students given tone bursts 50 msec in duration that could have two intensity levels (differing by db) and two frequencies (differing by 10 Hz from a mean frequency of 315 Hz). Tones were presented against background noise with approximately 25 db S/N ratio. The tasks used identical stimulus conditions, and the same average uncertainty. Set $b_1$, combines data from 3 long sessions with one subject, set $b_2$ from four sessions with 4 other subjects, all scoring approximately correct on both tasks. *Upper traces*: Solid line shows within set averaged evoked potential during intensity discrimination, with responses to all stimuli equally represented. Dotted line shows similar evoked potential during frequency identification task. Sweep duration 710 msec, traces negative upward. Stimulus presented at beginning of sweep. *Lower traces*: As an estimate of reliability of differences between potentials from intensity and frequency tasks, the $F$ statistic was calculated at 10 msec intervals, and plotted as a continuous function. Horizontal lines show 5.0, 1.0 and 0.1% confidence levels for $F$ for normal distribution. The two sets show similar configurations for identical tasks and similar differences between tasks, the most reliable changes occurring at longer latencies. (From Gardiner, 1969, with permission.)

wonders whether quite minor perturbations in the actual contour of the evoked potential may, indeed, significantly reflect ways in which the brain handles information.

## DISCRIMINANT ANALYSIS OF EEG DATA AQUIRED IN STRESSFUL QUESTIONING

These studies of evoked potentials took no account of subject mood. We have investigated this question of EEG concomitants of psychological stress in a series of 5 subjects tested in ways similar to the normative library method, using either audio-tape or video-tape (Berkhout, Walter and Adey, 1969). We compared auditory presentations with the effect of the "big-brother"-situation in which the examiner, recorded on video-tape, peered out at the test subject from a television screen. It turned out that merely hearing the voice was as alerting and, indeed, as stressful a stimulus as actually seeing the examiner on the screen.

The test questions were divided into 5 categories. Two classes of high stress questions were in the sexual sphere, and in matters of truthfulness. Low stress questions involved responses to the content of sexually oriented material read by the subject. A second low stress question was a simple query. The fifth class was non-stressful questions. The assessment of induction of high stress was based upon fluctuations in heart rate and pulse volume exceeding two standard deviations. Mild stress produced

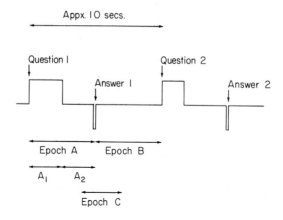

SCHEMATIC REPRESENTATION OF EPOCH DEFINITIONS

Fig. 4. Sequence of questions and answers in psychologically stressful testing. Two data analysis regimes were used, one involving separate question ($A_1$), decision ($A_2$) and anticipation (B) epochs, and the other using 5.0 sec of data before (A) and after (B) answering. (From Berkhout, Walter and Adey, 1969.)

TABLE 1

| Step | Parameter (3 Hz bandwidths) | Percent correct after step | Average values over 20 epochs | | |
|------|-----------------------------|-----------------------------|-------------------|------------------|----------------------|
| | | | Perception epochs | Decision epochs | Anticipation epochs |
| Subject 8 | | | | | |
| 1. | $T_5O_1 \times O_1O_2$ Coherence, 6 Hz | 54 | 0.34 | 0.12 | 0.23 |
| 2. | $T_5O_1$ Intensity, 12 Hz | 62 | 2.40 | 2.52 | 2.60 |
| 3. | $O_1O_2 \times O_2T_6$ Coherence, 6 Hz | 79 | 0.23 | 0.10 | 0.33 |
| 4. | $O_1O_2 \times O_2T_6$ Coherence, 18 Hz | 83 | 0.26 | 0.18 | 0.33 |

97% correct attained at Step 15.

less than one standard deviation. In non-stressful questions, no fluctuations in heart rate or pulse volume occurred.

The test situation involved the question epoch, an interval of decision making, the answer, and anticipation of the next question. Data were handled under two regimes (Fig. 4). In the first, separate perception, decision and anticipation epochs were analyzed. The second regime was used where subject response occurred within 1.5 sec of the end of the question. This second scheme simply used 5 sec of data before the answer and 5 sec after the answer. These were designated active and passive epochs. Both methods successfully separated categories of stressful questions.

TABLE 2

| Step | Parameter | Percent correct after step | Average values | |
|------|-----------|---------------------------|------------------|------------------|
| | | | Stress epochs | Non-stress epochs |
| Group A: | Non-reactive EEG | | | |
| 1. | $F_7T_3 \times T_5O_1$ Coherence 0–2 Hz | 67% | 0.48 | 0.38 |
| 2. | $T_3T_5$ Brandwidth 3–7 Hz | 68% | 2.2  Hz | 2.4  Hz |
| 3. | $O_1O_2 \times O_2T_6$ Coherence 8–12 Hz | 70% | +0.01 | 0.32 |
| 4. | $O_2T_6$ Bandwidth 8–12 Hz | 74% | 1.77 Hz | 1.9  Hz |
| 5. | $F_7T_3$ Intensity 20–30 Hz | 75% | 3.00 | 2.80 |
| 6. | $T_3T_5$ Phase 13–19 Hz | 84% | 0.12 | 0.02 |

92% correct at Step 12.

The following account of the discriminant analysis procedure illustrates its method for a single subject (Table 1). The first parameter selected was the coherence between temporo-occipital and bi-occipital leads at 6 Hz, and on that basis it was 54% correct in separating the 3 situations. It then selected as the second parameter the intensity at 12 Hz in the temporo-occipital lead, and it moved up to 62% correct. It then selected the bi-occipital to occipito-temporal coherence at 6 Hz. The fourth selection was the coherence between bi-occipital and occipito-temporal leads at 18 Hz, making an 83% correct selection. It was 97% correct at step 15 of this analysis. In this way, responsiveness of individuals was satisfactorily assessed by the character of the EEG alone in four subjects.

In the remaining 10 subjects, rapidity of reply to the questions made it necessary to use the active–passive epoch analysis described above. Again, it was possible to separate active and passive states with over 90% accuracy. In most cases the analysis utilized the parameters of intensity, bandwidth, coherence and phase angle.

Is it also possible to find patterns that show factors shared by a group of subjects for each of these categories of psychological stress? This proved possible when EEG records were first classified as "reactive" or "non-reactive", according to whether or not alpha spindling or alpha attenuation accompanied the presentation of questions (Table 2). Active epochs from 5 subjects with "reactive" EEGs were analyzed. All questions with high stress were combined in one set, and low stress questions in another. By restricting the discriminating procedure to these two classes, the parameter chosen as the basis of separation could be related to differential autonomic responses that defined the two sets. As discussed elsewhere (Berkhout, Walter and Adey, 1969), this does not imply a linear correlation of EEG and autonomic activity.

Over 90 percent of the epochs were correctly identified in this separation of high and low stress. The parameters selected may be tentatively considered an EEG index of stress. The EEG elements that appeared sensitive to the verbal presentation in ways that generalized across subjects were almost completely restricted to such cross-spectral derivatives as coherence and phase.

Thus, EEG criteria can indeed be used to separate behavioral epochs differing only in the nature of a verbal exchange, and this separation is valid for a series of subjects. It is scarcely conceivable that such a separation, based on parameters regionally organized and specific to a functional scheme of brain systems, would occur with strong similarities between individuals, if the EEG did not bear a close relation to transaction of information in cerebral systems.

### DISCRIMINANT ANALYSIS OF EEG SPECTRA IN CHIMPANZEES; CORRECTNESS OF DECISION MAKING

We have used the same pattern detection techniques in chimpanzees playing a game known in England as "noughts and crosses", and in the U.S.A. as "tick-tack-toe".

CASE 3                          Sample Size:  50

| Parameter in order of choice | Location | Band | Direction with performance |
|---|---|---|---|
| 1.  Sum of Spectra | L  T-0 | Beta-3 | Increased |
| 2.  COH | L  MBRF/ <br> L  Hipp | Theta | Decreased |
| 3.  Sum of Spectra | L  Hipp | Beta-1 | Decreased |
| 4.  COH | L  MBRF/ <br> L  Hipp | Beta-1 | Decreased |
| 5.  COH | L  Amyg/ <br> L  T-0 | Delta | Decreased |

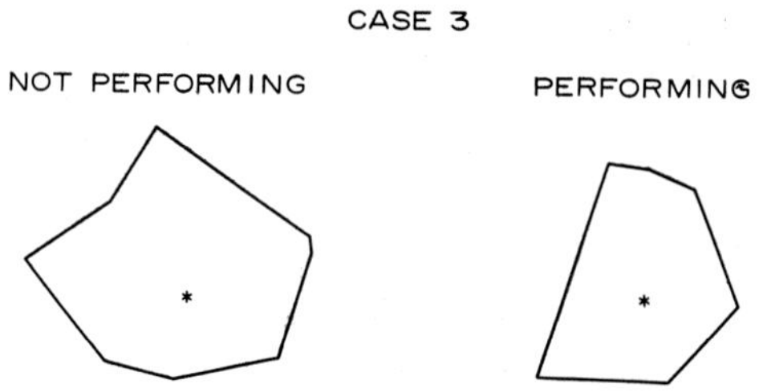

CASE 3

NOT PERFORMING                          PERFORMING

Fig. 5. Pattern recognition of separate EEG patterns characterizing non-performing and performing states in chimpanzee playing tic-tac-toe (see text). Stars located within polygons indicate means of multidimensional variables contributing to the separation; and distance between stars is a measure of the degree of separation of the data sets. (From Hanley, Walter, Rhodes and Adey, 1968.)

He plays with an opponent that may be the computer, or another chimpanzee, or the trainer, and has to make a line either horizontally, vertically or diagonally. These data were computed in a way that showed EEG characteristics when not performing, but attending to the game, awaiting his opponent's move; and performing with a response to the opponent's move (Hanley, Rhodes, Walter and Adey, 1968). The results of these analyses are presented in both graphic and tabular form (Fig. 5). The boundaries of the polygons enclose all the samples of the particular situation, and the asterisks indicate the position of the group means. In this display, a multidimensional plot has

CASE 5                          Before

| Parameter in order of choice | | Location | | Band | Comparison with correct and incorrect decision |
|---|---|---|---|---|---|
| I | Sum of spectra | Left ventral anterior thalamic nucleus | | Theta | Decreased in correct decision |
| | Coherence | Paracentral nuclei | Left caudate | Delta | Decreased in correct decision |
| II | Bandwidth | Left ventral anterior thalamic nucleus | | Alpha | Decreased in correct decision |
| | Phase | Left Hipp | Left Amyg | Alpha | Decreased in correct decision |
| III | Bandwidth | Left ventral anterior thalamic nucleus | | Alpha | Decreased in correct decision |
| | Phase | Left V.A. Nuc. Thal | Left Hipp | Beta-1 | Decreased in correct decision |

CASE 5

CORRECT                    INCORRECT

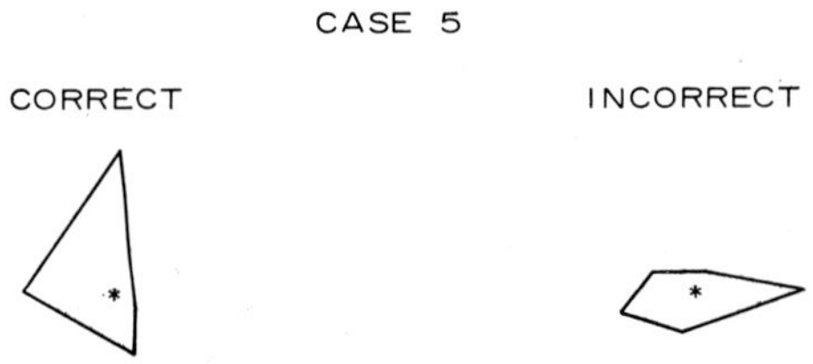

Fig. 6. Application of discriminant analysis (in similar way to Fig. 5) to chimpanzee EEG data immediately preceding correct and incorrect performances, showing complete separation of the two sets. (From Hanley, Walter, Rhodes and Adey, 1968.)

*References p. 62*

been reduced for purposes of reproduction to a bi-dimensional array. The "distance" between the means is obtained by calculating the sum of the products of the selected parameters, and their respective canonical coefficients. Where a large number of competing parameters entered into the discrimination, only those contributing to the best discrimination were chosen for the diagram. The parameters distinguishing the two situations were not detectable by visual inspection of the EEG, nor did they arise in muscle movement artifacts. Theta band frequencies again figured prominently in these separations, both in their amplitude characteristics in amygdala and hippocampus, and in high coherence between hippocampus and midbrain reticular formation.

It was also possible to separate EEG patterns accompanying correct and incorrect decisions (Fig. 6). A series of 5 incorrect responses was analyzed, the largest number of errors committed by one fully trained animal. They were successfully separated by analysis of both "before" and "after" epochs. Discriminant analysis of the decision making ("before") epoch also involved consideration of competing successful variables. In the "before" epoch, one parameter, the theta bandwidth in the thalamic nucleus ventralis anterior, survived the final competition; but in the "after" epoch, none of the first choices survived. In the "before" epoch, all parameters decreased with correct decisions. This also occurred in all but one parameter in the "after" situation. In both "before" and "after" epochs, there was a striking incidence in all sets of parameters from thalamic nucleus ventralis anterior. This invites consideration of the part played by the nucleus ventralis anterior in the thalamostriatal system described by Buchwald *et al.* (1961) as a caudate loop, and because the game included a willed motor act, draws attention to the evidence favoring subcortical structures, including the striatum, in the physiological basis of willed movements (Jung and Hassler, 1960).

## PLOTTING OF DENSITY CONTOURS THROUGH CONSECUTIVE SPECTRAL ANALYSES

Finally, there is the question of display methods for analyses of short data epochs recorded at intervals over long periods. These displays should retain most relevant details of trends over long periods, and also allow temporal compression of the total analysis. D. Brown and D. O. Walter showed in our laboratory about six years ago that it would be possible to take individual spectra and represent them in a 3-dimensional display with time along the abscissa for successive spectral analyses and to draw intensity contours through them (Walter, Rhodes, Brown and Adey, 1966). It takes about two minutes for the plotter to complete a typical display compiled from 30 to 50 separate spectral analyses.

In the chimpanzee, a single channel of data so analyzed over 20 min as the animal drifted from wakefulness to drowsiness, then to sleep, and finally back to the wakeful state clearly depicted these changes (Fig. 7). Typically, drowsiness and sleep were associated with sharply increased EEG low frequency components at around 2 Hz in hippocampal cortex.

In another example, taken from a simulation of the primate biosatellite flight, the

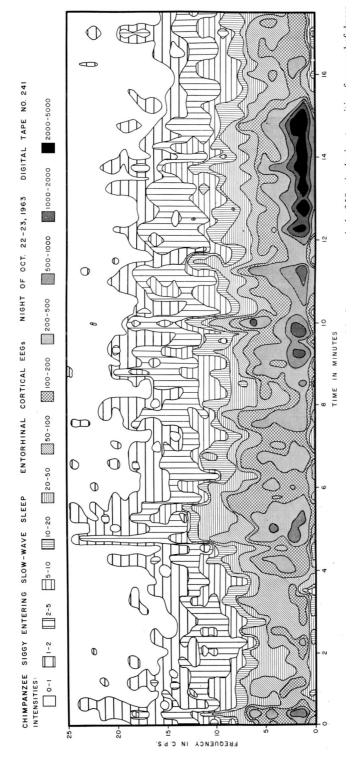

Fig. 7. Three-dimensional contour, plot of EEG spectral analysis from chimpanzee entorhinal cortex over period of 30 min during transition from wakefulness through a drowsy stage to slow wave sleep, and return to drowsiness. Plot shows spectrum 0–25 Hz on ordinate, and time on abscissae. Successive spectral analyses were performed on 20-sec epochs of data. Densities are expressed in $\mu V^2$/cycle/sec.

*References p. 62*

question was asked: if we acquired only 5.0 sec of data twice a day, and if they were acquired at the same time each day, could a shift in behavioral status be detected? We confined a monkey in a capsule for 30 days and fully simulated the flight situation. 5.0 sec of data were taken for 30 days at 1 : 30 a.m. and 1 : 30 p.m. In the autospectra from both surface and deep structures, their contours from day to day were very smooth indeed. In most leads the daily variance about the 30 day mean for each frequency of the spectrum was less than one standard deviation throughout that period. This uniformity was quite unexpected.

In summary, the method of contour display allows retention of much significant detail about the data, and yet compresses very long epochs into plots that can be held easily in the hand. These plots may cover periods from two minutes to several hours and any major perturbation can be clearly seen.

Another application of this technique involved studies on astronaut Frank Borman, the command pilot on the Gemini-7 flight (Adey, Kado and Walter, 1967). During the flight two EEG channels were recorded, one to the left of the midline and one in the midline, both spanning wide areas of cortex. These placements were not the most desirable, but were compatible with astronaut duties in the spacecraft. The recordings were made for 55 hours from launch.

Astronaut Borman was very cooperative, and participated in the normative library study, including the periods of visual discrimination and the auditory vigilance tasks. During the visual discrimination he still showed some $\alpha$-activity, enough to make dark peaks in the contour plot. When he performed the auditory task, he showed a dense $\alpha$-band and diminished power in the theta- and delta-bands. This was uniform across the posterior scalp regions.

From the normative laboratory tests in Houston, Dr. Kellaway and Dr. Maulsby followed Astronaut Borman to the Gemini simulator at the McDonnell Aircraft Company at St. Louis. He was in the Gemini space craft in a simulated space flight for about an hour. Now a rather different EEG pattern emerged. Although the low frequency cut off in the contour displays was at 3.0 Hz, much of the new activity was in the delta- and theta-bands, and was different from the frequency distribution when performing tasks in the laboratory. We interpreted this raised power in the theta- and delta-bands as a higher level of attention. In averages of the spectral contours over the whole test period, there was a persistent $\alpha$-peak, but also much power in the range from 3–7 Hz.

Flight records were gathered on a tape recorder in the spacecraft. The recording began on the launch pad, 15 minutes before lift-off. For those who may still doubt that the brain has any influence on the heart's activity, it may be profitable to examine the playback of the initial tape-recorded segments (Fig. 8). All the A-channels are from Borman, including his respiration, EKG, and two EEG channels. The B-channels show respiration and EKG from Lovell, the co-pilot. The next channel displays our timing code, put on after retrieval of the tape. The moment of launch is indicated by the start of the capsule clock. In anticipation of launch, Borman's heart speeded up, as did his respiration. It grew faster as the spacecraft lifted. Lovell, who was apparently more laconic, did not show such major changes in heart rate or respiration. All that

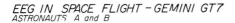

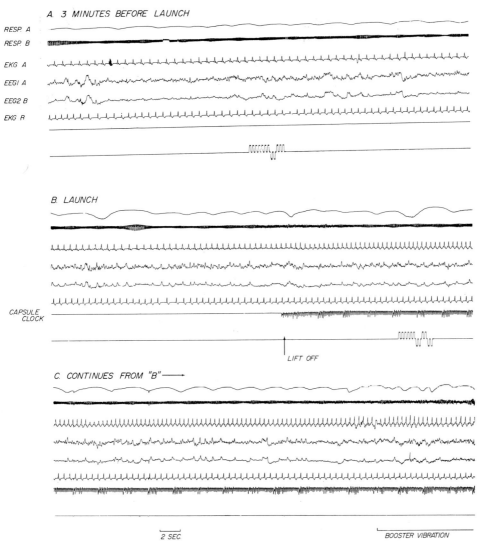

Fig. 8. Continuous physiological records from Astronauts Borman and Lovell immediately prior to launch and during booster acceleration at beginning of Gemini GT-7 flight. Channel designation A shows a 3-figure binary coded decimal (BCD) number applied to the tape recording during digitization for editing purposes. (From Adey, Kado and Walter, 1967.)

can be said from visual inspection of the EEG channels is that they show a very alerted record.

Contour displays of these prelaunch and launch EEG records were much more revealing (Fig. 9). Beginning about 15 minutes before launch, there was a gradual increase in intensity in all the bands from 5 through 7 Hz, then 7 through 9 to 11 Hz, in anticipation of the moment of launch. At that moment there was a veritable cataclysm

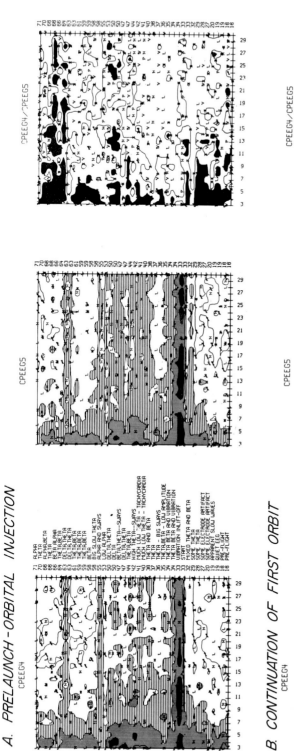

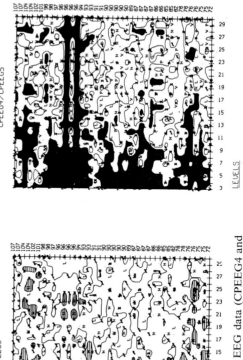

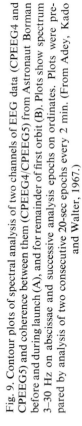

Fig. 9. Contour plots of spectral analysis of two channels of EEG data (CPEEG4 and CPEEG5) and coherence between them (CPEEG4/CPEEG5) from Astronaut Borman before and during launch (A), and for remainder of first orbit (B). Plots show spectrum 3–30 Hz on abscissae and successive analysis epochs on ordinates. Plots were prepared by analysis of two consecutive 20-sec epochs every 2 min. (From Adey, Kado and Walter, 1967.)

in the EEG, with enormous powers in all frequencies above 7 Hz up to 30 Hz. After a successful launch, they continued in the early stages of the first orbit. High powers in the theta band persisted throughout this period. Indeed, the EEG showed high theta intensities throughout all waking records in the two and a half days of data acquisition. Similar findings have been reported in Soviet cosmonauts. We do not yet know whether this is a specific response to weightlessness. At least we can say it is a very profound orienting reaction of the Pavlovian type induced by the reaction to novel situations.

If we look more closely at the prelaunch records, as the powers go up in the frequencies from 5 to 7 to 9 Hz, coherence between the two channels also increased to high levels. Immediately after launch it decreased to very low values. When he was safely in orbit, there was a broad band of high coherence from 3 to 11 Hz, running continuously for many minutes, showing that the records from these widely spaced parts of the head were almost completely synchronous over a wide frequency range. This was not seen in any of the preceding terrestrial baselines, and it did not occur again in flight. It appears to be a rebound which commonly occurs in the release from psychic stress. It exemplifies the fact that if we really wish to find out how people are reacting to physical and psychological stress, there are many situations that cannot be effectively simulated in the laboratory. Our sensing must be compatible with free movement of the individual in his working environment, and we must acquire data in a way that does not interfere with the subject in the performance of whatever tasks may be required of him. The non-interference instrumentation is a very important aspect of modern neurophysiology.

Borman's records showed only about a half hour of moderately deep sleep on his first night in space. On his second night, there were four cycles from light to deep sleep and a brief return to the waking state between each cycle, which lasted about 90 minutes. As far as one could tell, they were normal 90-minute sleep cycles that characterize sleep here on earth. So, to our colleague who said that he thought he could tell what sort of sleep a person is having by looking at him, I would encourage him to look a little closer. It is necessary that we understand the status of the sleep cycles as much as whether or not the subject is asleep. The normality of the sleep sequence is very important in the psychic well-being in the waking state.

In conclusion, we must face the question: Where do we go from here? In the future we will undoubtedly be dealing with non-linear components in the EEG. To this time virtually all our analyses are predicated on linearity of relationships. Non-linear analysis can be approached only indirectly. For example, complex demodulation allows assessment of the contributions at a point from a series of generators located elsewhere and is currently being evaluated in our laboratory by Dr. D. O. Walter (Walter and Adey, 1968). Another method might use matrix analyses to describe unique matrices that are as effective with non-linear parameters as with linear (Svoboda, 1964). These non-linear matrices would be based probably on computer statements rather than spectral analysis. Perhaps as many as 30 000 statements might be listed in the computer for comparison with the data. It should be emphasized that the value of these methods remains conjectural.

*References p. 62*

SUMMARY

It seems clear that there is a requirement for rapid, accurate and continuous assessment of physiological status in performing man, and in the sick patient. For this purpose, we may anticipate that a special purpose computer, simpler in its user interface than any now available, yet capable of carrying out the complex but essential calculations, and with special weighting factors to cover particular parameters, will achieve a reliable classification of states. Verification of states might well involve continuing comparison with a much larger library of data, and be declared in or out of limits in relation to the subject himself or a population of normal subjects.

ACKNOWLEDGEMENTS

Studies from our laboratory described here were supported by Grants NB-01883, NB-2503 and MH-03708 from the National Institutes of Health; by Contract AF-(49)638-1387 with the U.S. Air Force Office of Scientific Research; by Contract NONR 233-91 with the Office of Naval Research; and Contracts NsG 237-62, NsG 502, and NsG 1970 with the National Aeronautics and Space Administration. Our computations in the UCLA Health Sciences Computing Facility were supported by Grant FR-003 from the National Institutes of Health.

REFERENCES

ADEY, W. R., KADO, R. T. AND WALTER, D. O. (1967) Computer analysis of EEG data from Gemini flight GT-7. *Aerospace Med.*, **38**, 345–359.

BERKHOUT, J., WALTER, D. O. AND ADEY, W. R. (1969) Alterations of the human electroencephalogram induced by stressful verbal activity. *Electroenceph. Clin. Neurophysiol.*, **27**, 457–469.

BUCHWALD, N. A., WYERS, E. J., OKUMA, T. AND HEUSER, G. (1961) The "caudate spindle" I. Electrophysiological properties. *Electroenceph. Clin. Neurophysiol.*, **13**, 509–518.

DONCHIN, E. (1968) Average evoked potentials and uncertainty resolution. *Psychonomics Sci.*, **12**, 103.

GARDINER, M. F. (1969) Differences between human evoked potentials from the same acoustic stimuli during different stimulus-discrimination tasks. *Ph. D. Thesis, University of California*, Los Angeles.

HANLEY, J., WALTER, D. O., RHODES, J. M. AND ADEY, W. R. (1968) Chimpanzee performance: computer analysis of electroencephalograms. *Nature*, **220**, 879–881.

JUNG, R. AND HASSLER, R. (1960) The extrapyramidal motor system. In: *Handbook of Physiology, Section I, Neurophysiology*, J. FIELD, H. W. MAGOUN AND V. E. HALE (Eds.), American Physiological Society, Washington, pp. 863–928.

RAMSEY, D. M. (Ed.) (1969) *Image Processing in Biological Science*, University of California Press, Los Angeles.

SVOBODA, A. (1964) Behavior classifications in digital systems. *Information Processing Machines*, No. 10, Prague, pp. 25–41.

WALTER, D. O. AND ADEY, W. R. (1968) Is the brain linear? *Symposium of International Federation of Automation and Computing, Proceedings, Yerevan, Armenia*.

WALTER, D. O., KADO, R. T., RHODES, J. M. AND ADEY, W. R. (1967) Electroencephalographic baselines in astronaut candidates estimated by computation and pattern recognition techniques. *Aerospace Med.*, **38**, 371–379.

WALTER, D. O., RHODES, J. M., BROWN, D. AND ADEY, W. R. (1966) Comprehensive spectral analysis of human EEG generators in posterior cerebral regions. *Electroenceph. Clin. Neurophysiol.*, **20**, 224–237.

WALTER, D. O., RHODES, J. M. AND ADEY, W. R. (1967) Discriminating among states of consciousness by EEG measurements. A study of four subjects. *Electroenceph. Clin. Neurophysiol.*, **22**, 22–29.

# The Quantitative Analysis of EEG Data

H. PETSCHE

*Neurological Institute of the University, Vienna (Austria)*

The EEG, the origin of which is yet far from being elucidated, is a valuable tool for both clinical and brain research. The principal shortcoming in the interpretation of EEG records is the lack of knowledge of the physiological significance of the various measurable EEG parameters, *i.e.* amplitude, frequency and phase. Therefore, reading and interpreting EEG records has been a matter of personal experience. It is indeed astonishing to see, in spite of this limitation, to what degree conclusions drawn from the EEG may help the clinician to discover position and, sometimes, even type of a brain lesion. This intuitive handling of EEG data has left many scientists unsatisfied and has stimulated research to quantify EEG data. A vast amount of technical methods have been developed for this purpose. However, a real reduction of data could not be obtained by these means, the majority of them having not even been able to improve the EEG as auxiliary tool for the clinician. The rising computer technique, however, has contributed to these methods in several ways. Thus, it seems as if the interpretation of EEG records might be improved with the aid of computers even in the clinical field and a new blossoming era of electroencephalography might be initiated.

Applying computer technology to electroencephalography is closely connected to the many methods elaborated to quantify EEG data. Even if, with the increasing use of computers, these methods may become less and less important, they have to be reviewed briefly in order to understand the present situation.

Concerning "quantitative methods", it may be stated that they permit one or the other EEG parameter to be represented by numbers. The most efficient way to quantify all EEG parameters is of course to digitalize the analog EEG traces. By this procedure, the traces are replaced by series of equidistant bars, wherein the amplitude of each bar is expressed by a number. In this way, each trace may be represented sufficiently exactly by pairs of numbers giving both position and height of each bar. One can imagine what a vast amount of data would be needed to represent one 16-channel EEG record of half an hour's duration in this way. As in any kind of scientific research one of the main purposes is the reduction of data, it is necessary to ascertain significant parameters with regard to a thorough quantitative analysis. Therefore, quantitative methods should also include such techniques that bring into prominence one EEG parameter while neglecting the others. Such methods are useful, even if the parameter recorded does not come out with sufficient precision, since these methods may indicate which parameter should be studied more thoroughly with the aid of a computer. By these means true data reduction may be obtained.

*References pp. 85–86*

That is the reason why I prefer to deal also with some of the usual auxiliary methods of the EEG, though they do not really deserve the designation "quantitative methods" proper.

There are two principally different EEG phenomena that may be studied, namely (a) spontaneous electrical activity and (b) activities evoked by sensory or electrical stimuli. It is not too difficult to quantify evoked potentials, since they may be elicited repeatedly and summed up electronically. The methods for the detection and mathematical treatment of repetitive signals are well known and widely used today, and special purpose computers for this task are found in most neurophysiological laboratories. For this reason, a discussion of the technique of handling evoked potentials may be omitted. On the other hand it is useful to illustrate briefly to what other kinds of problems such special purpose computers may be applied if rhythmic spontaneous activities are to be studied. One example may suffice:

The pertinent problem is the origin of the regular hippocampus activity, called theta rhythm, in the rabbit. In this animal, the hippocampus is a big neuronal structure extending with two large wings between cortex and diencephalon. It produces, with sensory stimulation, a very regular activity usually of 4–7 c/s. Our studies (Petsche et al., 1962) have demonstrated that the theta rhythm depends upon the cellular activity of the dorsal part of Broca's nucleus of the diagonal band in the septum. Each unit of this nucleus discharges in bursts synchronous with a particular phase of the theta rhythm which, however, varies from one unit to the other. Histological techniques have demonstrated that the axons of these neurons project predominantly to the rostral part of the dorsal hippocampus whence the theta rhythm was found to spread symmetrically along the hippocampus as a travelling wave. The question arose how it was possible that the septum neurons, though discharging with different phases with respect to the theta wave, are able to give rise to such a highly synchronized activity as the theta rhythm.

This question could be answered by means of a Computer of Average Transients (CAT 1000 TMC). Two techniques of recording were used (Gogolák et al., 1968) (Fig. 1 A.) First, the phase relationship between the first action potential of each burst of a septum neuron and the theta wave was measured. The CAT was triggered externally by the first action potential of each burst, the hippocampus theta being fed simultaneously into the analog input of the CAT which was programmed for signal averaging. Because theta waves are phase-correlated to the bursts, a summation of theta waves gives an average value which permits to measure the average phase-relationship of that unit. The second technique was the following (Fig. 1 B): these experiments were recorded on tape. After each experiment, the average frequency distribution of firing of each neuron was recorded in form of a sequential histogram. Again, each burst was used to trigger the CAT. This time, however, the bursts themselves were added to give the average firing distribution curve.

Subsequently, each experiment was plotted in the following way: the sequential histograms of all septum units recorded during the experiment were arranged vertically one below the other according to their correct phase relationships to theta wave, the distances between time zero and the instants the neurons started firing being equal to

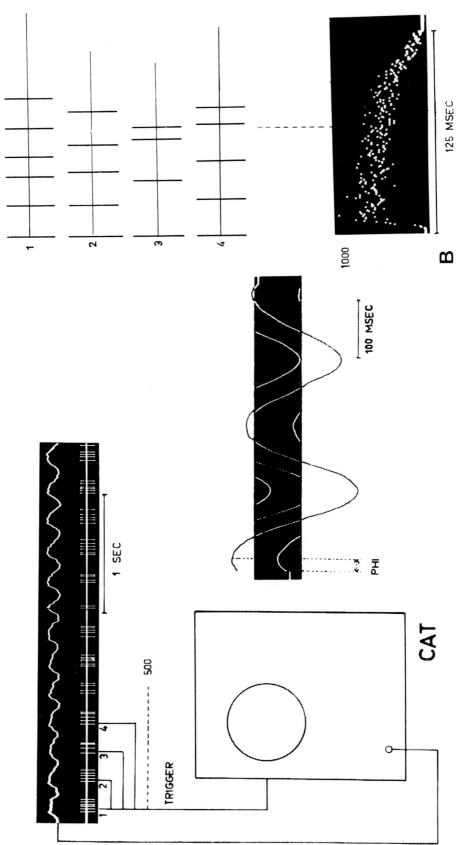

Fig. 1. A: measurement of phase relationship between burst and theta wave. B: determination of histograms (1000 bursts summed up) (Gogolák *et al.*, 1968).

their latencies. Summation of these histograms of all cells in each experiment gives an asymmetric curve with one peak. This curve represents the average firing distribution of septum cells with respect to the theta wave. Thus, the total output from the septum via hippocampus is pulsating. Analogous curves could be obtained from any experiment. An average of these curves from a total of 108 septum cells from five experiments yields a curve that is shown in Fig. 2, together with, and also in correct time relationship to the individual theta from the hippocampus. The surprising similarity between these two curves seems to support the assumption that the theta rhythm is formed by summation of postsynaptic potentials, the pacemaker of which is situated in the septum. The time difference of about 12 msec between the peaks of both curves can be accounted for by conduction time of the pulses along the septo-hippocampal fibers.

So far one example of how a special purpose computer, such as the CAT, may be used whenever cyclically recurring events are to be dealt with. In the following, I shall report on handling *non-repetitive* events, such as the EEG traces usually are. Let us first consider how the EEG may be treated if only a single trace is available and then, step by step proceed to more traces and finish by considering how a spatio-temporal approach to the brain activity may be made.

It is self-evident that any of the analyzing methods is affected by a certain loss of information. Valid new data may be obtained, indeed, but usually a great deal of information is deliberately sacrificed. In some laboratories, EEG records are fed directly into analyzers or other data-processing equipment without recording a primary trace. This practice is not recommendable. The electroencephalographer ought to see the EEG first before analyzing it any further. It is obvious that an optimum of information may be obtained if the EEG traces are stored on tape and different quantitative ap-

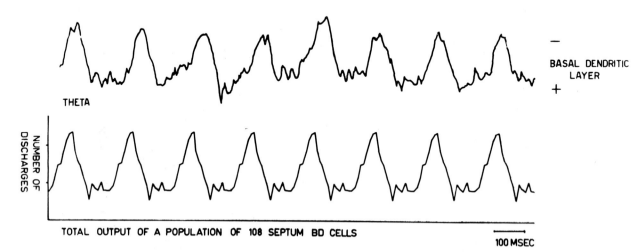

Fig. 2. Top: bipolar record of theta rhythm across pyramidal layer of hippocampus. Bottom: average of discharging curves of 108 septal cells, obtained by the phase-correct summation of the histograms of these cells. Note the correspondence between the total output of the septum cells and shape of theta wave (Gogolák *et al.*, 1968).

proaches according to the respective problems are made with different methods in succession.

One of the simplest methods of quantification of EEG data is a cumulative one, namely the amplitude integration, in which information upon frequency, wave shape and phase is lost. A long known device of this kind is that of Drohocki (1948). Different methods of amplitude integration are in use today. Only its two main types are to

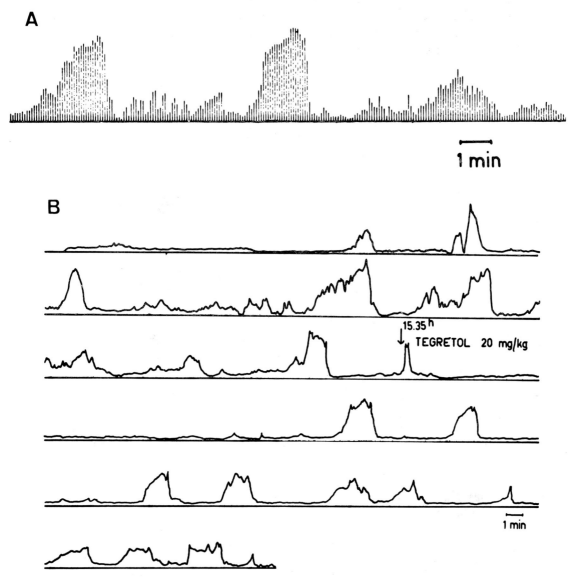

Fig. 3. A: constant reset time integrator curve. Every 5 sec a pen is deflected, the amplitude of this deflection being proportional to the integrated voltage of the past 5 sec. B: integrated activity of a status epilepticus produced by local application of ouabaine immediately before the start of the record. The contour of the integrated trace was inked in. The more or less regular occurrence of seizures is interrupted temporarily by an injection of Tegretol[R] (Geigy).

be mentioned here: the constant reset time integrator and the constant reset level integrator (Shaw, 1967). In the first type, the voltage of the EEG activity is represented by bars of different height but equal distance, in the second, the EEG voltage is proportional to the density of bars of equal height. Information about frequency is lost in both methods. Personally, we prefer the first type in which the amplitudes are rates of integrated voltage during constant periods of time. Fig. 3 may illustrate one possibility of its application. In this example, ouabaine was applied locally to a rabbit's cortex and a status epilepticus developed (Petsche and Rappelsberger, 1968). Seizures follow one another with intervals of a few minutes. This method seems to be particularly suited to test antiepileptic drugs. After intravenous injection of Tegretol® (Geigy)

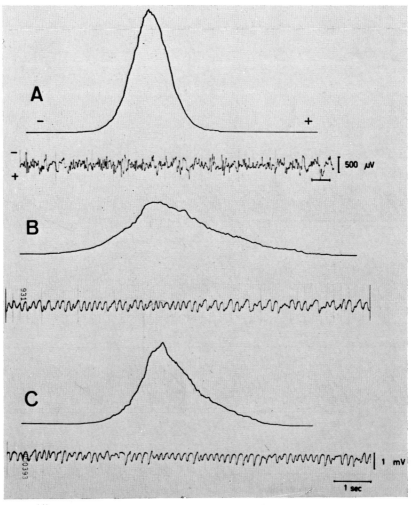

Fig. 4. Amplitude distributions. A: an almost normal distribution with spontaneous activity. B and C: skew distributions from seizure activities. Cortical records from area praecentralis agranularis of the rabbit.

the status stopped for nearly two hours (Fig. 3). This method is useful to represent long term changes in the EEG, its main field of application being the detection of drug effects and the monitoring of sleep. It is obvious that the method is too crude to elucidate finer details. It is also rather difficult to apply any further statistical analysis to this kind of traces.

If an answer is wanted to the question as to the symmetry of a given EEG pattern as to the zero line, in other words, as to its statistical amplitude distribution, the EEG may also be fed, after analog-to-digital conversion, into a Computer of Average Transients that will plot the distribution curve. The question as to the conditions of normality is still far from being decided. Spontaneous EEG activities recorded from humans usually show an almost normal distribution, though there are some doubts about normality (Prechtl, 1968). Obvious asymmetric amplitude distributions are obtained from cortical seizures (Fig. 4), an observation that confirms the assumption that positive and negative phases of the EEG are, functionally, not equivalent. There are still more observations to suggest that only one phase should be considered a physiological reality, whereas the other may be a rebound phenomenon. This question will be discussed later on. In any case, normal amplitude distributions seem to be an exception rather than a rule in EEG records.

An old and sometimes useful method to obtain the amount of a certain frequency band is to calculate its percentage time in a trace of given length. The concept "alpha-percentage-time" or "alpha-index" (Davis, 1937) respectively, was coined in the early days of electroencephalography. Morris (1956) measured alpha-percentage-time by feeding the EEG into an 8–13 c/sec filter. Thus the amount in the EEG of alpha waves may be roughly estimated. A more suitable method is the use of electronic frequency analyzers, but even these turned out to have only limited utility for clinical research. One representative of this group is the Baldock analyzer (Baldock and Walter, 1946), in which the resonance properties of electronic filters are used to select different frequencies. This technique is certainly less time-consuming than the calculation of spectrograms. It is much less exact, however. Because of the considerable loss of information due to the different inertias of the filter resonators and their different widths of Q, and also due to the difficulty to analyze these records by the naked eye, such methods are being used less and less today.

The same applies for Bekkering's method (Bekkering et al., 1958) in which the different frequency bands are arranged in lines, one below the other, the brightness of which indicates the amount of resonance in each filter. Although this method supplies an almost instantaneous spectrogram, these spectra may also be analyzed only visually. The same holds true for the majority of other methods such as wave-shape-coding, peak-point-coding etc. As useful as they may prove in several clinical EEG problems, they do not give data solid enough to be fed into computers.

Another method for the analysis of single traces is the autocorrelation, introduced into electroencephalography by Barlow and Brazier (1954). Its primary purpose is to ascertain whether or not a section of an EEG record contains periodic activities. In principle, an EEG trace of a certain duration, usually about 20 sec, is shifted in time step by step with a constant time lag in the millisecond range, the respective amplitudes being multiplied and summed up. Thus, in case of a pure sine wave, the auto-correlated function is a cosine of the same frequency. If the original trace is sinusoidal but noisy, the autocorrelogram will be of lower amplitude. Noise alone gives a sharp peak at the beginning of the correlogram, with more or less sharp decline. For extracting two or more periodic activities from a trace, however, the autocorrelogram alone will not give unequivocal results. A mixture of two or more correlograms, each starting with zero phase, will result, additional methods being necessary to interpret this pattern. Another considerable handicap in working with correlograms is that rather long sample lengths are needed if a correlogram is wanted to decline to negligible amplitudes. Walter (1963) stresses this fact in mentioning that the theory of correlographic estimates is very complicated. In this connection, he quotes Blackman and Tukey (1959): "Estimates of functions of lag have fluctuations which are so far from independence as to frequently fool almost anyone who examines tables or graphs of their values".

In spite of these limitations, autocorrelography may prove a useful method in ascertaining periodicity. On the other hand, correlograms may be used as a basis for computing power spectral density functions. This method seems to gain increasing importance. Autospectrograms may be thought of as analogous to optical spectra: they are functions relating intensity to frequency. This type of analysis is considered to be particularly effective in revealing response characteristics of systems subjected to random excitation. In autospectrography that is analogous to the filtering of EEG by electronic filters, the autocorrelograms are subjected to a Fourier transform with resulting spectral density function. Thus, the raw data that are filtered are correlograms instead of original EEG traces. Mathematical functions take over the role of electronic filters. One main difficulty that has to be overcome is to ascertain the proper shape of the weighting function. In case the Fourier transform of the correlogram is processed on a digitalized time series consisting of square pulses as spectral windows, a considerable amount of error may arise due to the fact that the Fourier transform of a square pulse is given by the function $\sin x/x$ representing a symmetric curve with several side bands. The error thereby introduced may be lowered by using, instead of a square function, other functions as spectral windows that do not give rise to side bands when Fourier-transformed. This can be achieved by "hanning" or "hamming" the time series (Kaiser and Petersén, 1966).

Dumermuth (1967) was one of the first clinical electroencephalographers who demonstrated the great value of power density functions in the analysis of background EEG activity. However, rather than calculating correlograms first, he calculates the Fourier transform which is then squared and averaged over frequency. This is a somewhat shorter procedure which may be recommended in case the autocorrelogram, the calculation of which is time-consuming, is not required.

Dumermuth's power density spectra of mono- and dizygotic twins demonstrate the genetical determination of statistical characteristics of the EEG. Fig. 5 shows, on the left, four spectra from both hemispheres of pairs of dizygotic twins, on the right, four pairs of homozygotic twins. Peak frequencies and peak shapes of alpha and its first harmonic are practically superimposable, as are the activities in other parts of the

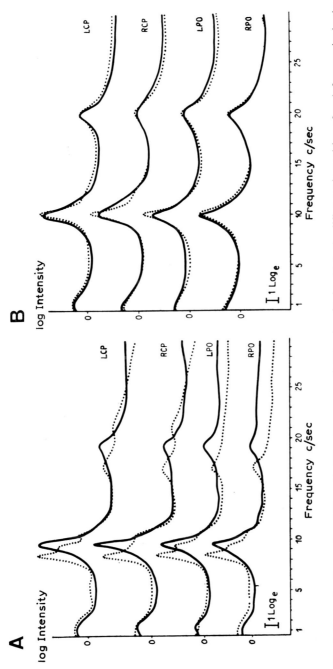

Fig. 5. Power density spectra of dizygotic (A) and monozygotic (B) pairs of twins. Note the difference in position of peak frequencies in the EEG records of dizygotic twins (Dunermuth, 1968).

CONSTRUCTION OF CONTOURS OF INTENSITY

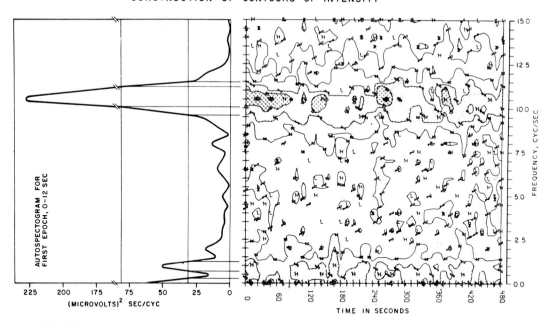

Fig. 6. Power density spectrum: on the left, in its usual form, on the right, written as a contour map, in 12 sec epochs. Bipolar posterior-occipital recording in man. The codes are used to distinguish the contour curves (Walter *et al.*, 1960).

spectrum. In sharp contrast, the power spectra of dizygotic twins show marked differences.

Walter *et al.* (1966) has programmed a computer to write out the power density spectrum (the "autospectrogram") as ordinate against time as abscissa. Fig. 6 demonstrates his representation of power density data as contour map. Time is indicated as periods of 12 sec each. The frequency band covers zero up to 15 c/sec. The left hand part of the figure gives the spectrogram in its usual form, with a maximum in the alpha band. The sample was recorded bipolarly in the parieto-occipital region. The various signs within the map are codes permitting the identification of contour curves.

These are the most usual methods of analyzing single EEG traces. If more than one EEG trace is available, several other questions may arise, chiefly concerning the features shared by two different traces and the best way of comparing the data in question.

The simplest method which has been used since the forties, is bipolar recording. The question whether the bipolar method or recording against a common reference should be preferred in routine EEG practice, was a matter of faith rather than of science for a long time. Today, it is generally agreed that each of the two methods has its merits but also its pitfalls. It is, however, surprising that a combination of both, simultaneous unipolar and bipolar recording, has been used so little up to now. Indeed, such a combination gives some clues to the coherence of two recordings (Petsche and Frühmann, 1966). In case two unipolar records have, on visual examination, nothing in

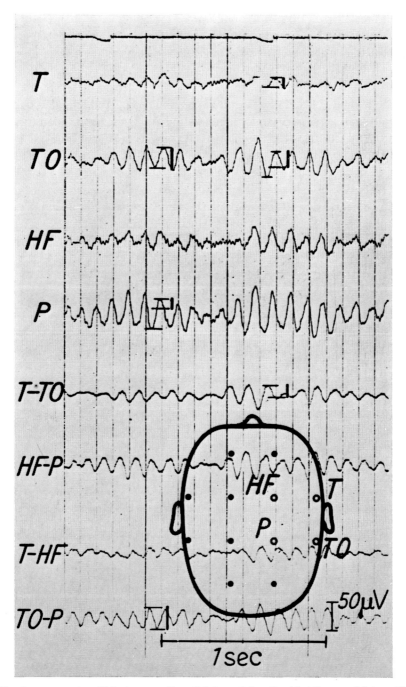

Fig. 7. Simultaneous uni- and bipolar recording of alpha activity of a girl at the age of sixteen. Channel 1–4: unipolar, channel 5–8: bipolar recordings. The difference in amplitude between two unipolar records should be identical to the bipolarly measured amplitude. Otherwise, phase differences are present.

common, it is obvious that additional bipolar recording will provide no further in-information. In so-called hypersynchronized activities, on the other hand, in which analogous patterns are observed over large areas—such as in seizures or in the alpha rhythm—bipolar recording may give additional information, as may be illustrated by an example. In the EEG of Fig. 7, the alpha rhythm was recorded from different electrodes uni- and bipolarly. The difference in amplitude between unipolar records from P (parietal) and TO (temporo-occipital) should equal the amplitude of the bipolar recording TO–P. In fact, the amplitude is at certain moments (marked by vertical dashes) much larger than expected. Such discrepancies are caused by a phase shift between the two recording sites. As was shown by toposcopic techniques (Petsche and Marko, 1955), the potential fields of most of the so-called hypersynchronous EEG waves are not stationary but move along the cortex at different directions so that the peak amplitudes are reached at different sites at different times.

Keeping this fact in mind, one may roughly estimate phase shifts from comparing

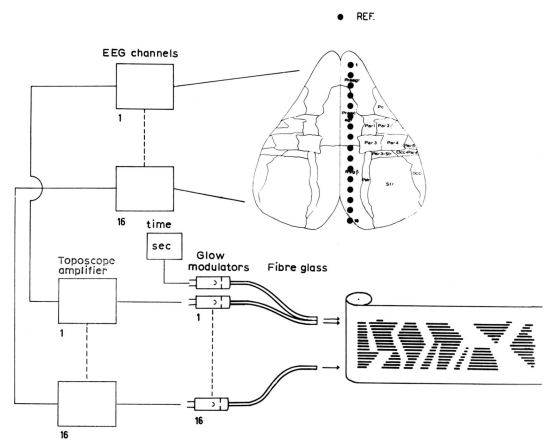

Fig. 8. Block diagram of the toposcopic technique of the author (Petsche, 1967). Travelling waves are made visible by (1) using straight rows of closely spaced electrodes, (2) transforming the EEG activities into corresponding alterations of brightness and (3) recording on a fast moving film.

simultaneous unipolar and bipolar recordings. Thus, difference in shape is not only to be ascribed to differences of amplitude but also of shape.

At this point it is necessary to discuss the question of a more exact quantitative analysis of the travelling phenomenon. Several methods have been developed (Walsh, 1958; Darrow *et al.*, 1958). Our own method (Petsche and Marko, 1955; Marko and Petsche, 1960; Petsche, 1967) has the advantage of giving not only an immediate survey of phase shifts, but also of direction and speed of the potential fields travelling along the cortex. The principle of this method is shown in Fig. 8. Sixteen unipolar recordings from equidistant cortical electrodes are amplified, brightness-modulated and recorded, by means of fiber glass guides, on a 35-mm film moving at 10 cm/sec. In this fashion, the 16 channels are compressed to give a band of 20-mm width on the film. Both the compression of a 16-channel record down to 20 mm and the elongation of the time scale (1 sec equals 10 cm) permit measurements of phase differences.

Fig. 9 shows an example of such a record. This topogram was obtained from the right hemisphere of a rabbit by means of two longitudinal rows of electrodes (electrode distance 1.5 mm). The seizure activity was produced by electrical stimulation. Above is the original EEG trace, below the topogram, recorded simultaneously. The EEG

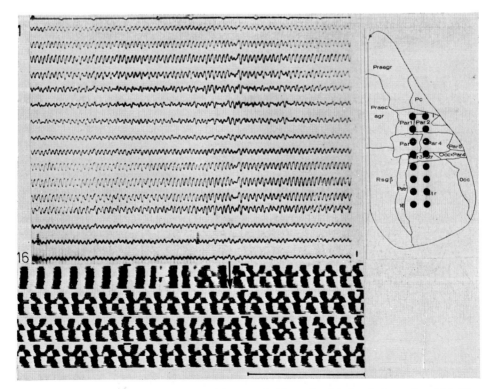

Fig. 9. EEG and topogram of a seizure activity recorded from the right hemisphere of a rabbit. Electrode 1 to 16 correspond to channels 1 to 16. The EEG record (10 sec) corresponds to the last ten seconds of the topogram (12 sec). Two distinctive activities, spreading into different directions, alternate in parietal areas and in the striate area. Calibration: 400 μV, 1 sec.

*References pp. 85–86*

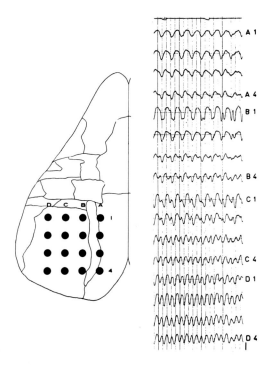

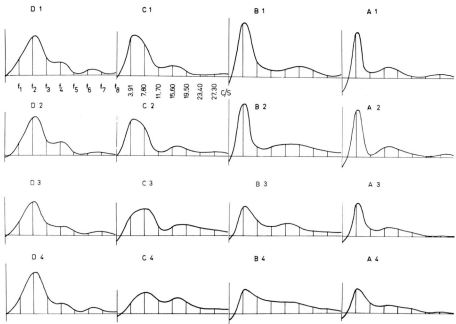

Fig. 10. Top: electrode position and EEG pattern that was Fourier-analyzed. Bottom: the 16 Fourier spectra were arranged according to the position of the 16 electrodes. On lateral regions, the second harmonic dominates, on medial regions, the basal frequency.

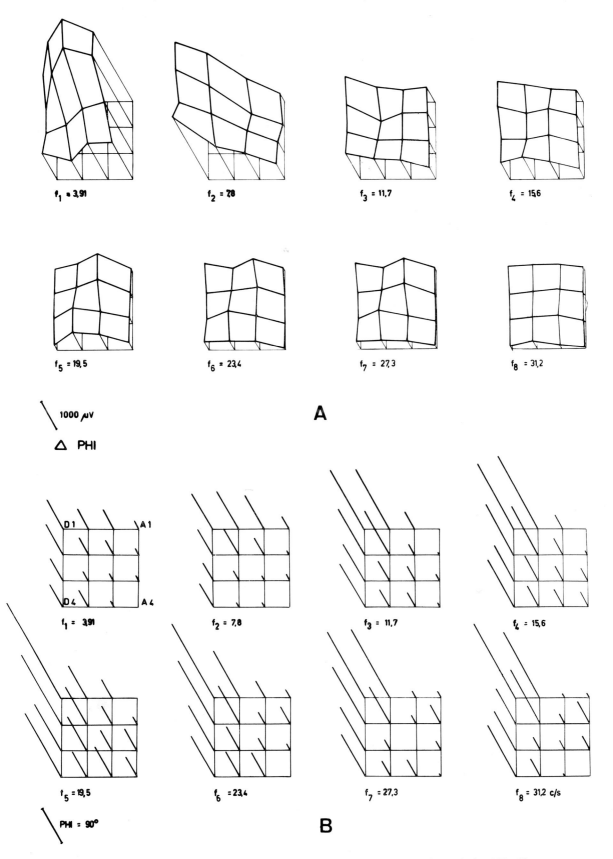

Fig. 11. A: distribution of amplitudes of the first eight harmonics of the Fourier analysis of Fig. 10.
B: relative phase angles.

starts, as indicated by the arrow, two seconds after beginning of recording the topogram. The first two seconds of the topogram display a rather uniform und regular
activity over the whole recording site. Subsequently, however, there begins an
alternating pattern that consists of two distinct activities in the parietal region and in
the striata, propagating into different directions. The slopes of the dark strips (dark is
positivity = downward deflection in the EEG) permit measurements of phase differences and, consequently, propagation velocities with respect to the electrode row. It
may also be seen that, at electrode 4 and 5, the activities are not sharply limited but
seem to merge for some millimeters before vanishing. This observation may be due to
the continuous transition from one cytoarchitectonic area to the other.

Such methods have not been made obsolete by computer techniques, as they do
supply information as to which channels ought to be chosen for refined analysis. In
this special case, for instance, we learned that discrepancies of phase, far better than
amplitude or frequency differences, do correlate with boundary zones between
cytoarchitectonically different areas.

One step further towards a still more thorough comprehension of wave shape and
phase is the Fourier analysis that can be processed by a computer from the digitalized
EEG record. To demonstrate the efficiency of this method, an example of an EEG
recorded during an epileptic seizure produced by local application of ouabaine was
chosen (Fig. 10 and 11). The trace is characterized by a very regular activity the frequency of which, in lateral regions, is double that near the midline. Intentionally only
a short period of about the length of the basal frequency was taken for sampling to
show the usefulness of Fourier analysis. The sampling length was 16 msec. Therefore,
according to Shannon's theorem, frequencies up to about 30 c/sec should be obtained
with sufficient reliability. Fig 11 A indicates that the basal frequency of about 4 c/sec is
clearest to be seen in medial regions and its first harmonic in lateral regions, whereas, in
the intermediate zone, a mixture of these two seems to occcur.

Fig. 10 demonstrates the Fourier spectra from the 16 electrodes up to the 8th
harmonic, in the same arrangement as the electrodes were placed. The amplitude rates
of the 8 frequencies were interpolated. At first glance, visual analysis confirms what
can be seen in the EEG record. The basal frequency dominates near the midline in
electrode ranges A and B, whereas laterally, the second harmonic is highest. The
intermediate region shows a mixture of $f_1$ and $f_2$: in the anterior part of the electrode
set, the basal frequency is preponderant, whereas, in C 3 and C 4, the second harmonic
is higher than the basal frequency. At this point, one may proceed to sketch the amplitude distribution of each of these eight harmonics (Fig. 11 A). In this figure, the difference of the potential fields of $f_1$ and $f_2$, with peaks at different sites, is striking. Whether
this difference has a physiological basis, being due to different neuronal populations
involved, is an open question.

Fourier analysis yields not only the amplitude spectra of harmonic sine compounds
but also their phase relationships. In Fig. 11 B, the phase differences were drawn for
each electrode and for each harmonic, with respect to that electrode with the lowest
value of phi in the basal frequency (A 4). This presentation indicates that, for $f_1$ and
most of the harmonics, the activity seems to start at A 4, in a posterior region near the

midline, and spreads laterally and anteriorly in a diagonal sense. Since the heights of these bars relate to phi and not to true time differences in milliseconds, the phase shifting of the higher harmonics seems to increase.

Cross-correlation is another way of comparing two EEG traces. These are obtained by the same procedures as auto-correlograms, the only distinction being that the traces to be compared and shifted towards each other are different. The peak of the cross-correlogram corresponds to the common main periodic and is shifted towards zero by a value equal to the phase shift between the two traces. Since, in cross-correlograms, only the main components are sufficiently well presented whereas higher harmonics do not come out clearly enough, the use of cross-spectrography is preferable. In cross-spectrograms, intensities are displayed as functions of common frequencies. Common waves are emphasized and phase relationships are quantified. The cross-spectrogram of two sinusoid activities of equal frequency has a sharp peak at that frequency. Its phase at that frequency equals the phase difference between the two records. If two traces share a sinusoidal activity whereas each contains in addition other unshared activities, their cross-spectrogram has a peak at the shared frequency only.

Ordinarily, cross-spectrograms will give more detailed information about the interrelationships of two traces than cross-correlograms, since the Fourier transform gives information on both intensity and phase with respect to frequency. If, therefore, activities of different periodicities and different phase relationships are present, cross-spectrograms will be a suitable way to analyze these relationships. Cross-correlo-

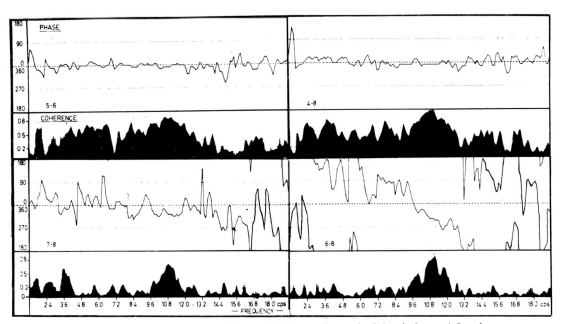

Fig. 12. Phase and coherence. 5–6: parieto-occipital recording on both hemispheres; 4–8: coherence between temporal and parietal region on the right side; 7–8: temporal regions on both hemispheres; 6–8: occipital and temporal region on the right side (Dumermuth, 1968).

grams, applied to such a case, would only give information about the basal frequency and its phase relationship.

To compare the degree of correlation of two records, a coherence function may be determined that is also presented as a function of frequency (Walter, 1963). Its magnitude lies between zero (none) and one (complete linear transformation of activity of one trace to the other). In each frequency band, the phase angle is that of the cross-spectrogram.

Another example taken from Dumermuth (1968) where phase and coherence were recorded at different sites of the skull, is illustrated by Fig. 12. Note the distinct phase shifts over nearly the whole frequency range between occipital and temporal areas (6–8 in Fig. 12), whereas almost no such differences are found between the temporal and the parietal areas (4–8). The highest degree of coherence is found in the alpha band. In the theta band, distinct coherence is present in the parieto-occipital region between both hemispheres (5–6), and little less also between temporal and parietal regions on the right side (4–8).

The coherence function may also be presented in the form of contour maps comparable to Fig. 6 (Walter et al., 1966).

Another way of studying the EEG is the spatio-temporal approach. Unfortunately, in thinking of the EEG, most electroencephalographers have in mind a group of one-dimensional traces displaying potential differences as amplitude against time as abscissa. Only a few of them try to interpolate, mentally, and to imagine an oscillating potential continuum extending over the whole surface of the skull. The best way of representing such a continuous activity would be a 4-parameter display with two parameters of space (length and width on the brain surface), one parameter of time and another, potential difference with respect to a common reference. Such a representation is, of course, not feasible. There are, however, different ways to approach this problem.

There are two main drawbacks preventing the complete representation of the potential continuum, namely (1) the necessity of using a large number of electrodes which does not only make the equipment bulky and expensive but also requires more computing work, (2) the abundantly folded human cortex is a very complicated structure in space. Since the site of the EEG generators in the cortex is established, any record from the skull represents the average activity of many millions of generators, with dipoles pointing at different directions, situated at different depths. It is obvious that recording under such conditions must yield equivocal results and thereby may give rise to misinterpretation. Nevertheless, it proved possible to define several spatio-temporal characteristics of gross electrical phenomena. For instance, it was found that a certain kind of regular spike-and-wave activity in humans is characterized by two semilunar shaped potential fields, the one representing the "spike", the other the "wave", spreading along the skull parallel to the midline with speeds in the meter-per-second range, as represented in the model of Fig. 13 (Petsche and Marko, 1959). Even in activities, however, which are apparently as simple as the alpha rhythm, the travelling pattern turns out to be extremely complicated (Rémond et al., 1962). Only so-

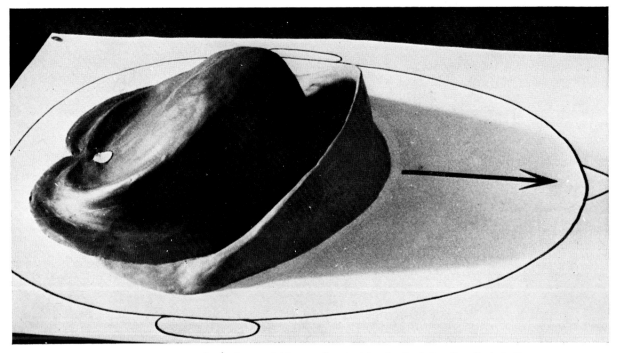

Fig. 13. Model of a regular spike-and-wave field, spreading in a longitudinal direction. Scale in the direction of spread shortened by 1 : 5 (Petsche and Marko, 1959).

called hypersynchronous phenomena, as occur in seizures, have been thus far amenable to toposcopic methods.

One way to obviate the difficulty of dealing with a generator that is a folded structure, such as the human cortex, is the use of a lissencephalic animal, like the rabbit.

Spatio-temporal studies have always to be planned from an economical point of view as a maximum of results should be obtained with a minimum of equipment and time of interpretation. Moreover, it is always advisable to record also the original EEG traces. Therefore, we did not go beyond the use of sixteen electrodes arranged in a square of four at distances of 2 mm each. Simultaneously with the EEG record, the activities are recorded on tape and also by the above mentioned toposcope. The tape is fed into an analog-to-digital converter. In the interest of economy, time lags of 16 msec were chosen. On the one hand, this time lag did not appear to be too long to suppress the highest frequencies observed in seizures and, on the other, is was not too short to supply too many data. Usually, only two or three characteristic waves are analyzed in this way. The computer was programmed by Dr. Trappl to print out equipotential lines at distances of 100 $\mu$V each.

Fig. 14 shows such a plot, recorded from the left striate area of the rabbit. It is a sort of a snapshot of the potential mountain at the moment it has reached its largest positivity. This method is best applicable to regular waves. It permits to study both the shape of potential fields and their alteration with time.

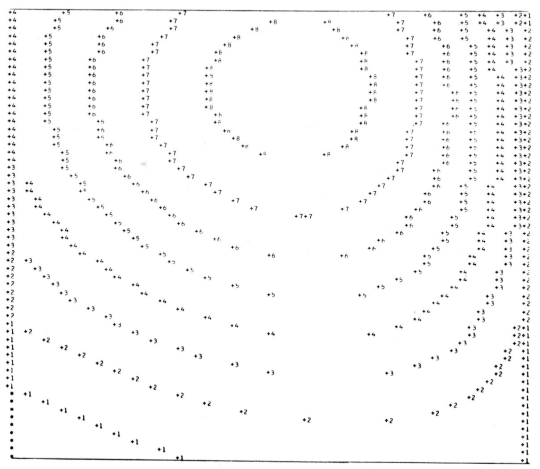

Fig. 14. Map of equipotential lines printed by an IBM 360 (Model 30). Distances between two adjacent lines are 100 μV. The rectangle corresponds to the electrode set of 4 × 4 electrodes and covers a region of 6 × 6 mm on the area striata. Seizure activity in the rabbit. The distortion of the square arrangement of electrodes into a rectangle is due to the dimensions of the type-writer of the computer.

In Fig. 15, somewhat less than half a second of seizure activity, elicited by electrical stimulation, was analyzed in the above described way. The potential maps are to be read from top left to bottom right. They were plotted at 16 msec intervals. One may see how the positive-going phases of the first wave (third plot from start at the left upper corner) is rising near the antero-lateral edge of the electrode array and is moving in the postero-medial direction. The same holds true for the second and the third wave (plot 12 and 19). The negative-going phases do not show this feature which adds weight to the previously mentioned assumption of a different physiological significance of the negative and the positive phase of the seizure EEG.

The evaluation of phase relationships enables us to correlate the morphology of the cortex with its electrical activity. Kornmüller (1935) was the first investigator who raised the question as to relationships between the morphology of the cortex and local-

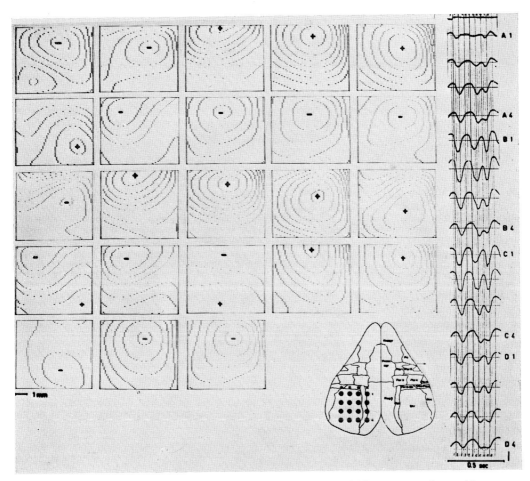

Fig. 15. Original EEG record (on the right) and maps of equipotential lines, presented every 16 msec. Maps to be read from top left to bottom right. Note the shifting of the positive summit of the potential field from antero-lateral to postero-medial regions. Seizure activity in the rabbit.

ly recorded electrical patterns. He particularly pointed out the differences, in EEG, between area retrosplenialis granularis beta (Rose, 1931), on the one hand, and area striata, on the other. The histological differences of these two areas are also very clear. In the following years, Kornmüllers hypothesis was completely abandoned though subsequent experimental data were lacking. In fact, no structure-dependent particularities of the EEG may be seen, if only the shape of gross electrical activities is studied by means of a few electrodes. If, however, attention is paid not only to the shape of the EEG trace but also to phase angles, boundaries of cytoarchitectonically homologous zones can be detected far better (Petsche and Seitelberger, 1967).

This fact is demonstrated by Fig. 16. As may be seen from the EEG trace that was recorded with 12 cm/sec, there is a distinct phase difference in the seizure activity between the two anterior and the two posterior recording rows in that row 1 and 2

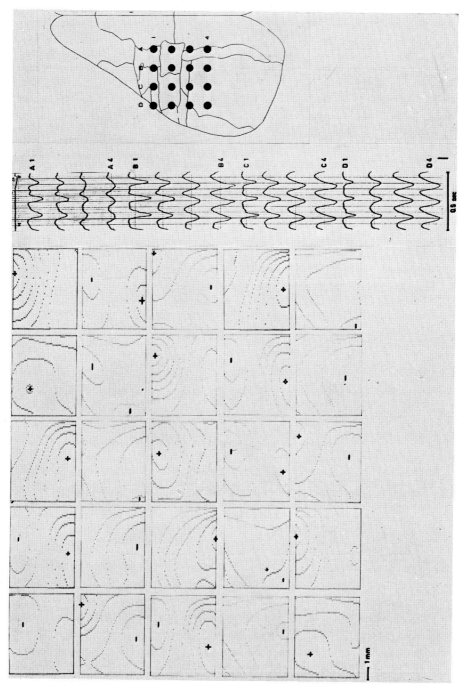

Fig. 16. EEG record and maps of equipotential lines from seizure activity in the rabbit. The set of electrodes was put on both the parietal region and the area striata. Although the EEG patterns are roughly the same in these two areas, the waves are clearly phase-shifted and the potential fields alternate in running from lateral to medial regions.

seem to oscillate nearly in phase as do row 3 and 4. There is, however, a marked phase difference between row 2 and 3. This may be accounted for by the fact that the anterior two recording rows were situated over the parietal area, whereas their posterior counterparts were placed on the striate area. Accordingly, the positive-going phases of the potential fields move, as can be seen from the plots, independently. Over both areas, spreading occurs asynchronously toward the midline.

When considering potential fields, one should bear in mind that current, not voltage, is the significant parameter of electrical brain activity, since currents are produced by the nerve cells. Our ultimate aim should, therefore, be to elucidate the topography of current generators and their alteration with time. This may be accomplished by calculating the second derivatives of the sets of equipotential lines. Finally, laminar analysis of the cortex by microelectrodes in different regions has to be performed to enlarge the realm of the observation into the third dimension.

## REFERENCES

BALDOCK, G. R. AND WALTER, W. G. (1946) A new electronic analyzer. *Electronic Engineering*, **18**, 339–342.

BARLOW, J. S. AND BRAZIER, M. A. B. (1954) A note on a correlator for electroencephalographic work. *Electroencephalog. Clin. Neurophysiol.*, **6**, 321.

BEKKERING, I. D. H., LEEUWEN, VA, W. S. AND KAMP, A. (1958) The EEG-spectrograph. *Electroenceph. Clin. Neurophysiol.*, **10**, 555.

BLACKMAN, R. B. AND TUKEY, J. W. (1959) *The Measurement of Power Spectra*, Dover, New York.

DARROW, C. W., VIETH, R. N. AND WILSON, J. P. (1958) Instrumental registration of EEG phase changes associated with stimulation, activity and learning. *Electroencephalog. Clin. Neurophysiol.*, **10**, 144.

DAVIS, H. (1937) The electrical activity of the human brain. *New Engl. J. Med.*, **216**, 97–98.

DROHOCKI, Z. (1948) L'Intégrateur de l'électroproduction cérébrale pour l'électroencéphalographie quantitative, *Rev. Neurol.*, **80**, 619.

DUMERMUTH, G. (1967) Variance spectra of electroencephalograms in twins. A contribution to the problem of quantification of EEG background activity in childhood. — *Proc. Intern. Symposium on Clinical EEG in Childhood, Göteborg, 1967*, Almquist & Wiksell, Stockholm, 1968, pp. 119–154.

DUMERMUTH, G. (1968) Der Computer in der Electroencephalographie. In: *Computeranwendung in der Hirnforschung, Beilage Technik, Neue Zürcher Zeitung* vom 3. April 1968, 15–23.

GOGOLÁK, G., STUMPF, CH., PETSCHE, H. AND ŠTERC, J. (1968) The firing pattern of septal neurons and the form of the hippocampal theta wave. *Brain Res.*, **7**, 201–207.

KAISER, E. AND PETERSÉN, I. (1966) Automatic analysis in EEG. *Acta Neurol. Scand.*, Suppl. 22, vol. 42.

KORNMÜLLER, A. E. (1935) Die bioelektrischen Erscheinungen architektonischer Felder der Grosshirnrinde. *Biol. Rev.*, **10**, 383–426.

MARKO, A. AND PETSCHE, H. (1960) The Multovibrator-Toposcope, an electronic multiple recorder. *Electroencephalog. Clin. Neurophysiol.*, **12**, 209–211.

MORRIS, G. W. (1956) A percent-time computer and associated band pass filter. *Electroencephalog. Clin. Neurophysiol.*, **8**, 705.

PETSCHE, H. (1967) Die Erfassung von Form und Verhalten der Potentialfelder an der Hirnoberfläche durch eine kombinierte EEG-toposkopische Methode. *Wien. Z. Nervenheilk.*, **25**, 373–387.

PETSCHE, H. UND FRÜHMANN, E. (1966) Die Analyse von lokalen EEG-Veränderungen durch gleichzeitige uni- und bipolare Ableitungen. *Arch. Psychiat.*, **208**, 447–461.

PETSCHE, H. AND MARKO, A. (1955) Über die Ausbreitung der Makrorhythmen am Gehirn des Menschen und des Kaninchens auf grund toposkopischer Untersuchungen. *Arch. Psychiat.*, **193**, 177–198.

PETSCHE, H. AND MARKO, A. (1959) Zur dreidimensionalen Darstellung des Spike-Wave-Feldes. *Wien. Z. Nervenheilk.*, **16**, 427–435.

PETSCHE, H. AND RAPPELSBERGER, P. (1969) Eine Methode zur Auswertung der corticalen anti-epileptischen Wirksamkeit eines Stoffes am Strophanthin-Status. *Arch. Exptl. Med.*, (in print).

PETSCHE, H. AND SEITELBERGER, F. (1967) Hirnelektrische Tätigkeit und Rindenstruktur. *Wien. Klin. Wochschr.*, **79**, 492–496.

PETSCHE, H., STUMPF, CH. AND GOGOLÁK, G. (1962) The significance of the rabbit's septum as a relay station between the midbrain and the hippocampus. I. The control of hippocampus arousal activity by the septum cells. *Electroencephalog. Clin. Neurophysiol.*, **14**, 202–211.

PRECHTL, H. F. R. (1968) Polygraphic studies of the full-term newborn. II. Computer analysis of recorded data. Studies in infancy. In: *Clinic in Developmental Medicine*, Vol. 27, BAX, M. AND MACKEITH, R. C. (Eds.), S.I.M.P./Heinemann, London, pp. 22–40.

RÉMOND, A., CONTE, C. ET ZARRIDJAM, M. (1962) Description de quelques aspects de l'organisation du rythme alpha à l'état de veille. *Rev. Neurol.*, **107**, 225–231.

ROSE, M. (1931) Cytoarchitektonischer Atlas der Grosshirnrinde des Kaninchens. *J. Psychol. Neurol. (Lpz.)*, **43**, 353–440.

SHAW, J. C. (1967) Quantification of biological signals using integration techniques. In: *A Manual of Psychophysiological Methods*, VENABLES, P. H. AND MARTIN, I. (Eds.), North-Holland Publishing Company, Amsterdam, pp. 403–465.

WALSH, E. C. (1958) Autonomy of alpha rhythm generators studied by multiple channel cross-correlation. *Electroencephalog. Clin. Neurophysiol.*, **10**, 121.

WALTER, D. O. (1963) Spectral analysis of electroencephalograms: mathematical determination of neurophysiological relationships from records of limited duration. *Exptl. Neurol.*, **8**, 155–181.

WALTER, D. O., RHODES, J. M., BROWN, D. AND ADEY, W. R. (1966) Comprehensive spectral analysis of human EEG generators in posterior cerebral regions. *Electroencephalog. Clin. Neurophysiol.*, **20**, 224–237.

# The Use of Correlation Analysis in Processing Neuroelectric Data

AAGE R. MØLLER

*Department of Physiology, Karolinska Institutet, Stockholm (Sweden)*

Recent technical developments of digital computers have made it possible to carry out various types of signal analysis which previously had been unrealistic because of the time required by manual performance.

Different forms of correlation analysis, such as auto- and cross-correlation analysis, mainly developed in the field of statistics, have lately proven to be important tools in various other types of signal processing (see, *e.g.* Blackman and Tukey, 1958; Davenport and Root, 1958; Rosenblith, 1962; Bendat and Piersal, 1966). This paper will give some examples of the use of correlation analysis of EEG signals and also of the use of a similar technique adapted to the study of unit activity.

## ANALYSIS OF EEG SIGNALS

### *Examples of the use of correlation analysis in experimental studies*

Fig. 1 shows some examples of records where correlation and spectral analysis have been used in the study of the ontogenetic development of cortical interhemispheric functions (Meyerson, 1968). The top records show the original EEG trace recorded from two homologous points on the exposed cortex of a sheep fetus, which show a marked periodicity. Below are the cross-correlogram (C) of two consecutive periods of recording and the power spectrum of each of the two channels (D). In the cross-correlogram a dominant periodicity is seen, indicating that this component is correlated in the two leads. It follows from the spectral analysis that the signal, in fact, contains two periodic components. One of these is thus not shown to be correlated in this experiment.

The tracings below are similar but the activity shown here is apparently of non-periodic type (E). Examination of the power spectrograms shows, however, that the signal does contain a periodic component. A marked peak in the spectrograms appears at about 15 c/sec. No periodicity is seen in the cross-correlogram indicating that the periodic component in the two leads is not correlated. Examination of the spectrograms shows that the frequency of the periodic component is slightly different for the two sides, thus explaining why the periodic component is not correlated in the two leads.

In the same study, cross-correlation analysis has been used to demonstrate the

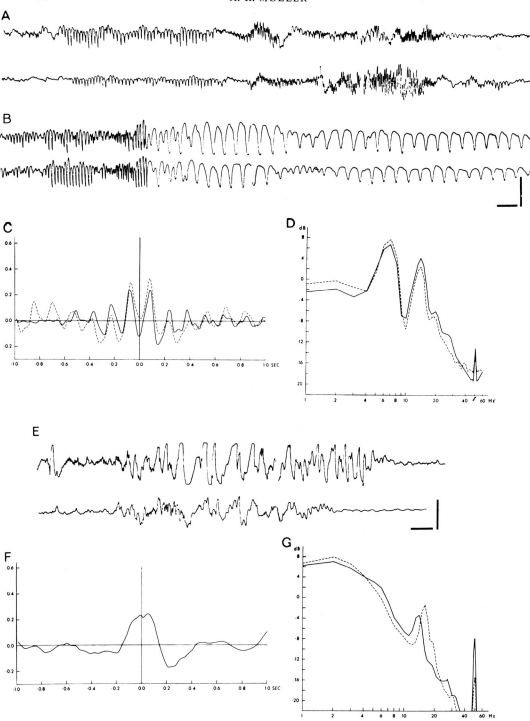

Fig. 1. Electrocortical activity in a 70-day-old sheep fetus. A and B are bilateral, monopolar recordings from the parietal area. C, cross-correlograms based on two consecutive periods of recording,
and D, spectrograms of bilateral activity illustrated in A and B. E, activity recorded from the anlage of
S. Suprasylvius. F, cross-correlogram; and G, spectrograms based on activity illustrated in E. Note,
right section of B recorded with high paper speed. Calibration, 50 μV, 1 sec, B right section, 0.25 sec.
(From Meyerson, 1968).

dependance of interhemispheric synchrony on fetal age, type of activity and certain structures in the brain (Meyerson, 1968).

### Autocorrelation

The autocorrelation function expresses the correlation of a signal with a delayed version of itself (Wiener, 1950). It is a function of the delay and its value at each delay interval is the sum of the product of the amplitude values of the signal and its delayed version. Such analysis enhances periodic components in a signal where periodic components are mixed with random components. Wiener (1930, 1950) demonstrated that the autocorrelation function contains all the information on the power density spectrum of the original signal, as the two functions were shown to be freely interconvertible through Fourier transformation. The power density spectrum represents the average intensity as a function of frequency but does not include phase information of the original signal. The data reduction which such an analysis implies is thus made at the expense of the phase information of individual frequency components in the original signal.

### Cross-correlation

A cross-correlation analysis provides a quantitative measure of the magnitude of the common components of two signals such as obtained in simultaneous EEG recordings from two points on the skull. It is calculated in a way similar to autocorrelation, the only difference being that two different signals are used. As in the case of autocorrelation, cross-correlation has its spectral analogy usually called cross-spectrum (Adey et al., 1961, Walter, 1963 and Dumermuth and Flühler, 1967).

### Correlation analysis compared with spectral analysis

Since the autocorrelation and the power spectrum carry the same information, it may just be a matter of convenience which one is used. The autocorrelation function may have the advantage of being more familiar to many people but if the data contain several periodic components with different frequencies, the autocorrelogram may be difficult to interpret and the spectrogram is superior. If only a single periodic component is present, the frequency and the stability of this component can be read from the autocorrelogram. In such cases this will show a damped oscillation, the frequency of which is equal to the frequency of the periodic component and the decay of the oscillation will be a measure of the frequency stability (or bandwidth) of the periodic component. This has been used by Daniel (1964) in study of human EEG.

### Methods of analysis

Both of these types of analysis can be carried out either by specially designed equipment (usually analog; see, e.g., Barlow and Brown, 1955) or by general purpose digital computers. The rapid development of digital computers with their speed, flexibility and accuracy make them preferable today for this type of analysis. Lately, accessories for auto- and cross-correlation analyses have also been made available for the small special purpose digital computers usually known as Computers of Average Transients. This development makes it possible to carry out an on-line computation of auto- or cross-correlation in laboratories which have no direct access to a large computer.

When power spectral analysis was performed on a general purpose digital computer it was almost always economically feasible to calculate the power spectrum on the basis of the autocorrelation, as compared to calculating it from the original signal. Recent development of mathematical methods employing Fourier transforms which are specially suited for use in connection with digital computers has, however, increased the speed of computation to such a degree that a direct spectral analysis of the signals in many cases will require less machine time than methods using autocorrelation as an intermediate stage. This special method for Fourier transform was developed by Cooly and Tukey (1965) and is usually known as the Fast Fourier Transform. It has recently been used in EEG analysis (Dumermuth and Flühler, 1967). If the autocorrelation function is wanted, it can be obtained by Fourier transformation of the computed power spectrum. The machine time for that computation is usually negligible compared with the requirements for spectral analysis.

There are other methods by which the power spectrum (and thus autocorrelation as well) of a signal can be determined. Recent developments in digital filtering have produced an economical alternative to spectral analysis using digital computers (Walter et al., 1966). In this case digital filtering is accomplished by using the computer as a series of spectral filters whose center frequencies are distributed over the frequency range of interest. Digital filters can be designed to have properties which are impossible to obtain in similar physical filters. This flexibility makes digital filtering superior in many cases to the conventional type of spectrum analyser, which works on the basis of electrical filters consisting of capacitance and inductance.

A further recent development employs spectral analysis and a special type of correlation (Reverse-Correlation, described by Kaiser and Petersén, 1966).

### Planning of correlation and spectral analysis of EEG

The autocorrelation function of stochastic (random) processes to which many neuro-electric signals may be referred is only defined for infinitely long duration of the signal. In practice, of course, only finite length of data can be processed and the resulting function is thus not the autocorrelation in its strict mathematical sense but an approximation to that. For a stationary stochastic signal (a signal where the statistics do not change with time) it is possible to calculate the length of sequences which have to be processed in order to obtain an autocorrelation function whose values fall within a certain confidence limit in relation to the signal's "theoretical" autocorrelation (see, e.g., Blackman and Tukey, 1958; Lee et al., 1950; Fano, 1950).

When the power spectrum is calculated on the basis of the autocorrelation, the spectral resolution is determined by the maximal delay in the autocorrelation function. The statistical stability of each spectral estimate increases with the length of the recording which is processed but it decreases when the resolution is increased. Thus a desired degree of spectral resolution has to be weighted against a less stable estimate for the same sample length (Hord *et al.*, 1965; Blackman and Tukey, 1958). Details describing the derivation of power spectra from autocorrelation funtions, including the averaging over frequency which is necessary to obtain a satisfactory stability of the spectral estimates can be obtained from Blackman and Tukey (1958) or Bendat and Piersal (1966).

In order to process an analog signal on a digital computer the signal has to be sampled in time and the amplitude values in each sample translated into numbers. The sampling rate determines the upper frequency limit which is included in the analysis. Since computational time increases rapidly with the number of samples, a too high sampling rate should be avoided. It should also be mentioned that the analog signal should be appropriate low pass-filtered before sampling so that the energy above a frequency equal to half the sampling rate is negligible. Energy above half the sampling frequency can introduce a serious error, since that spectrum is folded down into the frequency range of analysis by the sampling process, *i.e.*, components in the frequency range above half the sampling frequency cannot be distinguished from signals below that frequency. (This is called aliasing, see Blackman and Tukey, 1958).

A fact which can be readily overlooked in the planning of auto- and cross-correlation analysis is that the correlation between two signals is in general very resistive to amplitude distortion; this implies that the required accuracy of amplitude values of the signals which are analyzed is very moderate. One of the signals can, in fact, be infinitely clipped (*i.e.*, any positive amplitude value of the signal is represented by $+1$ and all negative values by $-1$) with only a small loss in accuracy of the computed auto- and cross-correlation function as a result. (The signals must have a zero mean value to make this statement valid.) This form of correlation is also called relay correlation (see, *e.g.*, Watts, 1961; de Boer and Kuyper, 1968). Even if both signals are subjected to such a drastic distortion, most of the properties of their correlation are retained compared to the case where the signal is not distorted. Thus, only a few amplitude values are required in order to give a correlation which is very close to that computed with a high amplitude resolution (Watts, 1961).

This circumstance ought to be of great advantage when executing correlation analysis on general purpose digital computers. In the case where one of the signals is infinitely clipped (represented by $+1$ and $-1$ depending on the signal's polarity) the multiplication of the two signals' amplitude values is very simple since it consists of multiplying the signal which is not clipped with $+1$ or $-1$. Thus multiplication can be replaced by a change of polarity of one of the signals in accordance with the polarity of the other signal.

Auto- and cross-correlation analysis is thus mainly reduced to a summing operation in contrast to the ordinary case, where a large number of multiplications have to be performed. Such a procedure is much faster to execute in most computers and more importantly the correlation analysis may be performed on much simpler machines like the Computer of Average Transients, without any accessories.

*References p. 98–99*

Another method which is based on the remarkable insensitivity of the correlation function to distortion of the signals is called triggered correlation. One of the two signals are replaced with a series of impulses which occurs either at times when the signal reaches a certain amplitude value or at the peaks of the signal. This principle of analysis is well suited for applications to average computers. No accessories are needed and the computer is used in its averaging mode. The sweep of the analyzer is triggered by pulses which are derived from one of the two signals while the other is fed into the ordinary input of the computer (Kamp *et al.*, 1965; de Boer and Kuyper, 1968).

### Effect of the scalp on EEG-recordings

The recordings shown in Fig. 1 were led off from the exposed surface of the cerebral cortex in the sheep with monopolar electrodes. In most cases where human EEG records are studied the recordings are made from the scalp and it has been shown that there is a substantial difference between the activity recorded from scalp and from cortex due to the spatial integrative action of the extracerebral tissues (deLucchi *et al.*, 1962; Hendrix, 1965; Geisler and Gerstein, 1961; Rayport *et al.*, 1966).

When recording directly from homologous points on the cortex a slight asymmetry of electrode arrangement reduces the correlation of the activity in the two leads nearly to zero. However, in recordings from the scalp, the symmetry in electrode arrangements is much less critical. This effect of spatial integration by the scalp is further illustrated when recording from neighboring points on the same hemisphere. When two leads are placed on the exposed cortex the electrodes have to be very close in order to show any significant correlation of the activity, while on the scalp high values of cross-correlation are found even with rather distant electrode placement.

### Machine time requirements

The analysis of EEG signals performed in the Department of Physiology and described above was made on an IBM 7090 general purpose computer, while the analog to digital conversion was performed on an IBM type 9 X 12 converter (Meyerson and Møller, 1968). It took 5.5 minutes to calculate auto- and cross-correlation of two channels of 9000 samples each and 100 delays. The computer time for spectral computation was only a few seconds.

### ANALYSIS OF SINGLE UNIT RESPONSES

In the analysis of activity recorded from single neurons the shape of the individual action potentials is usually of no interest and only the temporal pattern of the occurrence of spikes is considered. The simplest analysis is by counting the number of impulses during a certain time interval to obtain the average spike frequency. Since much information may be coded in the time pattern of the spikes, the average spike discharge frequency is in many cases an incomplete description of the sample of discharges.

*Interval histograms*

Because of the statistical nature of the firing of most units, the analysis must also be a statistical one. The basic form of statistical analysis is by determination of the interval distribution. For this purpose the spike intervals are sorted according to length and their numerical occurrence is plotted as a function of length of intervals. Such a graph is usually called an interval histogram. This type of histogram analysis can be carried out on the wired program computer of the type usually called Computer of Average Transients (see, *e.g.*, Clark *et al.*, 1961). In the interval histogram analysis the order of occurrence of intervals is lost. If, for instance, a long interval is usually followed by a short one, or a short interval by a long one, this cannot be seen in the interval histograms. The interval distribution thus characterizes the process under study completely only if individual intervals are statistically independent. Therefore, the information provided by interval histograms is in many cases limited and can be easily misinterpreted. There are several other methods of analysis where the time relation of intervals is preserved, but such analyses are usually much more complicated and, usually, cannot be done on the small wired program computers which are available.

The problem of statistical dependence of intervals is an important one and can be tested in several ways. Comparing the autocorrelation of a sequence of nerve impulses before and after a prolonged shuffling of intervals is one such test. This procedure destroys the original order of the intervals. The serial dependence can also be tested by making use of the fact that the autocorrelograms and the autoconvolution of the interval histogram are identical only if successive spike intervals are statistically independent (Rodieck, 1967). These methods serve to test the statistical independence of individual spike intervals, but they do not necessarily provide information about the character and degree of a dependence between individual intervals. (For further details about this matter the reader is referred to Gerstein and Kiang, 1960; Poggio and Viernstein, 1964; Moore *et al.*, 1966; Hyvärinen, 1966; Rodieck, 1967; Holmes and Houchin, 1967; and Perkel *et al.*, 1967.)

*Autocorrelation*

When general purpose computers became available and these were equipped with suitable input devices, it became feasible to carry out more complicated statistical analyses of sequences of nerve impulses. (For a review of some of these statistical methods see, *e.g.*, Gray, 1967; Rodieck, 1967; Gerstein and Kiang, 1960.) As in the analysis of EEG signals, autocorrelation analysis is a powerful tool in analysis of unit data, especially when hidden periodic components are of interest. In case of spike analysis the nerve impulses are replaced with short pulses of uniform amplitude triggered by the nerve impulses. The sequence of impulses is then sampled in similar manner to the analysis of analog signals, but the analysis of spike data is much simpler and it only comprises a computation of the number of spikes which coincide in the original and the delayed sequency of nerve impulses. In the analysis of spike data some confusion with regard to names has occurred. Several names, such as renewal density function, expectation density function, intensity functions and post-firing interval distribution has been used for essentially the same analysis as is called autocorrelation in this paper (see Moore *et al.*, 1966; and Perkel *et al.*, 1967).

### *Use of triggered correlation in study of unit responses*

The response of a general linear system when excited with a short impulse (the system's impulse response) can be derived from the cross-correlation between the output and the input signal, when this is of a broad spectrum (with the aid of the autocorrelation of the input, *cf. e.g.*, Bendat, 1958 or Lee, 1960). When a linear system is preceded by a non-linear one (which is not time-integrative) the cross-correlation mainly reflects the properties of the linear part of the system and thus mainly ignores those of the non-linear part (see above, p. 91 and Watts, 1961).

A special type of analysis which makes use of this circumstance was introduced by de Boer (1967) and de Boer and Kuyper (1968) with the purpose of resolving some of the neural excitatory processes in the cochlea. These authors made use of the fact that nerve impulses can be described as a triggering process, where an excitatory process is initiated when the amplitude of the stimulation exceeds a certain value. This method was applied to the responses of single units in the auditory nerve in order to recover the linear filter function of the cochlea. The resulting correlation function is assumed to be a close approximation to the impulse response of the linear part of the resonant function of the cochlea.

### *Examples of analysis*

In case of driven activity it is often desired to investigate whether the periodicity in the stimulus is preserved in the evoked spike trains. Fig. 2 shows examples of three types of analysis of the same spike data. The data which were analyzed were recorded from single excitable cells in the cochlear nucleus of rats, stimulated with pure tones which were amplitude-modulated with a sine wave. The frequency of the tone (5.5 kc/sec) matched the most excitable frequency (characteristic frequency) of the cell (for details on the experimental technique see Møller, 1969).

The frequency of the modulation ranged from 100 to 700 c/sec and is shown by numbers in Fig. 2. The periods of the modulation are indicated on the figure by inserted dots. It follows from this figure that the autocorrelation functions show oscillations with a frequency which is equal to the modulation frequency. The autocorrelation also shows quantitatively the degree of periodicity in the spike train. Furthermore, the autocorrelograms in this graph show that the investigated neuron is capable of following the amplitude variations in the stimulus tone up to a rate of about 500 c/sec which means that the spikes (or some of them) are time-locked to the modulation up to that frequency. The proportion of discharges which were time-locked begins to decrease at 300 c/sec and is essentially zero at 700 c/sec.

The location of the peaks in the interval histograms shown in the left column does not agree with the periodicity of the modulation especially at a modulation frequency

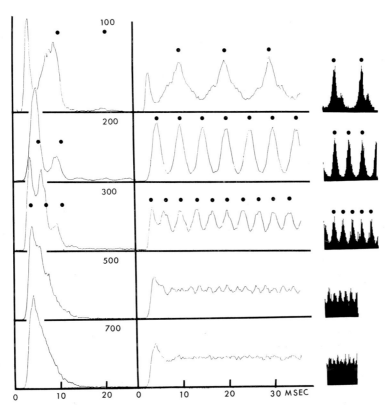

Fig. 2. Interval histograms (left column), autocorrelograms (middle) and "post-stimulus time histograms" (right column) of unit activity recorded in the cochlear nucleus of a rat. The stimulation was a continuous tone (5500 c/sec) which was amplitude-modulated by a sine-wave. The frequency of the modulation is indicated by numbers. The periods of the modulation are indicated with dots on the three upper rows of records. One minute of data was processed.

of 100 c/sec. This can be explained by the fact that the neural discharges occur in bursts which appear with the frequency of the modulation. The interval histogram, which does not take into account the serial dependence between intervals, thus has two peaks, one at short intervals representing the intervals between the spikes in each burst, and another at longer intervals which reflects the interval between the *end* of one burst and the *beginning* of another burst. This latter interval is different from the periodicity of the burst if more than one spike occurs in each burst. Thus, the second peak in the interval histogram appears at a time which is shorter than the period of the modulation when this was 100 c/sec. When the frequency of the modulation is increased, the shape of the interval histograms changes in accordance with whether more than one, one or less than one spike is evoked in each modulation period.

It is clear that the degree of periodicity in this case could have been determined equally well employing the phase relation of the modulation of the stimulus. This can be accomplished, for instance, by triggering a computer of average transients at a certain fixed point of the modulation wave and using the computer in its post-stimulus time histogram mode. Such an analysis is similar to that known as post-stimulus time histogram analysis and can be used to study to what degree the evoked nerve impulses are time locked to a given phase of the stimulus. The result of the analysis shows the distribution of nerve impulses over each modulation period and it thus expresses the probability of firing at different phases of the modulation wave (Gerstein and Kiang, 1960; Kiang, 1961). The result of such an analysis of the same data on which auto-correlation and interval histogram analysis was performed is seen in the right column in Fig. 2. These graphs very much resemble the autocorrelograms in that the peaks are separated with the same time as that of a modulation period and the height of the peaks is a quantitative measure of the degree of periodicity.

"Post-stimulus time histogram analysis" is similar to computing the cross-correlation between stimulus and response (Gerstein and Kiang, 1960). It is also seen in Fig. 2 that the "post-stimulus time histogram analysis" is more powerful in enhancing periodic information out of a random background than the autocorrelation analysis, which is in agreement with what is known from auto- and cross-correlation analysis of analog signals (Lee et al., 1950).

The activity of the neuron, whose responses were described above, showed no periodicity in its autocorrelogram when the unit was stimulated with a continuous steady tone. Some units in the cochlear nucleus do, however, show various degrees of periodicity when driven by a continuous tone. Interval histograms and autocorrelograms of the activity of such units to stimulation with a continuous tone having a frequency (21.5 kc/sec) equal to the characteristic frequency of the unit is seen in Fig. 3A. Since the interval histogram does not reflect the dependence between intervals, it is

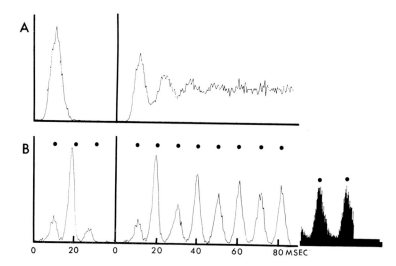

Fig. 3. A: Interval histogram (left) and autocorrelogram (middle) of unit activity recorded in the cochlear nucleus of a rat. The stimulation was a continuous tone with a frequency equal to the unit's characteristic frequency (21 500 c/sec). B: Interval histogram (left), autocorrelogram (middle) and "post-stimulus time histogram" (right) of the responses when the same tone was amplitude-modulated with a 100 c/sec sine wave. The dots indicate the periods of the modulation. One minute of data was processed.

not necessarily much different from histograms of non-periodic activity. On the other hand, the autocorrelogram differs markedly in units with periodic activity and in those with non-periodic activity. The decay of the periodicity in the autocorrelogram is an expression of the stability of the periodic component of the activity. Holmes and Houchin (1967) studied the periodicity in the activity of units in the cerebral cortex of the cat from autocorrelation analysis.

When such a unit with periodic activity is stimulated with a repetitive wave form, the spike train will contain two periodic components: the inherent one and that induced through stimulation. Interval histograms, autocorrelograms and "post-stimulus time histograms" of the activity of the same unit as in Fig. 3A are seen in Fig. 3 B, when the unit was stimulated with a tone which was amplitude-modulated with a sine wave having a frequency of 100 c/sec. The periods of the modulation are indicated in both graphs by dots. In this case, the interval histograms are not very valuable for the purpose of estimating the frequency of the two periodic components in the spike train, and the autocorrelogram is much more complicated. Instead of peaks with equal height, as was the case when only one periodic component was present, the peaks in the autocorrelograms originating from the stimulus periodicity vary in height as a result of superposition of the two components.

In the "post-stimulus time histogram" the periodicity which was inherent in the spike train is averaged out since it bears a random phase relationship to the induced periodicity. This histogram thus only reflects the induced periodicity. The post-stimulus time histogram must be considered an incomplete description of the information contents in the spike train, since the inherent periodicity is a significant feature of the spike train which cannot be ignored when the information content in the driven activity is considered. Of these three types of analysis, only the autocorrelogram conveys both these periodic components. It is thus clear from the given examples that the autocorrelation analysis is in many cases superior compared to interval histogram and post-stimulus time histogram in displaying important features of a sequence of nerve discharges.

*Analysis technique*

Autocorrelation analysis of spike data is obtained in a manner similar to that for analog data, such as EEG signals. The original sequence of data is sampled and the sample in which a discharge occurs is represented by a one, all other samples by zeros. The multiplication of the original and the delayed version becomes very simple since it can be replaced by counting the number of times a one in the original sequence coincides with a one in the delayed sequence.

While post-stimulus histogram analysis can be performed on small wired program computers (Computers of Average Transients), more complicated types of analysis are usually carried out on general purpose computers. Recently accessories for performing autocorrelation analysis have been made available for some of the wired program computers. These devices are, however, intended for autocorrelation analysis of analog signals, like the EEG recordings, but only a small modification is required in order to make it possible to perform autocorrelation analysis of spike data on these same devices. The autocorrelation analysis of spike data, examples of which are shown in Figs. 2 and 3, was performed on an IBM 7090 general purpose computer. A special program for this analysis was written in machine language in order to reduce the required computational time and to increase the maximal number of samples which could be processed at the time. Each word in the memory (36 bits long) contained 36 samples. With this programming the original sequence of data occupied less than half the memory space. The data was delayed and transferred to the other half of the memory and a comparison between the original and delayed version was done word by word to save computing time. This system enabled us to process data sequences of a maximum of 360 000 samples at a time and the computing time was less than 10 minutes for 100 delays (somewhat dependent on the number of spikes in each sequence).

## ACKNOWLEDGEMENTS

The research reported in this paper was supported by grants from the Swedish Medical Research Council (Grants B67-14X-90-02 and K67-14X-515-03B), Therese and Johan Andersons Minne and Magnus Bergvalls Stiftelse and by the Association for the Aid of Crippled Children. The author is grateful to Professor L. Leksell, Department of Neurosurgery, Karolinska Hospital for making the computer of average transients (TMC, CAT type 400 A) available. Mr. T. Jaeverfalk programmed the IBM 7090 for autocorrelation analysis of spike data. Computer time was made available by the Karolinska Institutet.

## REFERENCES

ADEY, W. R., WALTER, D. O. AND HENDRIX, C. E. (1961) Computer techniques in correlation and spectral analyses of cerebral slow waves during discriminative behavior. *Exptl. Neurol.*, 3, 501–524.

BARLOW, J. S. AND BROWN, R. M. (1955) An analog correlation system for brain potentials. *Mass. Inst. Tech. Res. Lab. Electron Tech. Rep.* 300.

BENDAT, J. S. (1958) *Principles and Applications of Random Noise Theory*, J. Wiley, New York.

BENDAT, J. S. AND PIERSAL, A. G. (1966) *Measurement and Analysis of Random Data*, J. Wiley, New York.

BLACKMAN, R. B. AND TUKEY, J. W. (1958) *The Measurement of Power Spectra*, Dover Publ., New York.

BOER, E. DE (1967) Cross-correlation studies applied to the frequency resolution of the cochlea. *J. Auditory Res.*, **7**, 209–217.

BOER, E. DE AND KUYPER, P. (1968) Triggered correlation. *IEEE Trans. on Biomedical Engineering*, BME-15, 169–179.

BRAZIER, M. A. B. (Ed.) (1961) Computer techniques in EEG analysis. *Electroenceph. Clin. Neurophysiol.*, Suppl. 20.

CLARK, W. A., GOLDSTEIN, M. H. JR., BROWN, R. M., O'BRIEN, D. F. AND ZIEMAN, H. E. (1961) The average response computer (ARC): A digital device for computing averages and amplitude and time histograms of electrophysiological responses. *Trans. IRE, BME-8*, No. **1**, 46–51.

COOLEY, J. W. AND TUKEY, J. W. (1965) An algorithm for the machine calculation of complex Fourier series. *Math. Comput.*, **19**, 297–301.

DANIEL, R. S. (1964) Electroencephalographic correlogram ratios and their stability. *Science*, **145**, 721–723.

DAVENPORT, W. B. AND ROOT, W. L. (1958) *Random Signals and Noise*, McGraw-Hill, New York.

DUMERMUTH, G. AND FLÜHLER, H. (1967) Some modern aspects in numerical spectrum analysis of multichannel electroencephalographic data. *Med. Biol. Eng.*, **5**, 319–331.

FANO, R. M. (1950) Short-time autocorrelation functions and power spectra. *J. Acoust. Soc. Amer.*, **22**, 546–550.

GEISLER, C. D. AND GERSTEIN, G. L. (1961) The surface EEG in relation to its sources. *Electroenceph. Clin. Neurophysiol.*, **13**, 927–934.

GERSTEIN, G. L. AND KIANG, N. Y.-S. (1960) An approach to the quantitative analysis of electrophysiological data from single neurons. *Biophys. J.*, **1**, 15–28.

GRAY, P. R. (1967) Conditional probability analyses of the spike activity of single neurons. *Biophys. J.*, **7**, 759–777.

HENDRIX, C. E. (1965) Transmission of electric fields in cortical tissues: A model for the origin of the alpha rhythm. *Bull. Math. Biophys.*, **27**, 2.

HOLMES, O. AND HOUCHIN, J. (1967) Analysis of the activity of one type of spontaneously discharging unit in the cortex cerebri of the anesthetized rat. *J. Physiol.*, **193**, 173–186.

HORD, D. J., JOHNSON, L. C., LUBIN, A. AND AUSTIN, M. T. (1965) Resolution and stability in the autospectra of EEG. *Electroenceph. Clin. Neurophysiol.* **19**, 305–308.

HYVÄRINEN, J. (1966) Analysis of spontaneous spike potential activity in developing rabbit diencephalon. *Acta Physiol. Scand.*, Suppl. 278, **68**, 1–67.

KAISER, E. AND PETERSÉN, I. (1966) Automatic analysis in EEG. 1. Tape-computer system for spectral analysis; 2. Reverse correlation. *Acta Neurol. Scand.*, Suppl. 22, **42**, 1–38.

KAMP, A., VAN LEEUWEN, W. S. AND THIELEN, A. M. (1965) A method for auto- and cross-correlation analysis of EEG. *Electroenceph. Clin. Neurophysiol.*, **19**, 91–95.

KIANG, N. Y.-S. (1961) The use of computers in studies of auditory neurophysiology. *Trans. Amer. Acad. Ophthalmol. Otolaryngol.*, **65**, 735–747.

LEE, Y. W. (1960) *Statistical Theory of Communication.* John Wiley & Sons, New York.

LEE, Y. W., CHEATHAM, T. P. AND WIESNER, J. B. (1950) Application of correlation analysis to the detection of periodic signals in noise. *Proc. IRE*, **38**, 1165–1171.

DELUCCHI, M. R., GAROUTTE, B. AND AIRD, R. B. (1962) The scalp as an electroencephalographic averager. *Electroenceph. Clin. Neurophysiol.*, **14**, 191–196.

MEYERSON, B. A. (1968) Ontogeny of interhemispheric functions. An electrophysiological study in pre- and postnatal sheep. *Acta Physiol. Scand.*, Suppl. 312, 1–108.

MEYERSON, B. A. AND MØLLER, A. R. (1968) Ontogeny of interhemispheric functions; Appendix. *Acta Physiol. Scand.*, Suppl., **312**, 109–111.

MOORE, G. P., PERKEL, D. H. AND SEGUNDO, J. P. (1966) Statistical analysis and functional interpretation of neuronal spike data. *Amer. Rev. Physiol.*, **28**, 493–522.

MØLLER, A. R. (1969) Unit responses in the cochlear nucleus of the rat to pure tones. *Acta Physiol. Scand.*, **75**, 530–541.

PERKEL, D. H., GERSTEIN, G. L. AND MOORE, G. P. (1967) Neuronal spike trains and stochastic point processes. I. The single spike train. *Biophys. J.*, **7**, 391–418.

POGGIO, G. R. AND VIERNSTEIN, L. J. (1964) Time series analysis of impulse sequences of thalamic somatic sensory neurons. *J. Neurophysiol.*, **27**, 517–545.

RAYPORT, M., SANDLER, B. AND KATZMAN, R. (1966) Observations on the passive electrical properties of the envelopes of cat brain. *Electroenceph. Clin. Neurophysiol.*, **20**, 513–519.

RODIECK, R. W. (1967) Maintained activity of cat retinal ganglion cells. *J. Neurophysiol.*, **30**, 1043–1071.

ROSENBLITH, W. A. (Ed.) (1962) *Processing Neuroelectric Data.* M.I.T. Press, Cambridge, Mass.

WALTER, D. O. (1963) Spectral analysis of electroencephalograms: Mathematical determination of neurophysiological relationships from records of limited duration. *Exptl. Neurol.*, **8**, 155–181.

WALTER, D. O. AND ADEY, W. R. (1966) Linear and non-linear mechanisms of brain-wave generation. *Ann. N.Y. Acad. Sci.*, **128**, 772–780.

WALTER, D. O., RHODES, J. M., BROWN, D. AND ADEY, W. R. (1966) Comprehensive spectral analysis of human EEG generators in posterior cerebral regions. *Electroenceph. Clin. Neurophysiol.*, **20**, 224–237.

WATTS, D. G. (1961) *A General Theory of Amplitude Quantization with Applications to Correlation Determinations*, IEE (London), Monograph 481 M.

WIENER, N. (1930) Generalized harmonic analysis. *Acta Mathematica*, **55**, 117–258.

WIENER, N. (1950) *Extrapolation, Interpolation and Smoothing of Stationary Time Series with Engineering Applications*, J. Wiley, New York.

# The Dynamic Response of a Photoreceptor

F. A. DODGE, JR.

*IBM Thomas J. Watson Research Center, Yorktown Heights, New York (U.S.A.)*

In this lecture I will discuss some research done by Jun-ichi Toyoda, Bruce Knight, and myself in the laboratory of Professor H. K. Hartline. Our problem is a classical one in neurophysiology: how can we understand the patterning of nerve impulses from a sense organ in terms of the basic neural mechanisms. In studying the dynamic response of the eye of the horseshoe crab (*Limulus*), we are taking advantage of much knowledge accumulated from the study of the steady-state response of this retina. In our research the digital computer has been an essential tool for the acquisition and processing of experimental data. Although I will not discuss it here, this computer played an equally important role in testing our mathematical models by simulating the responses of the eye.

Let me begin by introducing you to our experimental animal, Fig. 1A. According to the fossil record, the last of his family left Europe about a hundred million years ago to settle on the eastern shores of North America; and several of his cousins settled on the eastern shore of Asia. His unique place in visual physiology results from the large size of his eye and the simplicity of its retinal organization (Hartline, Ratliff and Miller, 1961). In an adult animal measuring 20 cm across the shell, the lateral eye (Fig. 1B) is about a centimeter wide. Because there are only about a thousand facets in this compound eye, it is fairly easy to optically isolate the individual photoreceptor elements, the ommatidia. The long optic nerve that conveys visual information to the central ganglion consists of one active axon from each of the ommatidia. Immediately behind the layer of photoreceptors (Fig. 1D), the axons give off numerous fine branches that form a plexus interconnecting the ommatidia at the specialized regions of synaptic contact, the neuropile.

By measuring single unit activity in axons teased out of the optic nerve, Hartline and his collaborators have assembled a beautiful story describing the response of this retina to patterns of steady illumination. If a single photoreceptor is illuminated by a step of light, there is an initial burst of impulses in its nerve fiber, which more or less quickly subsides to a steady repetitive discharge that is maintained for the duration of the stimulus. The steady-state spike train is usually quite regular, hence accurate measurements of the visual response can be made simply by counting the number of spikes which occur in some fixed interval. From such measurements it was found that the steady-state input–output relation for the isolated ommatidium is deceptively simple, the mean spike rate varies with the logarithm of the light intensity over a range of several orders of magnitude of illumination.

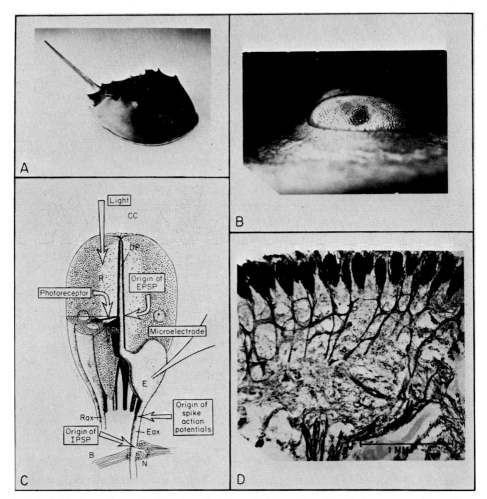

Fig. 1. A. The horseshoe crab, *Limulus polyphemus*. B. External surface of the compound lateral eye. The irregular dark area is the pseudopupil where much less light is reflected from those ommatidia whose optic axis is parallel to that of the camera. C. Schematic reconstruction of an ommatidium; CC, crystalline cone; DP, distal process of the eccentric cell E; Rh rhabdome of retinula cell R; N neuropile where inhibitory synaptic connections are made on axon of eccentric cell Eax. D. Micrograph of silver-stained section, perpendicular to cornea (cornea and lenses missing), showing darkly stained ommatidia, bundles of axons coming back to form the optic nerve, and transverse bundles of axonal branches forming a plexus of interconnections.

When neighboring ommatidia are illuminated the spike rate of the test ommatidium diminishes. The only interaction among the receptors is mutual inhibition. This inhibitory interaction was thoroughly investigated by Hartline and Ratliff (1958) who summarized their results by an empirical mathematical model of the eye. This model is a system of nearly linear algebraic equations of the form:

$$r_i = e_i - \sum_{\substack{j=1 \\ j \neq i}}^{n} k_{ij} (r_j - r^\circ_{ij})$$

which says that the steady-state spike rate of the $i$th ommatidium ($r_i$) is given by its local excitation ($e_i$), measured by the spike rate when only the $i$th ommatidium is illuminated, diminished by the sum of inhibitory terms due to the firing of spikes of the neighbors; each inhibitory term is the product of coefficient which depends only on the spatial separation of the ommatidia ($k_{ij}$) and a term that is the amount by which the rate of the $j$th ommatidium ($r_j$) exceeds a threshold value ($r^\circ_{ij}$). There are the obvious restrictions on the equations that all $r$'s and all terms in parentheses must be positive or zero. This model has held up to extensive tests, and it is a sufficient explanation for the functionally important visual property of enhancing contrast at the borders of patterns (Ratliff, Hartline and Miller, 1963; Ratliff, 1965).

There has been considerable success in explaining the form of Hartline–Ratliff equations in terms of the cellular mechanisms and structure of the photoreceptor. We can take a closer look at the structure in the schematic diagram of Fig. 1C which emphasizes the sensory cells of the ommatidium. Eleven retinula cells (R) are arranged like the segments of an orange around the optic axis of the ommatidium; the central borders of the retinula cells give off innumerable interdigitating microvilli which form the dense rhabdome (Rh) that is the photosensitive structure. The distal process (DP) of the eccentric cell (E) extends up the core, and it is the axon (Eax) of the eccentric cell which is the only active axon from the ommatidium. This diagram does not show the numerous small branches given off the axon to form the plexus, but it does indicate the convergence of several branches from the neighbors to the neuropile (N) where they mediate inhibition.

Reliable electrical measurements can be made when a micro-electrode impales the soma of the eccentric cell. Early recordings had shown that in response to illumination a slow maintained depolarization, the generator potential, underlie the spike discharge (Hartline, Wagner, and MacNichol, 1952). The intracellular recording (Fuortes, 1959) established that the steady-state spike rate is proportional to the amplitude of the generator potential, hence the logarithmic transduction takes place in the first electrical step. These experiments also showed that the generator potential was associated with an increased ionic conductance of the cell such that the generator potential is essentially similar to an excitatory postsynaptic potential (EPSP). The electrical signs of inhibition were difficult to observe because the site of inhibition lies some distance out of the axon and the electrical signals from the cell body is dominated by the light-induced conductance changes. Purple succeeded in making reliable measurements of the inhibitory postsynaptic potential (IPSP) and its associated conductance increase by the expedient of keeping the preparation in darkness and activating the inhibitory synapses by electrical stimulation of the optic nerve (Purple and Dodge, 1965). The linear dependence of the inhibitory effect on the spike rate of the neighbors in the Hartline–Ratliff equations thus appears to be the natural con-

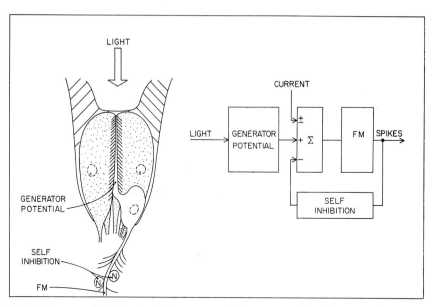

Fig. 2. Block diagram of the *Limulus* photoreceptor. FM represents the spike-generating mechanism by a voltage to frequency converter, and $\Sigma$ is the place in the cell where excitatory and inhibitory influences sum to drive the voltage to frequency converter.

sequence of its synaptic basis, each impulse adds its characteristic increment to the pool of inhibitory transmitter, which in turn decays at a rate proportional to its amplitude. In addition, the electrical separation of the site of inhibition and excitation explains why the inhibitory coefficients ($k$) in the model should be nearly independent of the level of excitation.

The possibility of self-inhibition was formally excluded from the Hartline–Ratliff model as its effect would not be observed in a steady-state experiment. Stevens (1964) demonstrated that the prominent transients in the spike rate associated with incremental current pulses could be explained simply by assuming that each impulse triggered an IPSP that acted back on its own axon. Subsequently, Purple demonstrated the linear summation of the self-inhibitory potential and of its associated conductance increase (Purple and Dodge, 1966). In magnitude the increment in self-inhibitory conductance associated with a spike in the test ommatidium is about equal to the increment in lateral inhibition resulting from a synchronous spike in *all* other axons. Hence, the self-inhibitory feedback must play a significant role in the dynamic response of the eye.

The established mechanisms for the transduction of light intensity to spike rate are summarized in the block diagram of Fig. 2. This diagram represents an optically isolated ommatidium since I neglect lateral inhibition from the neighbors. Following Stevens (1964) the spike generating mechanism of the axon (FM) is represented phenomenologically by a relaxation oscillator in which some internal variable integrates the input voltage to a criterion value, whereupon a spike fires and the integral is reset. The input voltage is the algebraic sum of the generator potential and the

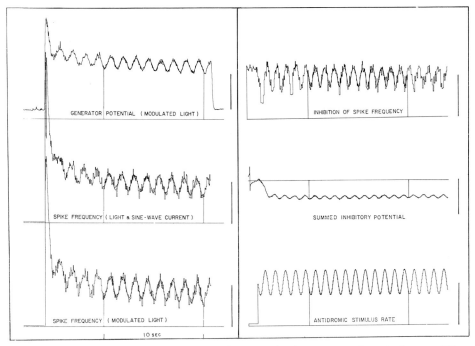

Fig. 3. (Left) Sample data records for the various transduction processes in a single ommatidium. Smooth curves show fit of data by our processing scheme. (Right) Sample records from experiment, not described in this paper, that measures the dynamics of lateral inhibition. Calibration marks are 20/sec for spike records and 10 mV for potential records.

summed self-inhibitory potential. Each spike increments the self-inhibitory potential with a waveform that rises instantaneously and decays exponentially. In an experiment extrinsic current can be injected through the microelectrode.

Our first question was whether this block diagram is sufficiently complete to explain the dynamic response of the ommatidium. Our approach to answering this question was to apply the powerful techniques of linear systems analysis, whereby we could see if the dynamics of the overall transduction can be synthesized from the dynamics of its components. Sample records of the data from an optically isolated ommatidium are shown on left of Fig. 3. The lower plot is a sample measurement of the overall transduction from modulation of the light intensity to modulation of the spike rate. The computer was programmed to measure the time interval between successive spikes to the nearest 0.2 msec, and to plot out the "instantaneous frequency" defined as the reciprocal of the preceding interspike interval assigned to the time of occurrence of each spike. The computer also measured the frequency of the sinusoidal modulation of the stimulus, then it fit the "instantaneous frequency" data by least mean squares to the sum of six functions, a constant, a linear ramp, the sine and cosine of the driving frequency, and the sine and cosine of twice the driving frequency. The coefficients obtained from this fit (which is shown superimposed on the records in Fig. 3) measure the mean response amplitude, its linear drift, the amplitude and phase of the driven response, and its harmonic content of the response.

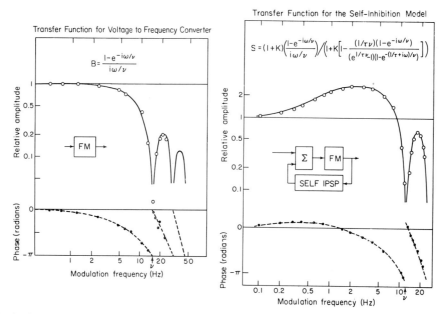

Fig. 4. Theoretical transfer functions for the phenomenological spike generator (left) and for the spike generator with self-inhibition (right). Smooth curves are plots of the analytical expressions and points are data from an electronic analog.

The component transduction from cell potential to spike rate is measured from data in the middle record. In this case the stimulus was a sinusoidal current injected through the microelectrode superimposed on a steady light of the same mean intensity as in the other records. The component transduction from modulation of light intensity to modulation of the generator potential is measured by data shown in the upper plot. For such records the spikes were blocked by treating the preparation with tetrodotoxin. The data in this case are measurements of the average value of the membrane potential over successive 20-msec intervals, but the data are processed in the same way.

Before showing the results of this experiment let me digress a moment to discuss what theory tells us to expect for the frequency response of the spike generator alone and with self-inhibitory feedback. In Fig. 4 the analytical expressions derived by Mr. Knight are compared to measurements on an electronic analog that replaced the preparation in our apparatus. This exercise proved valuable as it revealed bugs in our stimulator and in our data-processing program. Considering the isolated spike generator, left, we would expect that the instantaneous frequency would faithfully follow modulation of the stimulus as long as there were many impulses per cycle. On the other hand we would expect nulls in the frequency response when we could fit exactly one or two, etc., cycles of the stimulus in each mean interspike interval. The theoretical transfer function of such a frequency modulation device has one parameter, the mean spike rate ($\nu$). The idea behind the self-inhibitory feedback, right, is very simple, each impulse adds a unit IPSP that decays exponentially with a

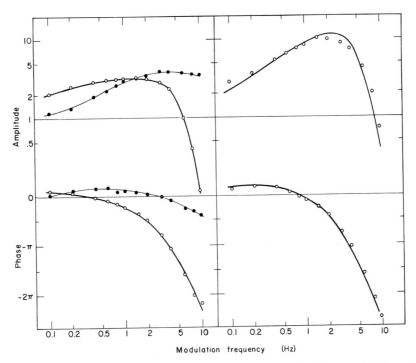

Fig. 5. Synthesis of the frequency response for the overall transduction from modulation of light to modulation of spike rate (right) in terms of the measured frequency responses (left) of the component transduction from light to generator potential (open circles) and from potential to spike rate (fitted circles).

time constant ($\tau$). At low modulation frequencies the summed self-inhibition keeps up with the modulation and the response follows the stimulus. At higher frequencies, the DC component of the inhibition remains constant because the average spike rate remains the same, but the slow time constant filters out the AC component of the inhibition and the gain of the system increases to the maximum set by the sensitivity of the *uninhibited* spike generator. Higher frequencies are cut off by the spike generator. The theoretical transfer function takes on this very complicated form because the inhibition is locked to the time of occurrence of the spike. There are three parameters in this function, the coefficient that measures the strength of the inhibition ($K$), the time constant ($\tau$), and the mean spike rate ($v$).

The results of an experiment on the *Limulus* photoreceptor are shown in Fig. 5. For these three curves the amplitudes were arbitrarily normalized to the incremental response at zero frequency. The two component transductions are shown on the left, the frequency response for the transduction from cell potential to spike rate (filled circles) fits very well the self-inhibition model with parameter values $K = 3$, $\tau = 0.5$ sec, and $v = 19$ per sec. The empirical frequency response of the generator potential (open circles) shows an optimum frequency, below which there is a gentle attenuation and above which there is a steep high frequency cut-off.

*References p. 112*

The answer to our first question is given on the right of Fig. 5. Here the smooth curve for the overall transduction from modulation of the light to modulation of the spike rate is predicted by the product of the amplitudes of the component transductions and the sum of their phase differences. There is strikingly good agreement between the smooth curve and the measured points. Equally good agreement was obtained in the several other experiments where we could collect all the required data, hence we are very confident that the block diagram is sufficiently complete and that we are not neglecting an important process that affects the dynamic response of the single photoreceptor.

In briefly presenting the frequency response of the generator potential I glossed over several remarkable features that are most important to the functioning of the eye. I mentioned earlier that the steady-state input–output relation of generator potential is that the mean amplitude of the potential varies as the logarithm of the mean light intensity. Such a relation makes it possible for the receptor to function over a wide range of ambient light intensities, but it makes the eye very insensitive to detecting moderate differences of intensity in stationary patterns, say, like a factor of two. On the other hand, the modulation of the generator potential is linear over a wide range of amplitudes and frequencies, and at the optimum frequency the modulation of the generator potential approaches direct proportionality to the modulation of the light. Our second question is what are the mechanisms underlying the generator potential?

To explain these features we have proposed a model of the generator potential which assumes it to arise from the superposition of discrete electrical shots whose amplitude adjusts to the ambient light intensity (Dodge, Knight and Toyoda, 1968). The bases of this model are the properties of the discrete potential fluctuations originally described by Yeandle (1958) and later studied by Fuortes and Yeandle (1964) and by Adolph (1964). When the preparation has adapted to darkness, one typically observes spontaneous, random occurrence of sub-threshold fluctuations of about 200 msec duration, widely distributed amplitudes, and somewhat variable shape that is generally an S-shaped rising phase and exponential decay. With dim illumination the mean rate of occurrence of the shots increases directly proportional with light intensity. During recovery from light adaptation it is the size of the shot that changes rather than the rate of occurrence (Adolph, 1964). To explain the generator potential we boldly extrapolate these findings to very much higher light intensities than were used in the study of the discrete events. The tests of our model must, therefore, be somewhat indirect.

The idea behind our test is that the same basic mechanism determines the frequency response to modulation of the light and the noisiness of the generator potential elicited by steady lights. The basic kinds of data are shown in Fig. 6. On the left are sample records of the generator potentials recorded at different light intensities; for a very dim light the record obviously looks like the superposition of shots, that occur more frequently than in the dark. Our model assumes that the rate increases directly with light intensity, but the size adjusts itself so that the mean potential varies approximately as the logarithm of the light intensity. Consistent with this idea we

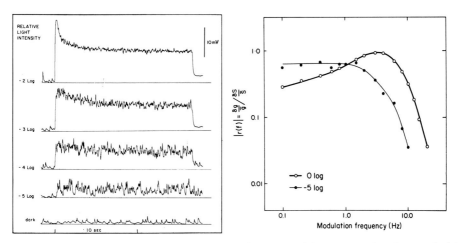

Fig. 6. (Left). Sample records of the generator potential measured in an eccentric cell treated with tetrodotoxin to block spikes, in response to 17 sec long steps of light of various intensities. (Right). Amplitudes of the frequency responses of the generator potential at two extreme light intensities.

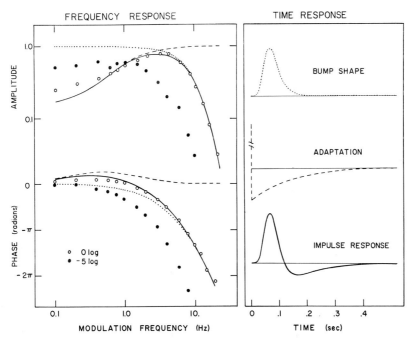

Fig. 7. Explanation of the frequency response in terms of the shape of the underlying electrical event and the adaptation of its size to variation of the light intensity.

see that the amplitude of the random noise actually decreases with increasing mean level. Note also the apparent absence of dark shots when the brighter lights go off. The change in shot size acts like an automatic gain control, and as shown by the transients, this gain control acts more quickly the higher the ambient light intensity. On the right in Fig. 6 are the amplitudes of the frequency responses measured at

References p. 112

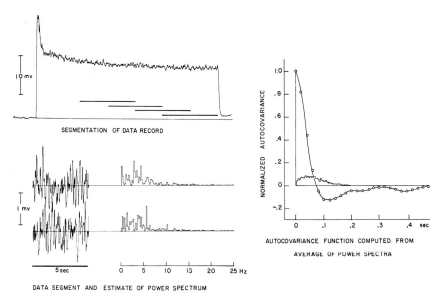

SEGMENTATION OF DATA RECORD

DATA SEGMENT AND ESTIMATE OF POWER SPECTRUM

AUTOCOVARIANCE FUNCTION COMPUTED FROM

AVERAGE OF POWER SPECTRA

Fig. 8. Method of estimating the power spectrum of the fluctuations of the generator potential as described in text.

extreme light intensities, normalized so that the fractional change in excitatory conductance is compared to the fractional modulation of the light. Our assumption that the shot rate goes directly proportional to light intensity demands that this maximum amplitude should not exceed unity, although it might approach it closely. We presume that the low frequency attenuation reflects adaptation at the shot size and, as expected, this feature becomes increasingly more prominent the higher the ambient light intensity.

How our shot model explains the frequency response is more fully described in Fig. 7. We presume that the high frequency cut-off results from the shape of the under-lying shot. Fitting the high frequency data to the measurements at high light intensities by the dotted curves yields the estimate of the shot (bump) shape shown on the right, which is obtained by the Fourier transform of the frequency response function. The zero frequency assymptote for the adaptation process is estimated from the slope of the steady-state relation between generator potential and light intensity, and a first order transition was fit to the data giving the dashed curves. At this high light intensity the time constant of adaptation was about 150 msec. Combining these two processes yields the solid curve whose Fourier transform shows that the response of the generator potential to an incremental brief flash of light (impulse response) should have a prominent undershoot. The comparison to the data shows some features that remain to be explained such as (1) the shot duration at high light intensities is about half the duration of the dark shot and (2) the low frequency attenuation is more complicated than a first order process.

Mr. Knight's mathematical formulation of this model suggested a more stringent test, namely, that the power spectrum of the fluctuation of the generator potential

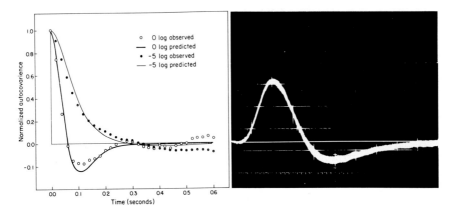

Fig. 9. (Left). Comparison of measured autocorrelation function of generator potential fluctuations with that predicted from the frequency response measured at the same mean light level. (Right). Several superimposed sweeps of the response of the generator potential to a 40 msec long bright flash superimposed on a bright background; sweep length 500 msec, amplitude of transient 4 mV, on steady-state generator potential of 16 mV.

should be proportional to the square of the amplitude of the frequency response function at that same mean light intensity. We have measured the power spectrum of the noise following the procedures of Welch (1967) using the fast Fourier transform. This procedure is shown in Fig. 8. The essentially flat part of the record was split into several 5 sec long overlapping segments. The mean and linear drift was subtracted from each segment and an estimate of the spectrum made by the absolute square of its Fourier coefficients. The ensemble average of about 20 such estimates yields the power spectrum shown on the right together with its Fourier transform, the auto-correlation function.

The comparison between the empirical autocorrelation functions of the noise in the generator potential with the autocorrelation function predicted from the frequency response measurements are shown on the left of Fig. 9. The agreement was indeed very good in this experiment. At the right we show a direct recording of the response to brief bright flash superimposed on a bright background, in order that the side by side comparison emphasize the point that the adaptation of the shot size results in a prominent negative correlation of the noise and a prominent undershoot in the driven response.

In summary, we have shown that both the driven response and the stochastic component of the response are adequately explained by a model which assumes the superposition of discrete electrical events whose mean size adjusts to ambient light intensity. The frequency response of the generator potential is enhanced by neural feedback, which quantitatively explains the remarkable sensitivity of this photo-receptor to flickering light. More recently Shapley (1969) has demonstrated that these mechanisms are a sufficient explanation of the stochastic component in the spike train.

This research was supported in part by grants NIH NB 864 from the United States Public Health Service and GB 6540 from the National Science Foundation.

## REFERENCES

ADOLPH, A. R. (1964) Spontaneous slow potential fluctuations in the *Limulus* photoreceptor. *J. Gen. Physiol.*, **48**, 297–322.

DODGE, F. A., KNIGHT, B. W. AND TOYODA, J. (1968) Voltage noise in *Limulus* visual cells. *Science*, **160**, 88–90.

FUORTES, M. G. F. (1959) Initiation of impulses in visual cells of *Limulus*. *J. Physiol.*, **148**, 14–28.

FUORTES, M. G. F. AND YEANDLE, S. (1964) Probability of occurrence of discrete potential waves in the eye of *Limulus*. *J. Gen. Physiol.*, **47**, 443–463.

HARTLINE, H. K. AND RATLIFF, F. (1958) Spatial summation of inhibitory influences in the eye of *Limulus*, and the mutual interaction of receptor units. *J. Gen. Physiol.*, **41**, 1049–1066.

HARTLINE, H. K., RATLIFF, F. AND MILLER, W. H. (1961) Inhibitory interaction in the retina and its significance in vision. In: *Nervous Inhibition*, E. FLOREY (Ed.), *Proceedings of an International Symposium*, Pergamon Press, New York, pp. 241–284.

HARTLINE, H. K., WAGNER, H. G. AND MACNICHOL, E. F. (1952) The peripheral origin of nervous activity in the visual system. *Cold Spring Harbor Symp. Quant. Biol.*, **17**, 125–141.

PURPLE, R. L. AND DODGE, F. A. (1965) Interaction of excitation and inhibition in the eccentric cell in the eye of *Limulus*. *Cold Spring Harbor Symp. Quant. Biol.*, **30**, 529–537.

PURPLE, R. L. AND DODGE, F. A. (1966) Self-inhibition in the eye of *Limulus*. In: *The Functional Organization of the Compound Eye*, C. G. Bernhard (Ed.), Pergamon Press, New York, pp. 451–464.

RATLIFF, F. (1965) *Mach Bands: Quantitative Studies on Neural Networks in the Retina*, Holden Day, San Francisco.

RATLIFF, F., HARTLINE, H. K. AND MILLER, W. H. (1963) Spatial and temporal aspects of retinal inhibitory interaction. *J. Optical Soc. Amer.*, **53**, 110–120.

SHAPLEY, R. M. (1969) Fluctuation in the response to light of visual neurones in *Limulus*. *Nature*, **221**, 437–440.

STEVENS, C. F. (1964) A quantitative theory of neural interactions; theoretical and experimental investigations. *Thesis, The Rockefeller University*, New York.

WELCH, P. D. (1967) The use of the fast Fourier transform for the estimation of power spectra: a method based on time averaging over short, modified periodograms. *IEEE Transactions on Audio and Electroacoustics*, AU-15, 70–73.

YEANDLE, S. (1958) Electrophysiology of the visual system — Discussion. *Amer. J. Ophthalmol.*, **46**, 82–87.

# Quantitative Data in Neuroanatomy*

HERBERT HAUG

*Department of Anatomy, University of Hamburg (Germany)***

## INTRODUCTION

By physiological measurement and by the development of cybernetical models an increasing amount of data was obtained during the last years. These more functional data must be supplemented by quantitative data of morphological parameters in neuroanatomy. Without such a supplement of quantitative morphological data physiological and cybernetical models may not agree with those derived from morphology. Moreover, the use of computers in quantitative morphology will become increasingly necessary, because the amount of data will increase.

Already during the last century, numerous macroscopical data were measured by simply evaluating weights and lengths. Until recently, no simple and at the same time exact methods have existed for the macroscopical measurement of volume fractions and folded surfaces, so that the published values are widely different. Neither have sufficiently exact microscopical methods been available for measuring density, volume fractions, surfaces and lengths of structures built in a complex way, such as the nerve cells.

During the last years, new simple methods have been introduced in quantitative morphology, solving the problem of such measurements. These new procedures were developed at the same time in different places in the world and in different disciplines. They are mostly based on integral mathematical reflection. The science dealing with such measuring methods is called Stereology. A short outline of its history has been given by Elias (1967) and by Weibel and Elias (1967a). In the year 1777, Buffon described the needle problem for the first time. His ideas about the needle problem are the key to the quantitative evaluation of complicated structures. His needle appears more or less distinctly with all integral procedures. Sometimes needles appear as lines, in other cases their ends are points. Buffon examined the mathematical possibilities of the position of a needle within a spatial structure only theoretically, without considering its practical use.

An integral procedure for the evaluation of volume was for the first time introduced by Delesse (1847), a geologist. Hundred years later Chalkley (1943) used for the first time the point sampling method in biology. Since 1950, Elias *et al.* (1955), Elias (1955),

---

\* This work was supported by Deutsche Forschungsgemeinschaft.
** Present address: *Department of Anatomy, University of Kiel (Germany)*.

*References pp. 125–127*

Haug (1956), Hennig (1956a and b, 1957), Weibel (1963) contributed to elaborating and introducing the new integral measuring procedures in biology. Thus, after 1960 we find an increasing amount of papers on the application of the new methods in biology.

## GENERAL VIEW

In the following, the four most important and well developed methods of morphometry will be described. Three of them have an integral basis. They deal with the estimation of the volume-fraction, of surfaces and of lengths of structures situated in a tissue. They cannot express values for single parts of the structure, but they give the total values for all examined parts of one structure very exactly. The fourth method consists in counting structures in sections, including the correction of error in evaluation. Such error arises from the thickness of a section. The practical evaluation of the count is restricted to the nerve cells.

Examples for the use of all described methods will be given in brief. These examples were taken from the macroscopical, light and electron-microscopical fields. The symbols to be used for the different parameters correspond to international standards and are listed in Table 1.

### TABLE 1

#### BASIC LIST OF SYMBOLS

| Symbol | Dimension | Definition |
|--------|-----------|------------|
| N | 1 | Number of objects |
| P | 1 | Number of points |
| L | cm | Length of linear element or test line |
| A | cm$^2$ | Planar area (transsection of object or test area) |
| S | cm$^2$ | Surface or interface area (not necessarily planar) |
| V | cm$^3$ | Volume of three dimensional object or test volume |
| T | cm | Section (slice) thickness |
| $N_V$ | cm$^{-3}$ | Number of objects per unit (test) volume (numerical density) |
| $L_V$ | cm$^{-2}$ | Length of line element per unit volume (line density) |
| $S_V$ | cm$^{-1}$ | Surface or interface area per unit volume (surface density) |
| $V_V$ | 1 | Volume of objects per unit volume (volumetric density) |
| $N_A$ | cm$^{-2}$ | Number of objects intersected (profiles) per unit area |
| $P_L$ | cm$^{-1}$ | Number of points per unit length of line |
| D | cm | Distance of parallel test lines |

With all these procedures certain basic rules must be observed in order to avoid errors in the evaluation, or to correct primary results into actual data. Namely, during preparation of the biological material, errors may inevitably arise, for example, due to swelling or shrinkage during fixation and embedding. The size of the alterations can be measured and thus the results can be corrected.

Insufficient observation of the physical data of the optical systems also leads to errors. By calibration of all optical data including the test planes used, such errors can be avoided. Using some of the new methods, errors can arise unless the thickness of the section is taken into account. Other methods do not depend on the thickness of the section. This problem will be discussed under the description of the various methods.

Structures orientated in a certain direction may give rise to errors. The possibility to avoid them will be discussed later on.

INSTRUMENTS

The question of which auxiliary instruments are desirable for fast and precise sampling of data should be considered. Counting with a list for classification with dashes is not effective enough. Counting instruments are preferred. Their size and speed are very different. Fischmeister (1967) gave a review on the latest development of instruments.

In this paper, a survey is given of a group of highly developed instruments for quanti-

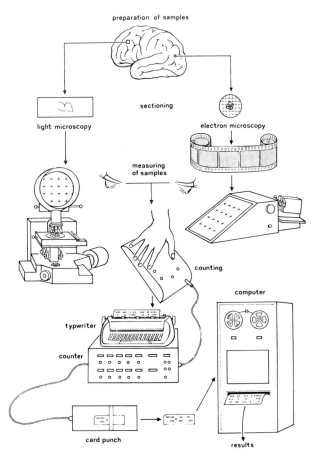

Fig. 1. Arrangement of instruments for counting in quantitative morphology (left for light microscopy and right for electron microscopy) altered according to Weibel (1967).

tative measurements on biological tissues. It was introduced by Weibel (1967). The combination of this group of instruments is shown in Fig. 1. This combination can be used for macroscopy as well as for light and for electron microscopy. Behind the counter there is a special construction with the scales of the counter. A type-writer automatically registers the result after the evaluation of each test area with the aid of a special switch. At the same time a card puncher is fed with the same data. The results punched on the cards are calculated with a computer. For every type of examination, the computer should be specially programmed.

INTEGRAL METHODS

The basis of integral methods will be described by an example in the chapter *measurement of the volume*. The methods of measuring surfaces and lengths are closely related. Special problems due to orientation will be discussed at the end of the chapter dealing with *measurement of the length of lines*.

*Measurement of the volume*

If we cut a structure in space, we see the distribution of the structure in the cutting plane. On the latter, a test area will be situated. The total distribution of the structure in this test area corresponds to the actual distribution of the structure in the entire volume, or the volume fraction. Obviously, it is necessary to measure a large number of cutting planes, so that random samples can be obtained.

In Fig. 2 the same cutting plane is shown three times. The left design presents the way first used by Delesse (1847). He evaluated the planes and found the volume fraction this way. This can be done by drawing the outlines of structures on paper as illustrated in the left area. The structure planes are gray. Then the total area of this paper is weighed and the gray areas of structures are cut out. The weight of these gray areas related to the weight of the total area corresponds to the area fraction and thus

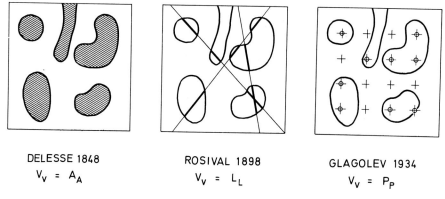

DELESSE 1848     ROSIVAL 1898     GLAGOLEV 1934

$V_V = A_A$     $V_V = L_L$     $V_V = P_P$

Fig. 2. Evaluation of the volume ratio by measurement of planes (Delesse, 1847), of lines (Rosiva. 1898), and of points (Glagoleff, 1933) according to Fischmeister (1967).

to the volume fraction. A more progressive way is planimetry. Both methods require a comparatively long time.

The next step was taken by Rosival (1898). He did not evaluate the planes but measured the fraction of the length of lines in the cutting planes (Fig. 2, middle). The fraction of length equals the fraction of volume. This procedure takes some time if measured by hand with a ruler. With the aid of an automatic procedure, for example by scanning in form of a flying spot microscope (Fischmeister, 1966), the linear analysis is optimal. Unfortunately, scanning procedures can only be used in structures that show a strong contrast. Such conditions actually do not occur in biology, as they do in metallurgy or geology.

The third step of simplification is the point sampling method introduced by Glagolev in 1933 and applied by Chalkley in biology in 1943. Glagolev, as well as Delesse and Rosival were mineralogists (Fig. 2, right). All evaluation points are sketched as crosses, and those additionally marked with small circles are situated inside the objects. The ratio between the points situated within the structure (sometimes called hit-points) and the total number of points corresponds to the volume fraction.

For all procedures described above the following relation is valid:

$$V_V = A_A = L_L = P_P \tag{1}$$

In the field of biology, point sampling is the most suitable method on account of the slight contrast between different structures. The question arises whether it is possible that the evaluation points could have a certain arrangement or whether they must be randomly distributed. Such a random distribution is only theoretically optimal, because we are unable to count an irregular arrangement of points systematically. Therefore a systematic arrangement is inevitable.

All test planes introduced by different authors during the last years have a systematic arrangement of measuring points and measuring lines (Sitte, 1967). Besides a good arrangement it is important that the lines and points should be sharply outlined so that unnecessary errors are avoided.

A further question has led to intensive discussions among experts. How many evaluation points should a test area have? Practice has shown that such test areas can be evaluated in a most convenient way and without needless errors if we count 2 to 20 points within the structure in a single test area, with an average of about 5 to 7 points. If we have a large volume fraction, a test area with 25 points is most favorable. In case the volume fraction is lower than about 5%, 100 evaluation points are preferable, for lower than about 1%, 400 points.

The number of evaluation points in a measuring area has no importance as far as the theory is concerned. The number of hit-points mentioned above is most convenient for two reasons: first, for statistical reasons, and second, because the subjective error in counting is very low. In a test examination we have to choose the best test area.

According to the theory, only real points in space should be evaluated. Each point of projection in a test area is an almost ideal point when dealing with opaque objects. In biology, we have translucent objects, therefore the points projected on the test area are in reality dashes that we can only see as points. This dash should therefore be as short as possible, or more exactly, it must be small in comparison to the diameter of structure.

The length of the dash in space depends on the focal depth of the microscopic optics. In case this is longer than the thickness of the section, the length of the dash is due to the thickness of section. Haug (1962) reported that the focal depth is dependent on the optical combination.

A focal depth of less than 1 $\mu$ can only be obtained with oil immersion. The evaluation point of dry, high-power objectives is at least 2 $\mu$ long. We obtain the shortest possible evaluation dash with oil immersion with an aperture of 1.3 and a total enlargement of 1300 $\times$. Its length is 0.3 to 0.4 $\mu$.

If the ratio between the diameter of a sphere and the depth of the evaluation point would be 1 : 1, 250% of the actual volume would be measured. This error in evaluation is called the Holmes effect (Hennig, 1956 b; Weibel and Elias, 1967 b). With a ratio of 5 : 1 between diameter and depth, the Holmes effect would still be 130%, or the evaluated result would be 30% too high. In case the ratio is higher than 7.5 : 1, the error in evaluation would remain below 20%. Under certain circumstances and on the condition that the smallest diameter of a structure has a ratio of 7.5 : 1, a safe limit of tolerance is obtained, because most structures would have diameters with a ratio of more than 7.5 : 1, so that the actual error would lie more or less below 20%.

In conclusion, we can state that using light microscopy with oil immersion, structures can only be evaluated by point sampling if their smallest diameter is greater than 3 $\mu$. Nearly all nuclei have diameters over 3 $\mu$. With dry objectives, this lower limit is raised to 15 $\mu$, so that the volume of dendrites of neurons cannot be satisfactorily evaluated.

In electron microscopy, the depth of space is only determined by the thickness of the ultra-sections, because the focal depth is greater than the thickness of sections. With the ultra-microtome a section thickness of 40–60 m$\mu$ can be reached. Therefore, the above mentioned lower limit of tolerance would be about 0.4 $\mu$.

*Measurement of surfaces*

The integral measurement of surfaces of structures was introduced only a few years ago, and the possibilities for neuromorphology are numerous. The method permits the rapid measurement of the surfaces of highly gyrencephalic brains macroscopically, as well as the surfaces of the cells, their processes and the synaptic membranes, by light- and electron microscopy.

Fig. 3 illustrates the procedure (Weibel and Elias, 1967 b). A number of parallel test-lines define the test structure that is lying on the cutting plane. All places where one of these lines cuts the surface of a structure are intersection points. The density of intersections equals the density of the surface itself. The development of this mathematical relation results in an equation with only 2 parameters, *viz.* the length of all test lines and the number of intersections:

$$S_V = 2 \cdot P_L \qquad (2)$$

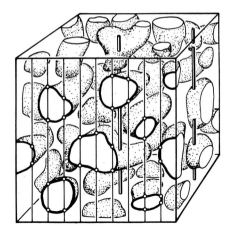

Fig. 3. Evaluation of the surface of structure in a volume. In front the points of intersection are marked with small circles (according to Weibel and Elias, 1967 b).

Within about the last ten years, the formula has been independently derived by several workers (Tomkeieff, 1945; Smith and Guttman, 1953; Duffin *et al.*, 1953; Horikawa, 1953; Hennig, 1956a; Saltykov, 1958). It is remarkable that in spite of the scientific explosion, there is a frequent exchange of new results among the various disciplines. That makes it evident how biologists were able to learn new procedures. At the same time, they also took advantage of methods that were 200 years old.

Formula (2) determines the surface per unit volume in general. It can be altered for the measurement of the surface of closed bodies in space, *viz.*:

$$S = 2 \cdot P \cdot T \cdot D \tag{3}$$

Such a closed body is the brain.

An error in evaluation can also arise due to the degree of orientation of the surface of the structure. Such error can be almost completely avoided by measuring each cutting plane three times, rotating the test lines after each measurement by 60°.

*Measurement of the length of lines*

It is possible to determine the length of a curved line in space with integral measurements. In this procedure the needles of Buffon are placed along the curved line. That way we can determine the position of needles in test areas.

In Fig. 4, the space with the curved line is cut by parallel test planes. The frequency of intersections of the curved line in these test areas corresponds to the total length of the line. The formula for the general solution is as follows (Smith and Guttman, 1953; Hennig, 1963; Blinkov and Moiseev, 1961):

$$L_V = 2 \cdot N_A \tag{4}$$

In practical use, the intersection of the curved line is counted within the test area. The

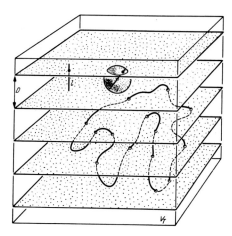

Fig. 4. Evaluation of the length of structure in a volume. In each equidistant plane the points of intersection are marked with small circles (according to Weibel and Elias, 1967 a).

result is the length of all lines in a certain volume. Here, a special formula has been
derived for limited lines, *viz.*:

$$L = 2 \cdot N \cdot D \tag{5}$$

The orientation of the lines must also be observed in surface measurements. It can be
done by a random distribution of the angles of cutting planes.

The simplest way to obtain such random distribution is to prepare many small
pieces of the tissues to be examined and to cut them without any orientation. This way
it is possible to eliminate a preferential angle between the cutting plane and the direction of the orientation of the structure. It is important that each little piece of tissue be
examined at the same frequency. In the example given later, these rules were observed
(Haug, 1967 d).

The thickness of sections has hardly any influence on the result of these procedures
for measuring surface and length (Weibel and Elias, 1967 b).

## COUNTING PARTICLES

The report on counting particles will be restricted to the theory and to the counting of
nerve cells by light microscopy. Counting particles in electron microscopy, for example, mitochondria and synapses, is highly complicated and therefore it is not discussed.

A section through a number of spheres of different sizes is seen in Fig. 5. Two sections
are made through the accumulated spheres: a thick one and a thin one. In the thin
section only sliced circles can be seen, marked by thick lines. These sliced circles are
mostly smaller than the diameter of the total spheres belonging to them. By microscopic observation it cannot be judged whether we have to deal with the actual largest
diameter or a smaller one, which leads to an error of evaluation. This error in the
evaluation of structures of different sizes is less in thick slices than in thin ones
(Haug, 1962, 1967 c; Hennig and Elias, 1966).

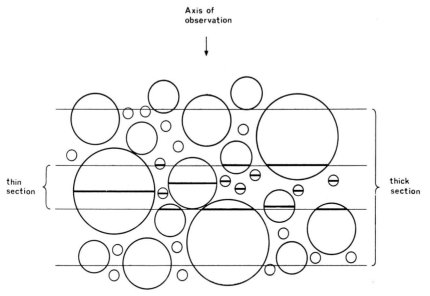

Fig. 5. The influence of the thickness of section on counting spheres of different thickness. The heavy lines within the thin section mark the diameters seen in the axis of observation.

The most serious error arises in counting spheres which are only partly situated in one section. This error in evaluation diminishes with increasing thickness of section or with diminishing size of structure. Therefore, a nearly mathematical dependence exists for the relation between size of structure and thickness of section.

In reality, there are neither ideal spheres nor homogeneous sizes in biological as well as in nervous tissues. How can we solve this dilemma? There are two possibilities: slices are to be either nearly infinitely thin or relatively thick. The method for the infinitely thin slices was developed by geologists. Their technique is very complicated and may possibly be adapted for very thin slices in electron microscopy (Schwartz, 1934; Bach, 1967; Haug, 1967 a; Underwood, 1967).

The problems are simpler for light microscopy on a thick section. Certain limitations are imposed by the methods of preparation. The optics and the quality of staining do not allow a slice thickness over 40 $\mu$. Counting large nerve cells, the relation between size of cells and thickness of section is therefore an unfavourable one (Haug, 1967 b).

In case a substructure of a structure occurs isolated, the substructure can represent the total structure in the counting. Most substructures are smaller than the total structures, therefore a more favourable relation is obtained for the correction. The nerve cells possess such single substructures in the form of nuclei and nucleoli. The nucleoli present an excellent relation between size of structure and thickness of section. Therefore, in most examinations the nerve cells can be counted by counting their nucleoli. In this case, we have to concentrate only on the presence of a nucleolus in the nerve cell.

The still remaining error in evaluation can be corrected with the aid of the improved formula of Abercrombie (1946) and Floderus (1944). This formula has been developed for the correction of the evaluation error in counting spheres in sections (Hennig, 1956 b; Haug, 1967 c).

$$N_V = N_A \frac{V}{A (D + T - 2k)} \qquad (6)$$

For symbols, see Table 1; $k$ is a correction factor for tiny inside callottes that are hardly or not at all visible in spheres lying outside the section. The value of $2k$ is mostly about 1/4th to 1/5th of the diameter in Nissl-stained nervous tissue.

In counting, the total depth of section thickness must be observed. Therefore, the fine adjustment screw of the microscope should be turned constantly. The reversal points of this movement indicate the upper and lower surface of the section.

Contrary to this procedure, the fine adjustment screw of the microscope should not be moved while the point samples in a measuring field are evaluated, because the focus should then have a minimal depth.

*Examples*

*Surface measurement*

For point sampling and surface measurement, the following example was derived by macroscopical examination. In brains from man, elephant and pilot whale,

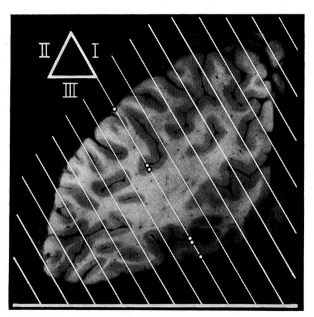

Fig. 6. A slice of elephant brain with the test lines for measuring the surface. On one test line, the intersection points are marked with small circles. I, II and III give the 3 directions of lines for the measurements, to avoid errors arising from orientation.

TABLE 2

MEASUREMENT OF SURFACE AND VOLUME OF CORTEX CEREBRI

|  | Elephant | Pilot whale | Man |
|---|---|---|---|
| Weight of total fresh brain, g | 4400 | 2600 | 1500 |
| Surface of cortex, cm² | 6300 | 5900 | 2500 |
| Volume of cortex, cm³ | 1460 | 1125 | 700 |
| Volume of cortex, % | 33.5 | 43.0 | 47.5 |
| Thickness of cortex, mm | 2.3 | 1.9 | 2.8 |

cortical surfaces and volume fractions were determined. The brains were dissected in slices of equal thickness of about 7 to 10 mm. One hemisphere was cut in frontal series, the other in horizontal slices in order to avoid errors due to orientation of the surfaces (Elias, Haug, Lange, Schwartz and Schlenska, in press, 1969).

Test planes made out of plexiglass were placed on the brain slices, as shown in Fig. 6. The results of the measurements are shown in Table 2. The volume fraction of the cortex referred to the whole brain is as high as 47% in man, *i.e.* nearly half of the human brain consists of cortex. In the elephant, the cortex amounts only to 33% of the whole brain.

It is interesting to state that the cortex of man is the thickest, while that of the pilot whale is only 60% thereof, and that of the elephant lies between the two values.

*Measurement of length*

The example for the evaluation of the length derives from electron microscopy. About 500 electron micrographs of the visual cortex of the cat were examined with the aid of a particle-size analyzer (TGZ 3 Zeiss), and the total length of myelinated fibres and the distribution of their diameters were measured. Comparison was confined to he upper third of the cortex and the white matter near the border of the cortex (see Fig. 7). In the white matter, the length of myelinated fibres per unit volume is 3 to 4 imes greater than in the upper cortex (Haug, 1967 e).

*Measurement of volume*

The volume ratio of all myelinated fibres was also determined by point sampling. In the white matter, it was found to be 78%, *i.e.* about 10 times higher than in the upper cortex. The volume fraction can also be defined by calculating the distribution of lengths and diameters, using the formula for evaluating the volume of a cylinder. The results of volume fractions obtained by the two methods of calculation are but slightly different, by less than 10%, which means that the results are highly reliable.

*Measurement of density*

The density of nerve cells in brain and cortex can be evaluated with the counting procedures described above. Counting was performed in the same brains as used for surface and volume fraction measurements. It was done in tissue sections embedded in

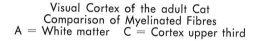

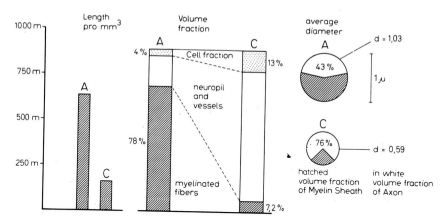

Fig. 7. Evaluation of length of myelinated fibres in the upper third of the visual cortex of the cat and in the white matter near the border of cortex. Left: length of fibres; middle: the volume ratio of fibres and all pericarya of cells; right: the ratio axon to myelin.

TABLE 3

DENSITY OF NERVE CELLS AND THEIR TOTAL AMOUNT IN CORTEX CEREBRI

(After elimination of the error due to shrinkage in paraffin)

|  | Elephant | Pilot whale | Man |
| --- | --- | --- | --- |
| Size of cortex, cm³ | 1460 | 1125 | 700 |
| Density of nerve cells per cm³ | 5800 | 8350 | 15 000 |
| Total amount of nerve cells, × 10⁹ | 8.5 | 9.4 | 10.5 |

paraffin. After counting the nucleoli and correcting the results with the aid of formula (6), the densities shown in Table 3 were found.

DISCUSSION

The four methods reported on are not the only possible ones for examining the nervous system morphometrically. Other procedures determine values that are, for the most part, related to single structures. Recently, the measurement of the length of dendrites and the frequency of dendrification have gained considerable interest. Following Sholl's studies (1956), these problems are being extensively investigated by the Dutch School (Schadé and Meeter, 1963; Loos, 1960; Colon, 1968; Smit, 1968).

Morphometric results are only important for the solution of scientific problems concerning function, development, comparison and pathological changes. For example, the total amount of nerve cells in the cortex can be calculated with the values reported above.

The approximate number of nerve cells in the cortex is calculated as follows: in man $10.5 \times 10^9$, in the pilot whale $9.4 \times 10^9$, in the elephant $8.5 \times 10^9$. In these figures, shrinkage of 50% due to fixation and embedding in paraffin have been taken into consideration. It is interesting to note that the cortex of the elephant, although 2.5 times larger than the human cortex, contains 20% less nerve cells.

The measurement of the length of myelinated fibres (Haug, 1967 e) together with the analysis of size and number of nerve cells (Sholl, 1956) can lead to an interesting model of the cortex (Haug, 1968).

It is to be expected that new and better conceptions about structure and function of the brain can be developed by morphometry, sometimes called stereology. For these developments, intense communication with other disciplines of brain research plays an important part.

## SUMMARY

The importance of quantitative methods in neuroanatomy is briefly described, and the history and basis of modern methods is outlined. Methods to avoid errors, and the use of various instruments are discussed. The principles of three integral methods are described: the measurement of volume ratio by point sampling, the measurement of surface per volume, and of length per volume, using mathematical formulas. Errors in counting structures and ways to avoid them are reported on. For this purpose, the ratio between the diameter of a structure and the thickness of the section should be as small as possible, and moreover, the results should be corrected by applying a mathematical formula. Examples for the use of all procedures are given.

## REFERENCES

ABERCROMBIE, M. (1946) Estimation of nuclear population from microtomic sections. *Anat. Rec.*, **94**, 239–247.

BACH, G. (1967) Kugelgrössenverteilung und Verteilung der Schnittkreise; ihre wechselseitigen Beziehungen und Verfahren zur Bestimmung der einen aus der anderen. In: *Quantitative Methods in Morphology*, E. R. WEIBEL AND H. ELIAS (Eds.), Springer, Berlin-Heidelberg-New York, pp. 23–45.

BLINKOV, S. M. AND MOISEEV, G. D. (1961) Die Bestimmung der Dichte der Kapillaren in den Organen und Geweben des Menschen und der Tiere, unabhängig von der Dicke des Schnittes (russisch). *Vortr. Akad. Wiss. UdSSR*, **140**, 465–468, quoted from WERNER, L. (1966).

BUFFON, G. LL. (1777) Essai d'arithmétique morale. Suppl. a, *l'Histoire Nature*, IV. Paris, quoted from WEIBEL, E. R. AND ELIAS, H. (1967b).

CHALKLEY, H. W. (1943) Method for quantitative morphological analysis of tissue. *J. Natl. Cancer Inst.*, **4**, 47–53.

COLON, E. J. (1968) Relation between dendritic patterns and position of nerve cells. *A quantitative study in the cerebral cortex of the rabbit, Thesis*, Amsterdam.

DELESSE, M. A. (1847) Procédé mécanique pour déterminer la composition des roches. *Compt Rend.*, **25**, 544.

DUFFIN, R. J., MEUSSNER, R. A. AND RHINES, F. N. (1953) Statistics of particle measurement and particle growth. *Carnegie Inst. Technol., Rept. No.* 32, CIT-AF 8 A-1 R 32, quoted from WEIBEL, E. R. AND ELIAS, H. (1967b).

126 H. HAUG

ELIAS, H. (1955) Contributions to the Geometry of Sectioning: III. Spheres in masses. *Z. Wiss. Mikroskopie*, **62**, 32–40.

ELIAS, H. (1967) Introduction: Problems of Stereology. Stereology, *Proc. Second Intern. Congr. Stereology, Chicago*, Springer, New York, Inc., p. 1–11.

ELIAS, H., HAUG, H., LANGE, W., SCHLENSKA, G. AND SCHWARTZ, D. (1969) (in the press) Oberflächenmessungen der Grosshirnrinde von Säugern mit besonderer Berücksichtigung des Menschen, der Cetacea, des Elefanten und der Marsupalia, *Anat. Anz.*

ELIAS, H., SOKAL, A. AND LAZAROWITZ, A. (1955) Contributions to the geometry of sectioning. II. Circular Cylinders. *Z. Wiss. Mikroskopie*, **62**, 20–31.

FISCHMEISTER, H. F. (1966) Scanning methods in quantitative Metallography. *Acta Polytechnica Scand.*, **56**, 1–50.

FISCHMEISTER, H. F. (1967) Apparative Hilfsmittel der Stereologie. In: *Quantitative Methods in Morphology*, WEIBEL, E. R. AND ELIAS, H. (Eds.), Springer, Berlin-Heidelberg-New York, pp. 221–249.

FLODERUS, S. (1944) Untersuchungen über den Bau der menschlichen Hypophyse mit besonderer Berücksichtigung der quantitativen mikromorphologischen Verhältnisse. *Acta Pathol. Microbiol. Scand.*, Suppl. **53**.

GLAGOLEFF, A. A. (1933) On the geometrical methods of quantitative mineralogic analysis of rocks. *Trans. Inst. Econ. Min. Moskau* (59), quoted from WEIBEL, E. R. AND ELIAS, H. (1967b).

HAUG, H. (1956) Remarks on the determination and significance of the gray cell coefficient. *J. Comp. Neurol.*, **104**, 473–492.

HAUG, H. (1962) Bedeutung und Grenzen der quantitativen Messmethoden. *Med. Grundlagenforsch.*, (G. Thieme), **4**, 302–344.

HAUG, H. (1967a) Number of particles per unit volume. Stereology, *Proc. Second Intern. Congr. Stereology, Chicago*, Springer, New York, Inc., p. 199–210.

HAUG, H. (1967b) Über die exakte Feststellung der Anzahl Nervenzellen pro Volumeneinheit des Cortex cerebri, zugleich ein Beispiel für die Durchführung genauer Zählungen. *Acta Anat.*, **67**, 53–73.

HAUG, H. (1967c) Probleme und Methoden der Strukturzählung im Schnittpräparat. In: *Quantitative Methods in Morphology*, WEIBEL, E. R. AND ELIAS, H. (Eds.), Springer, Berlin-Heidelberg-New York, p. 58–78.

HAUG, H. (1967d) Morphometrie der feinen Markfasern in der Sehrinde der Katze. *Z. Zellforsch.*, **77**, 416–424.

HAUG, H. (1967e) Quantitative examination of the myelinated fibers in electronmicrographs of the cat's visual cortex. *Proc. 25. Anniversary Meeting Electron Microscopy Society of America*, ARCENEAUX, C. (Ed.), Claitoc's Book Store, Baton Rouge.

HAUG, H. (1968) Quantitative elektronenmikroskopische Untersuchungen über den Markfaseraufbau in der Sehrinde der Katze. *Brain Res.*, **11**, 65–84.

HENNIG, A. (1956a) Bestimmung der Oberfläche beliebig geformter Körper mit besonderer Anwendung auf Körperhaufen im mikroskopischen Bereich. *Mikroskopie (Wien)*, **11**, 1–20.

HENNIG, A. (1956b) Diskussion der Fehler bei der Volumenbestimmung mikroskopisch kleiner kugeliger Körper und Hohlräume aus der Schnittprojektion. *Z. Wiss. Mikroskopie*, **63**, 67–71.

HENNIG, A. (1957) Zur Geometrie von Schnitten. 1. Bemerkungen zu ELIAS, E. R. *Z. Wiss. Mikroskopie*, **62** (1954). 2. Bemerkungen zu ELIAS, E. R., *Z. Wiss. Mikroskopie*, **61**, (1953) *Z. Wiss. Mikroskopie*, **63**, 362–365.

HENNIG, A. (1963) Länge eines räumlichen Linienzuges. *Z. Wiss. Mikroskopie*, **65**, 193–194.

HENNIG, A. AND ELIAS, H. (1966) Untersuchung von Kalottenanteilen an Kugelflächen aus Schnittbildern und Tangierproblem von Kernkörperchen. *Mikroskopie*, **21**, 32–36.

HORIKAWA, E. (1953) On a new method of representation of a mixture of several austenite grain sizes (in Japanese). *Tetsu to Hagane*, **40**, No. 10, 991. Quoted from WEIBEL, E. R. AND ELIAS, H. (1967b).

LOOS, H. V. D. (1960) On dendro-dendritic junction in the cerebral cortex. *Proc. II. Intern. Meeting Neurobiologists, Amsterdam, 1959*. Elsevier, Amsterdam, p. 36–42.

ROSIWAL, A. (1898) Über die geometrische Gesteinsanalyse. Ein einfacher Weg zur ziffernmässigen Feststellung der Quantitätsverhältnisse der Mineralbestandteile gemengter Gesteine. *Verh. KK. Geol. Reichsamt*, Wien, p. 143. quoted from WEIBEL, E. R. AND ELIAS, H. (1967b).

SALTYKOV, S. A. (1958) *Stereometric Metallography*, 2nd ed., p. 446. Metallurgizdat, Moscow. Quoted from WEIBEL, E. R. AND ELIAS, H. (1967b).

SCHADÉ, J. P. AND MEETER, K. (1963) Neuronal and dendritic pattern in the uncinate area of the human hippocampus. *Progress in Brain Research*, **3**, 89–110.

SCHWARTZ, H. A. (1934) The metallographic determination of the size distribution of temper carbon nodules. *Metals and Alloys*, **5**, 139.

SHOLL, D. A. (1956) *The Organization of the Cerebral Cortex*, Methuen, London; Wiley, New York.

SITTE, H. (1967) Morphometrische Untersuchungen an Zellen. In: *Quantitative Methods in Morphology*, WEIBEL, E. R. AND ELIAS, H. (Eds.), Springer, Berlin-Heidelberg-New York, p. 167–198.

SMIT, G. J. (1968) *Some quantitative aspects of the striate area in the rabbit brain. Thesis*, Amsterdam.

SMITH, C. S. AND GUTTMAN, L. (1953) Measurement of internal boundaries in three-dimensional structures by random sectioning. *Trans. Amer. Inst. Mining, Met. Petrol. Eng. Res.*, **197**, 81. Quoted from WEIBEL, E. R. AND ELIAS, H. (1967b).

TOMKEIEFF, S. I. (1945) Linear intercepts, areas and volumes. *Nature*, **155**, 24. Quoted from WEIBEL, E. R. AND ELIAS, H. (1967b).

UNDERWOOD, E. E. (1967) Quantitative evaluation of sectioned material. *Stereology, Proc. Second Intern. Congr. Stereology, Chicago*, Springer, New York, Inc., pp. 49–60.

WEIBEL, E. R. (1963) *Morphometry of the Human Lung*, Springer, Berlin-Göttingen-Heidelberg.

WEIBEL, E. R. (1967) A semi-automatic system for stereologic work in light and electron microscopy. *Stereology, Proc. Second Intern. Congr. Stereology, Chicago*, Springer, New York, Inc., pp. 275–276.

WEIBEL, E. R. AND ELIAS, H. (1967a) Introduction to stereology and morphometry. In: *Quantitative Methods in Morphology*, WEIBEL, E. R. AND ELIAS, H. (Eds.), Springer, Berlin-Heidelberg-New York, pp. 3–19.

WEIBEL, E. R. AND ELIAS, H. (1967b) Introduction to stereologic principles. In: *Quantitative Methods in Morphology*, WEIBEL, E. R. AND ELIAS, H. (Eds.), Springer, Berlin-Heidelberg-New York, pp. 89–98.

WERNER, L. (1966) Über die Kapillarlängenbestimmung nach Blinkov and Moiseev am Fadenmodell. *Z. Mikrosk.-Anat. Forsch.*, **74**, 321–329.

# Simultaneous Measurement of Quantitative Data in Neuroanatomy

G. J. SMIT AND E. J. COLON

*Central Institute for Brain Research, Amsterdam (The Netherlands)*

## INTRODUCTION

Haug (this volume) reviewed a number of methods to determine, with great accuracy, "the total values (of *e.g.* cell body volume and nuclear volume) for all examined parts of one structure". With such methods the distribution of parameters of the population of neurons cannot be investigated, nor the relation between different quantities, *e.g.* cell body volume and nuclear volume.

Measuring individual neurons permits the study of individual cells and of the distribution of their different quantities within the varying spectrum of the neuronal population. In this way it is, *e.g.*, possible to investigate whether one homogeneous population is present or whether there exists a multimodal population.

Simultaneous measurements of a number of quantities at individual neurons offer the advantage that the correlations between these quantities can be studied. The existence or non-existence of correlations constitutes an important element in understanding the design of the nervous system. Moreover, regression analysis can lead to estimation of one quantity from another and so to a reduction of measurements. When the form of the distribution and the correlations between the different quantities are known, realistic models of the anatomical structure can be generated. Such models will be of great use in testing hypotheses about function by means of computer simulation. The price for these advantages generally consists in a loss of accuracy with respect to the integration methods reviewed by Haug. In the analysis of individual neurons a model of the structure to be investigated has to be formulated. Simplification is necessary for such a model.

In this paper we will review our investigations* based upon simultaneous measurements of a number of neurological quantities in the striate area and the precentral area of the rabbit brain. One of our aims was a study of the dendritic tree. To obtain sufficient information about the spatial distribution of dendrites, thick sections are necessary. This necessity leads to one of the Golgi staining methods, since those only stain a low percentage of the neurons present. The Golgi–Cox technique (modification Van der Loos, 1959) we used, stains approximately 1 % of the neurons. The low staining ratio of the Golgi–Cox staining technique raises the question whether the stained neurons are a random sample of the total population of neurons. The best way to

---

* See Smit and Colon I, III, V and Colon and Smit II, IV and VI, 1970.

*References pp. 140–141*

investigate this is to compare the results for the cell body volume of Golgi–Cox-stained neurons with those of Nissl-stained neurons. With a Nissl-staining technique all neurons are stained and, therefore, no selection is present.

To create optimal conditions for the above-mentioned comparison both staining methods should be performed on material as equal as possible. Therefore, the Nissl counterstaining technique for Golgi–Cox stained sections developed by Van der Loos (1956) has been used. Fixation and dehydration are the same in both methods, therefore, no differences in cell body volume owing to differential shrinkage are to be expected.

The analyses have been constricted to a column with a small cross section (approximately 0.7 mm²). No differences, due to different location of the columns analysed, were present (*cf.* Smit and Colon I, 1970).

The quantities measured simultaneously at Golgi–Cox-stained neurons were the cell body volume, the number of first order dendrites and the structure of the dendritic tree (see later). Of the Nissl-stained neurons the cell body volume and the nuclear volume were measured simultaneously. Of each of the analysed neurons the depth below the pial surface was measured too. The depth of the neurons has been measured, since only the description of the changes as a function of depth gives a complete picture of the structural design of the architectonic field investigated. At the same time the relation between the qualitative architectonics and our quantitative data can be studied, since the different architectonic layers of the cerebral cortex are included in the analyses. To facilitate the depth measurements uncurved parts of the rabbit cerebral cortex have been selected (Bok, 1929).

### METHODS OF ANALYSIS

#### 1. Cell body volume and nuclear volume

There exist a great number of procedures for the evaluation of the nuclear volume. A review of these methods is given in *Karyometric Investigations* by Palkovits and Fisher (1968). Methods based on planimetric determination of the surface area of the nuclei in the section are the most accurate. These methods, however, are too time consuming to be useful in our analysis. Of the other methods the estimation of the nuclear volume by means of the rotation ellipsoid* gives the best results (Palkovits and Fisher VIII, 1963). In the most significant literature with respect to our investigations (Bok 1959, Van Alphen, 1945) this procedure has also been applied.

For the evaluation of the cell body volume the same procedure has been used. In general the rotation ellipsoid is a fair approximation of the cell body volume. The individual measurements, however, will be less accurate than with the nuclear volume. This is not a decisive objection, since these measurements are made mainly for a comparative purpose. The main reason for measuring the cell body volume is the

---

* Maximal height ($h$) and the maximal width ($w$) perpendicular to $h$ are measured and the nuclear volume estimated with $1/6 \, \pi h \, w^2$.

problem of aselectivity of the Golgi–Cox technique. This can be studied by comparing the values of $1/6\ \pi h\ w^2$ for Golgi–Cox and Nissl-stained neurons. Whether these values are an accurate approximation of the cell body volume is not important.

Moreover, the cell body volume is not an extremely interesting measure in itself, since cell body and nuclear volume of non-nervous tissue are strongly correlated. Bok (1959) also found a high correlation for the neurons of layers II and III of the area temporalis of the human cerebral cortex*. Finally, application of the same procedure to both nucleus and cell body is practical.

## 2. Dendritic tree

For a fruitful analysis of the dendritic tree the formulation of a model is of primary importance. E.g., the rotation ellipsoid as a model for nucleus and cell body of the neurons determined the accuracy of estimates and the measuring procedure.

The first, most fundamental step to a model of the dendritic system was made by Sholl (1953). He found for visual and motor cortex of the cat that the number of intersections of the dendrites of a certain neuron with spheres** with their centres in the centre of the cell body can be expressed by

$$I_r = a \times \exp(-k\ r) \times 4\ \pi\ r^2 \qquad (1)$$

where $r$        = radius of the sphere

$I_r$        = expected number of intersections with the sphere

$a$ and $k$ = parameters of the neuron concerned.

Before performing an analysis this model has, of course, to be tested for the animal species concerned. Therefore, we measured the $X$, $Y$ and $Z$ coordinates of all branchings and endings of a number of neurons. The number of intersections with spheres could now be calculated and the fit to the exponential equation examined. In both the striate area and the precentral area this fit was satisfactory (Colon and Smit II and VI, 1970).

The exponential model makes analysis of the dendritic tree possible. However, the technique is very time consuming, since spheres† cannot be visualized under the microscope. The $X$, $Y$ and $Z$ coordinates of every branching and ending of the dendrites have to be measured and the number of intersections found by calculation.

From the number of intersections with spheres, the model for the number of intersections with cylinders†† can be derived (Colon and Smit II, 1970).

---

* Bok also used the rotation ellipsoid to estimate nuclear and cell body volume. The regression coefficient differs from that in non-nervous material.
** In case of a pyramidal neuron by "dendrites" will be meant the "basal dendrites" only. The intersections are considered to be randomly distributed over the spheres.
† To estimate the 2 parameters the number of intersections with at least 2 spheres is necessary. By counting at more spheres the accuracy of the estimates is increased.
†† A cylinder can be easily visualized in the microscope by means of a circle in the eye-piece.

$$I_R^+ = 2 \pi a R^2 \times \left( \int_0^d \frac{\exp(-k\sqrt{R^2 + x^2})}{\sqrt{R^2 + x^2}} dx + \int_0^{\mu - d} \frac{\exp(-k\sqrt{R^2 + x^2})}{\sqrt{R^2 + x^2}} dx \right) \tag{2}$$

where $R$     = radius of the cylinder
$I_R^+$    = expected number of intersections with the cylinder
$\mu$       = thickness of the section
$d$       = depth of the neurons below the surface of sectioning
$a$ and $k$ = parameters of the particular neuron.

This equation can be solved numerically for any configuration of $R$, $\mu$ and $d$ used in a particular analysis*. The variable $d$ proved to be of little importance. Moreover, $d$ is very difficult to measure. Therefore, the mean values of the parameters $a$ and $k$ over a meaningful range of $d$** were taken as estimators.

In our analyses we used 2 cylinders with radii of 20 $\mu$ and 80 $\mu$ respectively. These cylinders are favourably located with respect to the majority of dendritic fields in the rabbit. The relations for these two cylinders between number of intersections and the parameters $a$ and $k$ are:

$$I_{20}^+ = a \times \exp(-k \times 26.96 + 8.8170) \tag{3}$$

$$I_{80}^+ = a \times \exp(-k \times 84.10 + 10.544) \tag{4}$$

Apart from these 2 cylinders we also used the number of first order dendrites to estimate $a$ and $k$. This number is considered as the number of intersections with a sphere with a diameter equal to the geometric mean of height ($h$) and width ($w$):

$$I_{fd} = a \times \exp(-k \times \sqrt{\tfrac{1}{4}h^2 + \tfrac{1}{4}w^2}) \times 4 \pi (\tfrac{1}{4}h^2 + \tfrac{1}{4}w^2) \tag{5}$$

The estimation of $\ln(a)$ and $k$ from (3), (4) and (5) is the solution of a linear regression problem. The countings of number of first order dendrites and intersections does not present special difficulties (*cf.* Colon and Smit II, 1970).

Once the estimated values of $a$ and $k$ are known, the total length ($L_{tot}$), the total surface ($S_{tot}$) and the radius of the dendritic tree ($R$) can be estimated.

$$L_{tot} = c \times \int_0^\infty a \times \exp(-kr) \times 4 \pi r^2 \, dr \tag{6}$$

$$S_{tot} = c \times \int_0^\infty a \times \exp(-kr) \times 4 \pi r^2 \times \pi \Phi_r \, dr \tag{7}$$

The radius of the dendritic tree ($R$) is defined as the diameter of the sphere in which 95% of $L_{tot}$ is contained and is, therefore, given by

---

* These calculations (Colon and Smit II, 1970) apply only to the particular analysis configuration we used.
** The values of $d$ were limited to the range from 10 $\mu$ to 70 $\mu$, since the section thickness was 80 $\mu$ and the distance between a neuron and the surfaces of sectioning had to be at least 10 $\mu$ to meet the requirements of our analysis (Smit and Colon I, 1970).

$$1/20 \times L_{\text{tot}} = c \times \int_{R}^{\infty} a \times \exp(-kr) \times 4\,\pi r^2 \, dr \tag{8}$$

Partial integration, followed by numerical evaluation gives

$$R = 6.296/k \tag{9}$$

In these formulae 2 new parameters are introduced. The first $(c)$ is the correction for winding of the dendrites, the second $(\Phi_r)$ is the perpendicular diameter of the dendrites as a function of the distance $(r)$ to the cell body. Measurements in striate and precentral areas of the rabbit (Colon and Smit II and VI, 1970) demonstrated that

$$\Phi_r = 3.82 \times r-.225 \text{ and} \tag{10}$$
$$\Phi_r = 13.2 \times r-.76 \quad \text{respectively} \tag{11}$$

Correction for winding is necessary, since integration of the number of intersections assumes that the dendrites are orientated along the radials. When the angles of deflection from the radials are the same in every plane of projection, they can be measured in the microscope with the plane of sectioning as the plane of projection and

$$c = \sum_{i=1}^{n} \sum_{j=1}^{n} \sec \alpha_i \times \sec \alpha_j/n^2$$

where $\sec \alpha$ is this angle of deviation of $n$ randomly selected points. In the striate area (Colon and Smit II, 1970) a correction factor of 3.24 has been found.

Sholl (1953) assumed that no preference of the dendrites for a certain direction was present. Recently, measurements demonstrated that this assumption is not completely justified for stellate cells. Colonnier (1964) found that in the visual cortex of cat, rat and monkey the pyramidal cells generally have circular dendritic fields. Those of the majority (approximately 75%) of stellate cells, however, were elongated. The long axis of these fields showed a preference for the direction of the vertical axis of the projection of the retina on the visual cortex. Wong (1967) investigated the auditory cortex of the cat in this respect. He obtained practically the same results. The dendritic fields of the pyramidal cells were generally spherical. Approximately 50% of the stellate cells showed an elongated field, but Wong could not demonstrate a directional preference. When examining the validity of the model of Sholl for the rabbit, we found that the stellate cells often show a deviation from the exponential decay for greater distances from the cell body. This is caused by a relatively long dendrite* (i.e., an elongated dendritic field). This aspect of the stellate cells is, of course, of great importance for the spatial reconstruction of the dendritic tree and certainly needs further investigation.

This applies also for the apical dendrites of the pyramidal neurons**.

---

* It is possible that this dendrite could be compared with the apical dendrite of the pyramidal cells.
** Sholl (1953) proposed for the apical dendrites $I_r = a \times \exp(-k \times \ln(r)) \times 4\pi r^2$ for spheres centered in the principal branching point of the apical dendrite. Of course, the length of the apical shaft would be an additional parameter. A careful evaluation of this model is in progress at the moment.

## TABLE 1

### LEAST SQUARES ESTIMATES OF REGRESSION AND CORRELATION COEFFICIENTS

| | Precentral area | | | | | | | | Striate area 1 rabbit only | |
| | Rabbit No. 1 | | Rabbit No. 2 | | Rabbit No. 3 | | All rabbits pooled | | | |
| | a | b | a | b | a | b | a | b | a | b |
|---|---|---|---|---|---|---|---|---|---|---|
| **Nissle stained neurons** | | | | | | | | | | |
| cv on nv (1) | 3.08 | 0.72 | 2.07 | 0.88 | 1.96 | 0.90 | 2.52 | 0.81 | 3.42 | 0.67 |
| nv on cv | 1.45 | 0.61 | 1.64 | 0.63 | 1.65 | 0.61 | 1.36 | 0.64 | 2.08 | 0.54 |
| corr. coeff. | 0.67 | | 0.74 | | 0.74 | | 0.72 | | 0.61 | |
| **Golgi–Cox-stained neurons (3)** | | | | | | | | | | |
| cv on fd (2) | 6.58 | 0.15 | 7.33 | 0.04 | 7.29 | 0.04 | 7.13 | 0.06 | 6.91 | 0.08 |
| fd on cv | 1.20 | 0.52 | 2.49 | 0.30 | 1.91 | 0.33 | 2.09 | 0.35 | 1.47 | 0.42 |
| corr. coeff. | 0.28 | | 0.11 | | 0.12 | | 0.15 | | 0.18 | |

(1) cv on nv means ln(cell body vol.) = a + b × ln(nuclear vol.).
(2) cv on fd means ln(cell body vol.) = a + b × ln (number of first order dendrites).
(3) The data of the Golgi–Cox-stained neurons refer to the pyramidal cells only.

RESULTS

## 1. Regression analysis

The results for cell body volume* and nuclear volume* of the Nissl-stained neurons and for cell body volume* and number of first order dendrites of the Golgi–Cox-stained neurons are given in Table 1. Figs. 1 and 2 are two examples of the correlation diagrams. The correlation diagrams were plotted in a standard way. The bisectrix of the 2 regression lines makes an angle of approximately 45° with the plot frame. The other data of the Golgi–Cox material all show essentially the same picture. Therefore, only the correlation coefficients are given (Table 2).

TABLE 2

GOLGI–COX-STAINED NEURONS

Least squares estimates of correlation coefficients between ln(cell body volume) and several parameters of the dendritic tree.

|  | Precentral area all 3 rabbits* pooled | Striate area all 5 rabbits* pooled |
|---|---|---|
| ln($a$) | —0.40 | —0.30 |
| $k$ | —0.28 | —0.22 |
| ln($L_{tot}$) | 0.11 | 0.10 |
| ln($S_{tot}$) | 0.02 | 0.06 |
| ln($R$) = ln(6.296/$k$) | 0.32 | 0.25 |

* The rabbits 1 and 3 for the striate area are identical to the rabbits 1 and 2 for the precentral area.

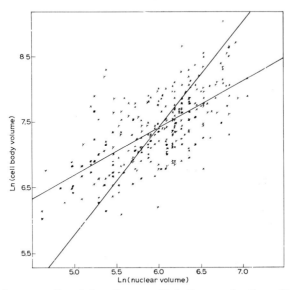

Fig. 1. Nissl-stained neurons. Correlation diagram with both regression lines of ln(cell body volume) and ln(nuclear volume) in the precentral area of rabbit No. 1 ($r = 0.67$).

* The natural logarithms of the volumes have been used throughout, since these show a better fit to the normal distribution.

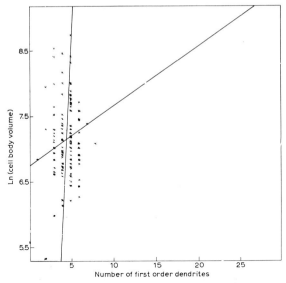

Fig. 2. Golgi–Cox-stained neurons. Correlation diagram with both regression lines of ln(cell body volume) and number of first order dendrites in the striate area of rabbit No. 2 ($r = 0.18$).

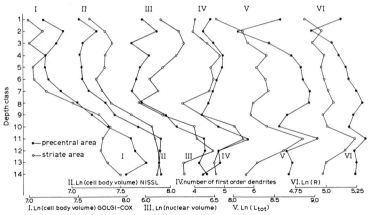

Fig. 3. The general means of the material, pooled with respect to rabbits and left or right hemisphere, in the various depth classes in both the striate and the precentral area:

I    ln(cell body volume) (Golgi–Cox-stained neurons)
II   ln(cell body volume) (Nissl-stained neurons)
III  ln(nuclear volume) (Nissl-stained neurons)
IV   number of first order dendrites (Golgi–Cox-stained neurons)
V    ln(total length of the dendrites) (Golgi–Cox-stained neurons)
VI   ln(radius of dendritic tree) (Golgi–Cox-stained neurons)

## 2. Course against depth

By course against depth the pattern of increases and decreases with depth will be meant. Since a complete account of our results has already been given elsewhere (see footnote pag. 137), we summarize our results by means of Fig. 3. For clarity's sake *a* and $k$ have been omitted. $\text{Ln}(R) = \ln(6.296/k)$ and both $a$ and $k$ are represented in $\ln(L_{tot})$.

For comparisons of the course against depth a uniform representation of depth is essential. Variations in thickness between different sections, different animals and different areas make standardization necessary. Therefore, the distance from the border of layers I and II* to the margin of gray and white matter was standardized to 2000 arbitrary units ($E$). The mean thickness in $E$ of (layer I + pia) was added to the depth values. For comparison's sake the value found in the striate area (183 $\mu$ = 298 $E$) was also used for the precentral area (226 $\mu$ = 219 $E$)**. To obtain a more uniform distribution of the neurons over the depth a (natural) logarithmic representation of depth was taken and 14 equidistant depth classes of a width of 0.15 were used.

## DISCUSSION

### 1. Aselectivity

A conclusion about randomness of the Golgi–Cox staining technique is important, since a low staining ratio is necessary for analyses of the dendritic tree. The best-method of investigation is comparison of cell body volumes measured in Golgi–Cox stained sections with those measured in Golgi–Cox/Nissl-stained sections (*cf.* INTRODUCTION).

In the striate area 5 rabbits were used for the analysis of the Golgi–Cox-stained neurons and a 6th rabbit for the analysis of Nissl-stained neurons (detailed results in Smit and Colon I, 1970). For this reason our conclusion could not be final, since we could not discriminate between a possible preference of the Golgi–Cox technique for smaller neurons (especially in the first 7 depth classes) and individual variation (*cf.* Fig. 4). In the precentral area the Nissl-stained neurons were analysed in the same 3 rabbits as the Golgi–Cox-stained neurons, but of course not in the same sections (detailed results in Smit and Colon V, 1970 and Colon and Smit VI, 1970). A good agreement generally exists between the values for Golgi–Cox and Nissl-stained neurons (*cf.* Fig. 5). The number of observations contributing to the means of the Golgi–Cox values is sometimes low. E.g., the outlying observation for rabbit no. 1 (o———o) in depth class No. 3 is based on 3 neurons only. On the basis of the data of the precentral area alone, one could conclude, however, that the Golgi–Cox technique shows some preference for larger neurons. Especially for rabbit No. 2 (□———□) relatively high values are present in the depth classes 6 through 9. This conclusion would be the opposite of the possibility we could not exclude for the striate area. All rabbits used in both investigations are from the same batch of animals and were all processed in the same way. Therefore, it can be concluded that our Golgi–Cox staining technique does stain a random sample of the neurons present.

---

\* Layer I was excluded from the standardized range, since it scarcely contained any neurons and could be well distinguished.

\*\* The mean thickness of the gray substance in the precentral area is much larger (2305 $\mu$) than in the striate area (1388 $\mu$).

*References pp. 140–141*

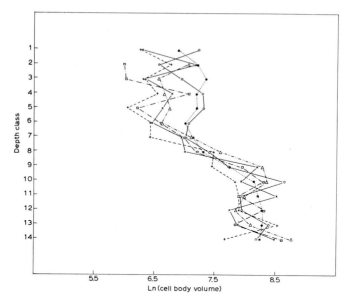

Fig. 4. Area striata. The mean ln(cell body volume) in the various depth classes for the 5 different Golgi–Cox-stained rabbits and the 1 Nissl-stained rabbit (● . . . . . ●).

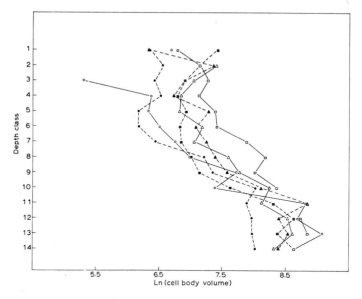

Fig. 5. Area precentralis. The mean ln(cell body volume) in the various depth classes of the Golgi–Cox neurons (continuous lines) and of the Nissl-stained neurons in the same 3 rabbits.

## 2. Course against depth

Fig. 3 shows that a great measure of correspondence exists in the course against depth of the different quantities. In all cases 3 different phases can be distinguished. In the first 7 to 8 depth classes a constancy or a decrease (only significant for the first order dendrites) is observed. It is followed by an increase in approximately the depth classes 8 through 11*. This increase is followed by a constancy or a decrease**. The correspondence between cell body and nuclear volume is confirmed by the high degree of correlation (see Table 1). On the other hand, the correlation between cell body volume and the different parameters of the dendritic tree respectively is rather low (see Table 2). Whether this is caused by different behaviour or is inherent to our method of analysis of the dendritic tree is difficult to elucidate. It is possible that the increase in the second phase sets in later here. It could also be that the pronounced discrete nature of the numbers of intersections causes important estimation errors and nivellation. In each case the value of the correlation coefficient between the cell body volume and the number of first order dendrites is very limited, since for the last quantity practically only 4 different values occur.

### 3. Interareal correspondence

The close correspondence between the area striata and the area precentralis is not only surprising, but also very clear. The only difference present is a shift for the parameters of the dendritic tree (*cf.* Colon and Smit VI, 1970). Apart from this shift all differences observed between striate and precentral area are largely within the observed individual variation (*cf.* Smit and Colon V, 1970). The correspondence is stressed by the fact that in both areas practically the same number of neurons was found in columns with the same surface area[†]. The numbers of neurons in the different depth classes were also practically equal. Moreover, the margins between the different architectonic layers also showed a close correspondence, when expressed in $E$ (*cf.* Table 3). The difference between the general means for the total dendritic length of striate and precentral area is equal to a multiplication factor of 1.70. This is practically the same as the quotient of the thicknesses of the gray substance of both areas, namely $2305 \, \mu / 1388 \, \mu = 1.66$.

It seems that the essential difference between the striate and precentral area is a difference in total thickness and that the one can be formed out of the other by simple stretching or shrinking. If such a relationship could be proved to exist for all architectonic areas, this would be of great importance. It would imply that a model of the anatomical structure of the cerebral cortex could be formulated dependent on 1 (area-specific) parameter only[††]. The principal aim of our current investigations is to subject this hypothesis to a thorough analysis.

---

* No significant increase in this range has been found for $\ln(R)$ and $\ln(L_{tot})$ in the precentral area.
** A significant decrease in the depth classes 11 through 14 has been found in the striate area for $\ln(L_{tot})$ and $\ln(R)$.
† In the Nissl-stained material we found below a surface area of $17040 \, \mu^2$ in the striate area 1195 neurons and in the precentral area 1206 neurons.
†† Already in the 1930's Bok (*cf.* Bok, 1959) formulated a model for the anatomical structure of the cortex with only 1 area-specific parameter. The thickness of the cortex in this model was a function of this parameter. Bok's model, however, does not show a satisfactory fit to his or our data (*cf.* Smit and Colon III, 1969).

*References pp. 140–141*

TABLE 3

THE MEAN DISTANCES FROM THE MARGIN BETWEEN
LAYERS I AND II TO THE LOWER BORDERS OF THE
DIFFERENT LAYERS

| Layer | Precentral area distance in E | Striata area distance in E |
|-------|-------------------------------|----------------------------|
| II | 345 | 418 |
| III | 688 | 673 |
| IV | 981 | 1007 |
| V | 1395 | 1453 |
| VI | 2000 | 2000 |

SUMMARY

Methods suitable for simultaneous measurements on individual neurons are outlined, especially with respect to the analyses of the dendritic tree.

For analyses of the dendritic tree a Golgi staining technique is necessary. The techniques only stain a small percentage of the neurons and, therefore, thick sections can be analysed. The random selection of the modification we used (Golgi–Cox mod. v. d. Loos) is demonstrated.

A review of our investigations in the striate and precentral area of the rabbit cerebral cortex is given. The analysed quantities were cell body and nuclear volume in Nissl-stained neurons and cell body volume, number of first order dendrites and parameters of the dendritic tree of Golgi–Cox-stained neurons. The pattern of increases and decreases as a function of depth of a number of neuronal quantities is described. Moreover, we concluded that the only essential difference between the striate and precentral area is a difference in cortical thickness.

REFERENCES

BOK, S. T. (1929) Der Einfluss der in den Furchen und Windungen auftretenden Krümmungen der Grosshirnrinde auf die Rindenarchitektur. Z. ges. Neurol. Psychiat., 121, 682–750.
BOK, S. T. (1959) Histonomy of the Cerebral Cortex, Elsevier, Amsterdam, New York.
COLON, E. J. AND SMIT, G. J. (1970) Quantitative Analysis of the Cerebral Cortex, II. A method for analysing basal dendritic plexuses, in press.
COLON, E. J. AND SMIT, G. J. (1970) Quantitative Analysis of the Cerebral Cortex, IV. Analysis of basal dendritic parameters in the area striata, in press.
COLON, E. J. AND SMIT, G. J. (1970) Quantitative Analysis of the Cerebral Cortex, VI. Dendritic parameters in the area precentralis of the rabbit, in press.
COLONNIER, M. (1964) The tangential organization of the visual cortex. J. Anat., 98, 327–344.
PALKOVITS, M. AND FISHER, J. (1963) Über die Fragen der kernvariationstatistischen Methoden, VIII. Bedingungen der Bewertung der Messergebnisse bei unterschiedlicher Gewebestruktur und Zellkernform. Z. Mikr.-Anat. Forsch., 69, 410–424.
PALKOVITS, M. AND FISHER, J. (1968) Karyometric Investigations, Akadémiai Kiadó, Budapest.
SHOLL, D. A. (1953) Dendritic organization in the neurons of the visual and motor cortices of the cat, J. Anat., 87 387–406.

SMIT, G. J. AND COLON, E. J. (1970) *Quantitative Analysis of the Cerebral Cortex.* I. Aselectivity of the Golgi–Cox staining technique, in press.

SMIT, G. J. AND COLON, E. J. (1970) *Quantitative Analysis of the Cerebral Cortex.* III. Nuclear volume and first order dendrites in the area striata of the rabbit, in press.

SMIT, G. J. AND COLON, E. J. (1970) *Quantitative Analysis of the Cerebral Cortex.* V. Nuclear and cell body volume in the area precentralis of the rabbit, in press.

VAN ALPHEN, G. W. H. M. (1945) Measurements of nuclear volume in the human neocortex (in (Dutch). *Thesis, Leiden,* Eduard IJdo, Leiden.

VAN DER LOOS, H. (1956) Une combination de deux vieilles méthodes histologiques pour le système nerveux central. *Monatschr. Psychiat. Neurol.*, **132**, 330–334.

VAN DER LOOS, H. (1959) Dendro-dendritic connections in the cerebral cortex (in Dutch). *Thesis, Amsterdam,* H. Stam, Haarlem.

WONG, W. C. (1967) The tangential organization of dendrites and axons in three auditory areas of the cat's cerebral cortex. *J. Anat.*, **101**, 419–433.

# Applications of Computer Simulation to the Study of Neurochemical Behavior

DAVID GARFINKEL

*Johnson Research Foundation University of Pennsylvania, Philadelphia, Penna. 19104 (U.S.A.)*

## INTRODUCTION

Many of the other papers in this volume show clearly that present-day neurophysiology is very heavily dependent on the appropriate usage of computers, both for the acquisition of data, and for their interpretation or reduction to usable form. In contrast, computer applications to neurochemistry are still quite novel. Many neurochemists may not even be aware of what applications have been made, let alone what may reasonably be expected in the near future. This paper is concerned both with existing accomplishments in this area and with possible future applications.

The work summarized here commenced as a compartmentation study, a type of investigation in which computer usage is fairly routine (*e.g.*, Berman *et al.*, 1962). "Compartmentation", as generally used in the biological literature, implies a matter of physiological rather than of biochemical scale: one is usually concerned with a large system divided into several large compartments (often the whole body divided into spaces such as the blood, the muscle mass, etc.). There are exceptions: the red blood cells may collectively constitute a compartment in spite of their small individual size. Here we appear to be concerned with a compartmentation at the cellular level, of the kind where certain types of cells or parts of cells are in one compartment, whereas other parts of the same cells may be in another compartment.

In addition to the usual compartmentations between mitochondria and cytoplasm, the long processes characteristic of nerve cells, such as axons, may constitute a compartmentation barrier because diffusion down their length is necessarily slow.

## METHODOLOGY

The computer methodology used in the construction of the models here discussed has been described in detail elsewhere (Garfinkel *et al.*, 1961; Garfinkel and Hess, 1964; Garfinkel, 1968). The following is therefore intended only to help orient the reader, rather than as a definitive description.

Models of this type are written in the language of the biochemist rather than the mathematician. They are structured in terms of chemical reactions of the form

$$A + B \rightarrow C + D$$

## TABLE 1

### LABELING OF AMINO ACIDS AFTER INPUT OF $^{14}C$

Expressed as specific activity ratios relative to glutamate

| Labeled substance and time (min) | Glutamine | | Aspartate | | Alanine | | GABA | | Glutathione | |
|---|---|---|---|---|---|---|---|---|---|---|
| | Exptl. | Calc'd. | Exptl. | Calc'd. | Exptl. | Calc'd. | Exptl. | Calc'd. | Exptl. | Calc'd. |
| [U-$^{14}$C]Glucose (intraperitoneally) | | | | | | | | | | |
| 5 | 0.47 | 0.51 | 0.58 | 0.68 | | | | 0.273 | | |
| 10 | 0.55 | 0.58* | 0.68 | 0.73* | 3.8 | 3.9* | 0.45 | 0.45* | | |
| 15 | 0.68 | 0.714 | 0.79 | 0.72 | | 3.3* | | 0.55 | | |
| 30 | 0.83 | 0.85 | 0.86 | 0.74 | | 2.0 | ca. 5 | 0.72 | | |
| 40 | 0.905 | | | | 1.9 | 1.4 | ca. 6 | 0.78 | | |
| [U-$^{14}$C]Glutamate (into CSF) | | | | | | | | | | |
| 1 | 1.3 | 1.85 | | | | | 0.25 | 0.21 | 1.1 | 1.2 |
| 2 | 3.8 | 3.45 | | | | | | 0.51 | | |
| 5 | 5.2 | 5.5 | | | | | ca. 8 | 0.85 | | |
| 15 | 5.0 | 5.0 | | | | | 0.86 | 1.2 | | |
| 30 | 3.5 | 3.9 | | | | | | | | |
| [U-$^{14}$C]Glutamine (into CSF) | | | | | | | | | | |
| 2 | 13 | 13.6 | 0.6 | 0.55 | | | 0.7 | 0.59 | 1.7 | 1.9 |
| [U-$^{14}$C]Aspartate (into CSF) | | | | | | | | | | |
| 2 | 5 | 4.5 | 34 | 63 | | | 0.11 | 0.14 | 0.17 | 0.4 |
| 5 | 5 | 5.3 | 12.5 | 11.4 | | | 0.37 | 0.34 | 0.58 | 0.88 |
| [1-$^{14}$C]GABA (into CSF) | | | | | | | % orig. cts. still in GABA | | | |
| 2 | ca. 4.5 | 2.2* | ca. 10 | 12* | | | 91 | 93* | | |
| 5 | | | | | | | 58 | 59* | | |
| 27 | | | | | | | 16 | 7* | | |

Sources of the experimental data:

For *glucose* input, Van den Berg *et al.* (1966 and personal communication) for glutamine and aspartate; Machiyama (1965) for alanine and GABA except for the last 3 GABA points, which are from Minard and Mushahwar (1966).

For *glutamate, glutamine* and *aspartate*, Berl *et al.* (1961) except the 30-min GABA point, which is from Roberts *et al.* (1958).

For *GABA*, Roberts *et al.* (1958), and Baxter (1968 and personal communication). Probably, the glutathione experimental values are the least reliable.

\* Values obtained using slightly different sets of rate constants from that used for the main body of results.

where substances *A* and *B* are consumed in the reaction unless otherwise specified (provision is also made to specify *how many* of *A*, *B*, . . . are produced or consumed). To each reaction corresponds a flux, determined by the expression

$$\text{Flux} = k\,(A)\,(B),$$

where *k* is the rate constant. The differential equation for one of the substances *A*, *B* . . . is formed by summing the fluxes of the reactions in which it is involved, with appropriate sign according to whether it appears or disappears. For each set of chemical reactions, a computer program is automatically constructed to numerically solve the corresponding differential equations (the simpler the method of solution the better) starting from an appropriate set of initial concentrations, rate constants, etc. The process of varying these to obtain the best possible fit to a given set of experimental data (optimization) can be automated, as have been the processes of error-checking the input, putting the output in a form convenient to the user, etc. Selecting the right sets of initial conditions is unfortunately still an art and difficult to describe; it is made easier by close interaction of the user with a suitable computer. The current version of the program to do this is described in Garfinkel (1968), and copies are available for distribution through the SHARE organization.

## MODELS

It was originally noticed by Berl *et al.* (1961) that when [$^{14}$C]glutamate was injected into the cerebrospinal fluid (CSF) of the rat, the glutamine of the brain became labeled within 5 minutes so that its specific activity was about 5 times as great as that of the glutamate in the same brain at the same time (Table 1). This is anomalous; the specific activity of a product is here greater than that of its precursor. This unusual ratio of specific activities was *not* observed if the labeled glutamate was injected into the blood instead of the CSF. It *was* observed if other radioactive substances, such as glutamine, aspartate, and γ-aminobutyric acid (GABA) were injected into the CSF. O'Neal and Koeppe (1966) subsequently found that a number of other substances, such as acetate, could yield glutamine/glutamate specific activity ratios of more than 1, although glucose does not. Table 1 is a compendium of some of the ratios of specific activity observed in the brain when various substances are injected into the blood or CSF; this set of data is being explored quantitatively with suitable computer models of neurochemical behavior, with the intention of extracting all the information inherent in it.

This sequence of models originally started out (Garfinkel, 1962) as a linear model, primarily of compartmentation. This has since become non-linear and has included many other things, but with various important parts being omitted as they are finished with and no longer needed. Thus, the second model in the sequence (Garfinkel, 1966) was strongly concerned with nitrogen metabolism, and a $^{15}$N-labeled version was constructed based on the work of Berl *et al.* (1962). In the third generation of the model nitrogen metabolism is no longer considered (this is assumed to operate at constant rates and normal steady-state levels) but glucose metabolism is considered in much greater detail. In both the second and third models the interaction of compartmentation with metabolism has been considered; identification of the compartments (in morphological terms) and the determination of their physiological function is also attempted. In a fourth model version, now under construction, the radioactivity is traced through the system atom-by-atom rather than by average labeling of molecules, as in the others (this is important because a molecule of given origin that has been around the Krebs cycle twice will be quite differently labeled than when it had been around only once).

All of these models (excepting the first) are based on the experiments of more than one group of workers with all the resulting problems of differing experimental errors and biases, etc., and real biological differences due to differences in conditions, different strains of experimental animals, etc., no single source of data being complete enough to determine a model. Fortunately the disagreements between different groups of workers are not particularly bad. In compiling Table 1 data were selected; the values used are the single values deemed most reliable by the author rather than averages of those obtained by several workers (in large part this is because there is no appropriate statistical procedure for combining such data from different sources in this way).

As these models were originally an attempt to understand a compartmentation which required at least two glutamate compartments, they were built with a large compartment and a small compartment. The small compartment must contain between 14 and 20% of the total glutamate (Garfinkel, 1962), with the most probable figure being about 18%, and is in communication with the CSF. The model has kept this general form since, although many other substances, structures, and pathways have been added and the aspartate and glutamate content within each compartment has been subfractionated again so that there are four pools of each (in addition to the content in the CSF). It was necessary to assume (Garfinkel, 1966) that the Krebs cycle itself is compartmented also, with comparable fluxes in the two compartments, because radioactivity is otherwise not transmitted between glutamate and aspartate at the proper rate. This indicates that there are mitochondria in each compartment, and it is in fact observed that there is more than one population of mitochondria within the brain, those within the nerve endings differing from the others (Salganicoff and De Robertis, 1965), but in comparable amount, in agreement with the model.

An overall diagram of this model, which is still in a state of continuous evolution, is shown in Figs. 1 and 2 (as of the date of writing). It is impossible to explain here every step and nuance in the evolution of the model, owing to its complexity (as of the time of writing it includes 66 molecular forms and 131 reactions involving them) and the fact that several cubic feet of paper were required to print out the calculations required in its development. It will therefore be possible to describe only some "highlights".

Overall matches to experimental data starting with [14]C labelling are shown in Table 1; those for [15]N labelling are also shown in Table 2. A fairly good match to the experimental data is obtained, even allowing for the wide scatter of the [15]N data; this is especially gratifying in view of the complexity of the model. (It should be noted that not all the [14]C matches had been obtained with the same initial conditions, owing to

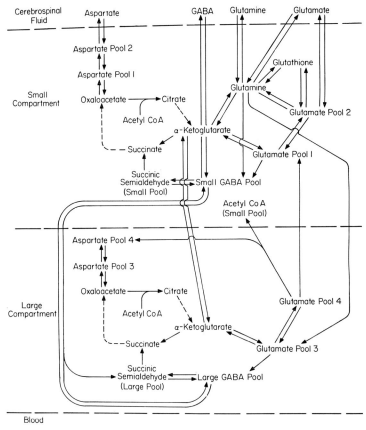

Fig. 1. Overall structure of the brain metabolism model as of the time of writing. The sources of the acetyl-CoA groups are detailed in Fig. 2.

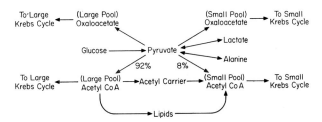

Fig. 2. Detailed metabolism of glucose in the model.

the continuing evolution of the model.) Further attempts to improve the fitting of the data, and to include additional data, are in progress.

## INTERPRETATION OF MODELS

Models of this type are not constructed solely to secure good matches to the data. They are intended both to indicate things about the structure and organization of the

TABLE 2

BEHAVIOR OF MODEL WHEN SIMULATING INTRAVENOUS INFUSION LABELED AMMONIUM ACETATE INTO CATS[a]

| Substance | Amount observed (μmoles/g of brain tissue) | | | Amount calculated (μmoles/g of brain tissue) | | | | Relative specific activity observed | | | | Relative specific activity calculated | | | | |
|---|---|---|---|---|---|---|---|---|---|---|---|---|---|---|---|---|
| | 10 min | Maximum | Minimum | Run 3[b] | Run 5[c] | Run 6[d] | Run 1 (revised)[e] | 10 min | Minimum | Maximum | Trend with time | Run 3 | Run 5 | Run 6 | Run 1 (revised) | Trend with time |
| Glutamate | 8.9 | 9.7 | 8.0 | 8.8 | 8.8 | 8.7 | 8.7 | 1[f] | 1 | 1 | | 1 | 1 | 1 | 1 | |
| Glutamine | 7.6 | 9.6 | 7.6 | 6.7 | 6.6 | 6.2 | 5.9 | | | | | | | | | |
| α-Amino | | | | | | | | 9 | 3.3 | 13.5 | Interdeterminate | 7.2 | 8.4 | 5.1 | 4.7 | Rises |
| Amide | | | | | | | | 30.5 | 10 | 67 | Falls | 10 | 19.7 | 12.5 | 13.2 | Falls |
| Aspartate | 2.1 | 3.1 | 2.0 | 2.2 | 2.1 | 2.2 | 2.2 | 0.48 | 0.34 | 0.7 | Rises | 0.53 | 0.24 | 0.47 | 0.53 | Rises |
| Glutathione | 2.4 | 2.4 | 1.7 | 2.1 | 2.1 | 2.1 | 2.1 | | | | | | | | | |
| Glutamate moiety | | | | | | | | 0.12 | 0.08 | 0.3 | Rises | 0.24 | 0.2 | 0.14 | 0.18 | Rises |
| GABA | 1.3 | 2.1 | 1.2 | 1.7 | 1.4 | 2.0 | 2.1 | 0.275 | 0.25 | 0.94 | Indeterminate | 1.27 | 0.95 | 0.98 | 0.93 | Rises |
| Ammonia | 5.5 | 13.0 | 1.8 | 4.7 | 5.8 | 6.2 | 4.9 | 55 | 13.5 | 122 | Falls | 25 | 24 | 28 | 17 | Falls |

[a] From Garfinkel (1966), reproduced by permission of the *Journal of Biological Chemistry*. Experimental data (for both amounts of substances and $^{15}N$ labeling) from eight experiments of varying time duration (8 to 25 min) (Berl et al., 1962) are compared with four simulation runs, for which data are presented at 10 min only. Specific activities are expressed relative to that of glutamate as 1.

[b] Run 3, Rate(s) 96 = $1 \times 10^{-1}$, Rate 100 = $3 \times 10^{-4}$ (Rate 96 is rate of glutamine disappearance from brain; Rate 100, ammonia-catalyzed $CO_2$ fixation into oxaloacetate).

[c] Run 5, Rate(s) 96 = $6 \times 10^{-2}$, Rate 100 = $3 \times 10^{-4}$, amount of glutamic dehydrogenase = 0.25.

[d] Run 6, Rate(s) 96 = $5 \times 10^{-2}$, changed to $7 \times 10^{-2}$ after 15 min; Rate 100 = $1 \times 10^{-4}$.

[e] Run 1 (revised) is identical with Run 6 except that the handling of ammonia by Reaction(s) 96 is changed.

[f] The range of observed specific activities is from 0.41 to 5.9 atom % excess.

system being studied that are not obvious from direct examination of the experimental data, and to suggest new experiments. Part of this type of result is included in the description of each model (*e.g.*, the pool and connection structure) and part is described below.

The second version of this model (Garfinkel, 1966) was heavily concerned with ammonia metabolism in the brain, and therefore included many related features (*e.g.*, ammonia-handling enzymes such as glutamic dehydrogenase) that have since been omitted. These were used to explore such possibilities as that hepatic coma may be due to elevated blood ammonia levels depleting the Krebs cycle intermediates in the brain (it was impossible to get the model to behave in this way) and that glutamine may be an excretory product of ammonia (its efflux from the brain increases sharply at high ammonia levels).

The third version of this model is particularly concerned with the metabolism of two substances, GABA and glucose. The metabolism of GABA was examined particularly in the light of the experiments of Wood *et al.* (1963) and of Machiyama (1965). They both found that GABA made externally available to the brain (either by intraperitoneal injection followed by transport through the blood, or by addition to the medium surrounding brain slices) could be taken up and then metabolized; and upon examination of their data it appears not to be metabolized very rapidly. The original data of Berl *et al.* (1961) which indicate rapid rates of GABA labeling, would seem to contradict this, indicating that GABA is compartmented between the large and the small compartment as with the other substances considered. The rate of GABA metabolism in the small compartment is rapid compared to that in the large one (in the second model (Garfinkel, 1966) these rates were comparable, but much of the experimental data was not then available, or was erroneous). The apparent rate of metabolism of GABA in the small compartment is approximately 80 $\mu$moles/kilogram wet weight brain/minute; that in the large compartment is perhaps a quarter as much, so that the total is 10–15% of the Krebs cycle flux. However the content of GABA in the small compartment may be 1/8 to 1/10 to that of the large compartment, as this proportion gives the best fit to the data of Berl *et al.* (1961). There are some (preliminary) indications in the work of Baxter (1968 and personal communication), that GABA may effectively flow from the small to the large compartment, there being immediately converted into something else (presumably the large pool of succinic semialdehyde; see Fig. 1) without mixing freely with the GABA of that compartment. This would be consistent with the picture of the inhibitory synapse (with GABA as a transmitter) presented by De Robertis (1967). Other flows of GABA between compartments are indicated by the model, as are flows of glutamate, a substance whose physiological action is opposite to that of GABA; perhaps their opposed pharmacological actions partly cancel out. This model is compatible with the idea that GABA is the inhibitory neurotransmitter, although it does not constitute a proof, in part because there is insufficient experimental evidence to satisfactorily determine GABA movement.

Failure to consider the GABA compartmentation properly may yield strange results in analyzing the behavior of GABA (as with the other brain constituents). For exam-

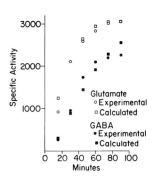

Fig. 3. Comparison of calculated and experimental points for the experiments of McKhann *et al.* (1960), as described in the text.

ple, McKhann *et al.* (1960) came to the conclusion that GABA metabolism in the brain was very rapid, perhaps 40% of the Krebs cycle flux, because they neglected GABA compartmentation. It is seen in Fig. 3 that a fairly good fit to their results can be obtained with this model, modified primarily to compensate for differences in gross chemical analysis (the GABA content of their preparations is three times that assumed for this model) but with the GABA flux nearly unchanged.

The flow of the carbons derived from glucose has been represented in some detail in the third version of the model, as shown in Fig. 2. Glusose metabolism appears to be carried on primarily in the large compartment; about 92% of the glucose conversion into acetyl-CoA takes place there, and presumably almost all the glycolysis; the metabolism of the smaller compartment is therefore primarily oxidative rather than glycolytic. This behavior appears to be largely related to permeability properties, because the isolated nerve endings do in fact contain glycolytic enzymes (C. Moore, personal communication). This would leave the nerve endings in particular highly sensitive to anoxia, as they cannot use glycolytic energy with which to stay alive. Since the Krebs cycle flux seems to be comparable in the two compartments whereas the primary metabolic fuel for the brain (glucose) is first processed exclusively in the large compartment, what does the small compartment use as its immediate source of fuel? Identification of the acetyl source for the small compartment Krebs cycle is presently a major source of difficulty, as no acetyl transport or carrier system is clearly indicated by the $^{14}C$ data. For a while *N*-acetyl aspartate appeared a likely source (D'Adamo and Yatsu, 1966; Minard and Mushahwar, 1966) but it then turned out to have no turnover of the acetyl moiety in adult rat brain (Minard, personal communication). At the moment it appears that the small compartment burns lipids, proteins, such small molecules as $\beta$-hydroxybutyrate, such acetyl groups as are somehow transported from the large compartment, and an appreciable amount of glutamate, but this definitely requires further investigation. It has been shown in accord with this idea that glutamate is the principal endogenous substrate of brain mitochondria (Cohen, 1964), and that it does serve as an acetyl carrier in brain (D'Adamo and D'Adamo, 1968). The small compartment would then be at the end of a long fuel "pipeline" which tends to isolate if from changes of blood concentration of substrates, especially glucose. One may regard the small compartment as the innermost of a series of nested homeostatic mechanisms which include the blood–brain barrier and the body's regulatory mechanism for glucose.

The overall structure of this model indicates that the nerve-endings, which are the message-originating side of the synapses, are contained within the small metabolic compartment. This is based on such evidence as distribution of enzymes, amino acids, and total protein, permeability to substances like glutamine, patterns of metabolism of possible transmitter substances, etc. (Garfinkel, 1966).

The structure of the model is in some disagreement with enzyme distribution studies because the model calls for some activities to be present in or around the nerve endings, whereas only a few percent of the total of such enzymes is in fact present in the isolated nerve endings. This few percent is nevertheless sufficient to provide the absolute amount of activity required by the model. This type of evidence must in any event be taken with caution because isolated enzymes in the test tube behave quite differently from the way they behave in a composite multi-enzyme system, especially *in situ* (Garfinkel *et al.*, 1968).

Physiological evidence for this overall structure is provided by the experiments of F. Jöbsis and M. Rosenthal (personal communication) in which they were able to separately study the metabolic behavior of the synapses and of the rest of the brain by following fluorescence levels. In one instance in which a cat died of anoxia they found that the synapses died first, which is exactly in accordance with this model. Additional supporting evidence from a variety of sources is available. It is found (*e.g.*, Lowry, 1966) that the brain dies of anoxia before it has exhausted its supply of glycolyzable substrate. It is also found by Berl (1965) that this compartmentation as a whole appears in the maturing brain at the stage of development (the critical period, about 3 to 4 weeks of age in the cat) when the great sensitivity to anoxia of adult mammals appears.

A key phrase in the preceding paragraph is *from a variety of sources*. Superficially the contributions of Jöbsis and Rosenthal, of Lowry (1966) and of Berl (1965) would appear to be unrelated to each other, but they are all united into a common picture by this model. This illustrates an important application of this type of simulation: it permits one to unite data from different fields and from different laboratories, which is difficult to do otherwise. Having done this, one can then proceed to design experiments, perhaps in yet another experimental field, which would not have been at all obvious without such a model. It is anticipated that the design of experiments will become an important function of this type of computer simulation.

## POSSIBLE (AND PERHAPS SPECULATIVE) FUTURE APPLICATIONS OF THE MODELS

There do exist medical conditions in which the brain's sensitivity to anoxia is troublesome, especially where blood circulation to the brain is interrupted, when death results in about three minutes. If the compartmentation could be broken down so that glycolytic energy would be available to the small compartment this period of time might be extended, saving a fair number of lives in appropriate clinical situations. Thus far, any artificial breakdown of this compartmentation has been obtained only by cooling brain slices during preparation (Berl, Nicklas and Clarke, 1968). Extrapolating this to cooling the brain *in situ* (perhaps as a first aid measure) is probably less likely than the development of a drug to change the compartmentation by altering membrane permeabilities (a common behavior of drugs), or perhaps one to stimulate the general glycolytic rate (if a fixed proportion of this can get into the small compartment). Predicting arrests of brain circulation (since a drug for this purpose must be administered in advance) is often (though not always) possible.

The model thus indicates that it may be worthwhile to try to develop a drug to alter a situation which thus far has appeared to be a fact of nature. Perhaps development of other drugs, such as anti-convulsants, stimulants, etc., may be suggested by the model also, although appreciable further simulation will be required before this is ready for experimental testing and no amount of simulation will substitute for the usual clinical testing of any drugs developed.

Another possible application of this type of simulation studies is to alcoholism, if its effects are actually due to hypoglycemia, as has been suggested by some workers (reviewed by Madison, 1968). In this situation the brain is relatively short of glucose but well-provided with acetate resulting from ethanol oxidation. Since some anti-convulsant drugs increase the affinity of the brain for acetate they might be applied to help to make up for the glucose lack.

Another type of application to which this type of simulation can be extended is rather close to the neurophysiological. We usually think of neurons as all-or-none affairs, but they are in fact made of membranes containing enzymatic ion pumps drawing power from other enzyme systems, and their behavior may respond to the properties of these subunits. Thus, it may be possible to calculate how the threshold level of a given neuron or the length of its refractory period is a function of its metabolic state, and perhaps how this might be altered by drugs or changes in membrane properties. By putting together enough biochemical data one would thus have a model of a neuron that could help explain the physiology in terms of the biochemistry, and could perhaps be combined with other physiological simulations (*e.g.*, those of Farley, 1965) to assist in the better understanding of the functioning of neurons, both singly and in combination.

It appears that the construction of models of this type, by permitting the combination of large numbers of quantitative items about the brain, permits us to extract information from experiments from several different fields which was not originally obvious to the people who did them. Computer modeling thus allows us to better understand and perhaps even to manipulate somewhat the complex biochemical system which is the basis of brain behavior.

### ACKNOWLEDGEMENTS

This work was supported by a Research Career Development Award (GM 5469) from the National Institutes of Health. Most of the simulation described herein was supported by grants FR-15 and GM-AM 16501 from the National Institutes of Health.

## REFERENCES

BAXTER, C. F. (1968) Intrinsic amino acid levels and the blood-brain barrier. *Prog. Brain Res.*, **29**, 429–450.

BERL, S., LAJTHA, A. AND WAELSCH, H., (1961) Amino acid and protein metabolism VI. Cerebral compartments of glutamic acid metabolism. *J. Neurochem.*, **7**, 186–197.

BERL, S., TAKAGAKI, G., CLARKE, D. D. AND WAELSCH, H. (1962) Metabolic compartments *in vivo*. *J. Biol. Chem.*, **237**, 2562–2569.

BERL, S. (1965) Compartmentation of glutamic acid metabolism in developing cerebral cortex. *J. Biol. Chem.*, **240**, 2047–2054.

BERL, S., NICKLAS, W. J. AND CLARKE, D. D. (1968) Compartmentation of glutamic acid metabolism in brain slices. *J. Neurochem.*, **15**, 131–140.

BERMAN, M., SHAHN, E. AND WEISS, M. F. (1962) The routine fitting of kinetic data to models: A mathematical formalism for digital computers. *Biophys. J.* **2**, 275–287.

COHEN, H. P. (1964) Some factors involved in the use of glucose and hexokinase as a trap for ATP in cerebral mitochondrial studies. In: *Morphological and Biochemical Correlates of Neural Activity*, M. M. COHEN AND R. S. SNYDER (Eds.), Harper and Row, New York, pp. 212–224.

D'ADAMO, A. F., JR. AND YATSU, F. M. (1966) Acetate metabolism in the nervous system. *N*-Acetyl-L-aspartic acid and the biosynthesis of brain lipids. *J. Neurochem.* **13**, 961–965.

D'ADAMO, A. F. JR. AND D'ADAMO, A. P. (1968) Acetyl transport mechanisms in the nervous system. The oxoglutarate shunt and fatty acid synthesis in the developing rat brain. *J. Neurochem.*, **15**, 315–323.

DE ROBERTIS, E. (1967) Ultrastructure and cytochemistry of the synaptic region. *Science*, **156**, 907–914.

FARLEY, B. G. (1965) A neural network model and the "slow potentials" of electrophysiology. In: *Computers in Biomedical Research*, R. W. STACY AND B. WAXMAN (Eds.), Academic Press, New York, pp. 265–294.

GARFINKEL, D., RUTLEDGE, J. D. AND HIGGINS, J. J. (1961) Simulation and analysis of biochemical systems, I. Representation of chemical kinetics. *Commun. Assoc. Computing Machinery*, **4**, 559–562.

GARFINKEL, D. (1962) Computer simulation of steady state glutamate metabolism in rat brain. *J. Theoret. Biol.*, **3**, 412–422.

GARFINKEL, D. AND HESS, B. (1964) Metabolic control mechanisms VII. A detailed computer model of the glycolytic pathway in ascites cells. *J. Biol. Chem.*, **239**, 971–983.

GARFINKEL, D. (1966) A simulation study of the metabolism and compartmentation in brain of glutamate, aspartate, Krebs cycle, and related metabolites. *J. Biol. Chem.*, **241**, 3918–3929.

GARFINKEL, D. (1968) A machine-independent language for the simulation of complex chemical and biochemical systems. *Computers Biomed. Res.*, **2**, 31–44.

GARFINKEL, D., FRENKEL, R. AND GARFINKEL, L. (1968) Simulation of the detailed regulation of glycolysis in a heart supernatant preparation. *Computers Biomed. Res.*, **2**, 68–91.

LOWRY, O. H. (1966) Metabolic levels as indicators of control mechanisms. *Federation Proc.*, **25**, 846–849.

MACHIYAMA, Y. (1965) Relation of carbohydrate metabolism in the brain to amino acid metabolism. Some aspects of $\gamma$-amino acid metabolism in isolated cerebral tissue *in vitro*. Thesis, *University of London*.

MADISON, L. (1968) Ethanol-induced hypoglycemia. In: *Advances in Metabolic Disorders*, R. LEVINE AND R. LUFT (Eds.), Academic Press, New York, pp. 85–109.

McKHANN, G. E., ALBERS, R. W., SOKOLOFF, L., MICKELSEN, O. AND TOWER, D. B. (1960) The quantitative significance of the gamma-aminobutyric acid pathway in cerebral oxidative metabolism. In: *Inhibition in the Nervous System and Gamma-Aminobutyric Acid*, E. ROBERTS, C. F. BAXTER, A. VAN HARREVELD, C. A. G. WIERSMA, W. R. ADEY AND K. KILLAM (Eds.), Pergamon, New York, pp. 169–181.

MINARD, F. N. AND MUSHAHWAR, I. K. (1966) The effect of periodic convulsions induced by 1,1-dimethyl hydrazine on the synthesis of rat brain metabolites from [2-$^{14}$C]glucose. *J. Neurochem.*, **13**, 1–11.

O'NEAL, R. M. AND KOEPPE, R. E. (1966) Precursors *in vivo* of glutamate, aspartate and their derivatives of rat brain. *J. Neurochem.*, **13**, 835–847.

ROBERTS, E., ROTHSTEIN, M. AND BAXTER, C. F. (1958) Some metabolic studies of $\gamma$-aminobutyric acid. *Proc. Soc. Exptl. Biol. Med.*, **97**, 796–802.

SALGANICOFF, L. AND DE ROBERTIS, E. (1965) Subcellular distribution of the enzymes of the glutamic acid, glutamine, and γ-aminobutyric acid cycles in rat brain. *J. Neurochem.*, **12**, 287–309.

VAN DEN BERG, C. J., MELA, P. AND WAELSCH, H. (1966) On the contribution of the tricarboxylic acid cycle to the synthesis of glutamate, glutamine, and aspartate in brain. *Biochem. Biophys. Res. Commun.*, **23**, 479–484.

WOOD, J. D., WATSON, W. J. AND CLYDESDALE, F. M. (1963) Gamma-aminobutyric acid and oxygen poisoning. *J. Neurochem.*, **10**, 625–633.

# A Primer for Writing Medical Data Base for the Clinical Decision Support System

H. FALLON, G. GOERTZEL, G. E. MARLER AND R. W. PULVER

*IBM, Advanced Systems Development Division, Yorktown Heights, N.Y. (U.S.A.)*

## INTRODUCTION

The Clinical Decision Support System (CDSS) consists of a group of computer programs. The system has the following goals:

    A. to aid in the acquisition of the patient data,

    B. to present the data in a summary form, and

    C. to suggest appropriate decisions on the basis of the data.

These decisions may be concerned with further data needed, procedures required, diagnoses, treatments, or the basis of presenting medical findings.

The system operates as a repetitive process. The data are entered. Decisions are made. More data are entered, etc. The early decisions needed in patient care are concerned with questions as to what tests are to be performed and what additional data are to be required.

The patient record is a basic component of any system for computer-assisted patient care. It is the file which contains the information about the patient. Decisions calculated by the computer for this patient on the basis of this information are also part of the patient record. This record is displayed as desired on a printer or other device.

### Data acquisition

The collecting of the patient information for the patient record is the data acquisition process. It is the activity which will, in many cases, take the most time. The data to be acquired for a given patient may include:

    1. Routine history

    2. Routine physical

    3. Routine laboratory results

    4. Routine x-ray results

    5. Special work-ups

    6. Results of procedures.

It is the complexity of the data acquisition process that makes a computer a useful tool. Although the data are obtained by answering previously prepared questions, the direction the questioning takes is based on the answers. For example, a patient who says he has a cough may be asked about the cough. The computer can generate the branching instructions, greatly increasing the depth of branching that is practical. Since the computer is directing the branching, the detailing of cough, for example, need not occur immediately after the question about cough is answered. Furthermore, special work-ups of procedures can be called for on the basis of decisions made during the process.

A variety of terminals are available for input. For the more routine portions of data acquisition, where the branching is simple, forms may easily be used. Such forms will most likely be prepared as optical mark-sense forms, so that they are computer-readable with an optical mark-sense reader. Alternatively, the forms may go to a keypunch operator, who converts the data into punched cards for entry into the computer.

The computer-controlled typewriter is a common input device. However, its printing speed is too low to permit effective use for both questions and answers. If the questions to be asked are mainly contained in a preprinted booklet at the typewriter, the answers are readily entered at the keyboard for computer processing. Or an optical image terminal, which is a computer-controlled slide projector, can serve as an automated page turner for the questioning procedure while the typewriter is used to enter the answers.

The most flexible device available for input is the cathode ray tube type of terminal. Here, the computer communicates with the user via a television-like screen. In some such devices (highly expensive), drawings may also be displayed. In the ones likely to be used in the clinic, only some 500 characters are displayed at any one time. There is clearly a great flexibility in being able to compose the questions to be asked on the basis of the previous data obtained. The price of this flexibility is the need to transmit the questions from the computer to the display while the display is being used. This data transmission will require a significant fraction of computer time and will thus tend to limit the capacity of the system.

It is expected that the cathode ray tube type of terminal will be needed in certain areas, such as radiology, and in later stages of the diagnostic process, where the data acquisition is becoming highly specific to the patient at hand. In the early stages, one of the other terminals will be more suitable.

*Data base*

The procedures to be used, from a medical standpoint, in acquiring the data are specified in the data base. That is, the questions to be asked (questionnaires) and the branching logic (protocols) are specified. It is not necessary that the physician concern himself with what device is to be used. Any protocol suitable for use on forms can be converted to the cathode ray tube terminal (unless drawings are extensively used as part of the forms).

In the data base the nodes or items of medical information are arranged in a structure called a hierarchy. This hierarchy is physician-supplied and will be in the order of the systemic review in many cases. The hierarchy is used to structure the patient record for display. It also indicates language relations as needed for inference. If the hierarchy is well structured, synonyms will tend to be adjacent within it. This is highly desirable since it makes the identification of synonyms within the system fairly straightforward. This, in turn, is a useful tool in the development of the standard nomenclature needed for decision making.

The heart of CDSS is decision making. The decision criteria for a given decision can be described in terms of which data are needed to make the decision and in what manner they are used. Each decision is described separately by the data base writer. The same data may be used in many decisions—in different manners.

As the patient data are collected a number (specified in the data base) is added to an accumulator and measured against an arbitrary limit of 100. It has been our experience that this method of specifying decision criteria can be readily learned and applied by physicians. It seems to be a fairly natural language in which to describe the decisions precisely.

*Summary*

CDSS is a tool to aid the physician in patient care
... in data acquisition,
... in decision making, and
... in patient summary presentation.
   To do this, CDSS uses a physician-supplied data base consisting of
... protocols and questionnaires, (III)
... hierarchy, and              (IV)
... decision criteria.          (V).
   In order to proceed, part II (How To Start Writing Data Base) should be studied along with the appropriate part listed above.

## II. HOW TO START WRITING DATA BASE

To start writing data base, the physician must learn a few basic concepts. The first concept is "the computer has no knowledge of medicine". You have to identify all medical terms you wish to use in a language by which the physican, the computer, and the system can communicate. You also have to instruct the computer how it is to use the information. You convey this knowledge to the system by use of three forms:
   CDSS QUESTIONNAIRE SPECIFICATION FORM (M61-0194),
   CDSS NODE HIERARCHY (M61-0195), and
   CDSS DECISION MODULES (M61-0196).
Instructions on the completion of these forms and their usage are presented in part III, IV, and V, respectively. General considerations are discussed in this part.

## *Node*

To convey medical knowledge to the computer, you have to identify all medical findings, diseases, treatments, etc. Arbitrarily, these items are called "nodes". Each node in the system may have a value after the patient data are collected (i.e., yes, no, 98.6 degrees). The physician, however, has to create a "node identifier".

## *Node identifier*

Each of the forms has a series of fields called a node identifier. It must be completed on one of the forms. You may then cross-reference it with the other forms by use of a label (see below). The requirements for transcribing the information into the five fields are as follows:

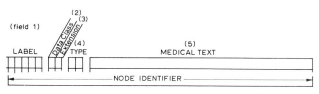

Fig. 1

## *Medical text (field 5)*

Write the name of the node in free form. "Free form" means that you write as many words as you can fit into the field. You may use as many lines as you require.

The medical text should be clear to the reader "out of context". This is the text to be read when writing the patient summary or displaying the system's decisions. "Pain" would mean little, for example. "Chest pain" is more clear "out of context".

Structure your text as much as practical. This will add clarity and uniformity to your reports. You will probably want particular groupings of medical findings in your summary. Medical terminology lends itself nicely to classification. Example:

DYSPHAGIA, MILD

DYSPHAGIA, INTERMITTENT

DYSPHAGIA, FOUR WEEKS OR LONGER

etc.

The computer can, without any further effort from the physician, convert to a phrase, such as:

DYSPHAGIA: MILD, INTERMITTENT, AND FOUR WEEKS OR LONGER.

## *Type—2 Columns (field 4)*

"Columns" are the boxes on the forms. In each column you can put only one letter or number unless described as free form. "Type—2 Columns" means that the field TYPE allows 2 columns.

Type is designated by two letters. We have assigned a few types which might be meaningful to a physician. Below are these types and sample text for each:

| Type | | Sample text |
|---|---|---|
| DS | = Disease | "Pneumonia" |
| RX | = Treatment | "Aspirin" |
| DO | = Doctor's Order | "Barium swallow" |
| IN* | = Intermediate Decision (part II) | "Hiatus hernia, suspected" |
| SG | = Sign | "Red throat" |
| SM | = Symptom | "Headache" |
| LB | = Laboratory Test | "Hematocrit" |
| XR | = X-ray | "Chest X-ray normal" |
| HX | = History | "Age" |

Further types may be assigned at the convenience of the physician.

### Data class—1 Column (field 2)

Nodes are of three classes. These classes are determined by the type of patient data you receive as an answer to your question. B, N, or T are the proper entries.

B "Boolean nodes" have an answer (value) of yes or no. An example, DYSPHAGIA (yes, the patient complains of dysphagia).

N "Numeric nodes" have numbers for their value. Examples are age, weight, hematocrit, etc.

T "Textual nodes" have free text. Such nodes will include name, address, or a variety of descriptive material, as required.

### Extension—1 Column (field 3)

"Extending" the definition of the data class, we have four possible entries:
(with Numeric of Text nodes)

S Single entry is when a new value replaces any previous value.

M Multiple entries are retained for comparison or reporting. (e.g., TEMPERATURE)
(with Boolean nodes)

R Repeated groups of nodes. This node would be the title. For an example, if the patient had several growths, his questioning might be a special work-up called, DESCRIBE THE GROWTH.

Questions: SIZE? LOCATION? etc.
(Blank) The routine yes or no answer.

### Label—5 Columns (field 1)

Any combination of letters and numbers may be used. At least one letter must be part of a label (e.g., TEST, LAB23, XYZ). As we have discussed, the node identifier is present on all three forms. The physician must complete it on at least one form. You may then cross-reference the other entries with a common label (e.g., one form MF3 B SM DYSPHAGIA, another MF3 ........., etc.).

### Identification fields

Another group of fields which is common to all forms are the I.D., PAGE, and LINE fields. They must be used on all forms for general identification of your work.

*I.D.—3 Columns*

Write any combination of letters or numbers to identify your work. (e.g., LAB, JJ, G 8).

*Page—2 Columns*

Number the pages (e.g., 02, 2, 2).

*Line—3 Columns*

These columns are prenumbered for your convenience. They may be overwritten if required.

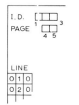

Fig. 2

### III. QUESTIONNAIRE SPECIFICATION

We require the same steps as any organized acquisition of patient data. The physician must specify: What questions are to be asked? Under what conditions are they asked? In what sequence are they asked? How does he translate the answers to standard medical terminology?

*What questions are to be asked?*

The intelligibility of questions to be asked of a patient is dependent on various factors, including:

(a) Who is reading the questions: a patient or parent seeing the question for the first time, or a doctor or paramedical person who reads the question and elicits the answer from the patient.

(b) The background of the reader of the question: a person unfamiliar with well-specified medical terminology and a physician would see different questions; patients will have different understandings of terms; differences in educational level require different ways of expressing questions, maybe a different language.

*Under what conditions are the questions asked?*

The direction that questioning takes is based on the answers received. An answer of "yes" to a symptom suggests exploration in depth of the symptom—when it began, its duration, frequency, intensity, location; circumstances which may have a bearing on the diagnosis. Similarly, a "no" answer suggests that different questions should be asked.

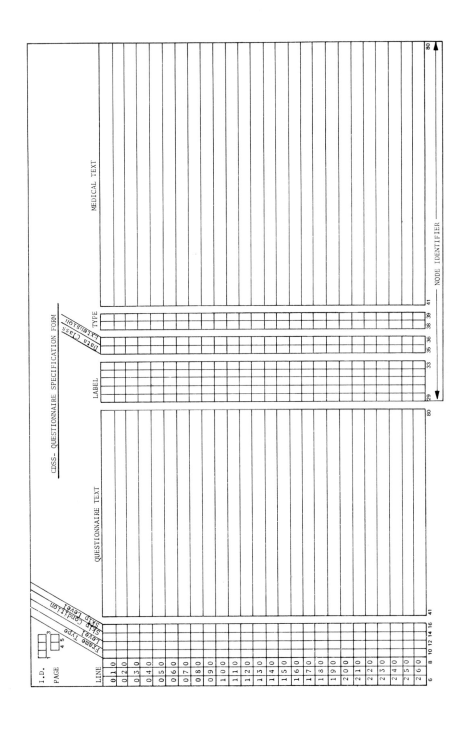

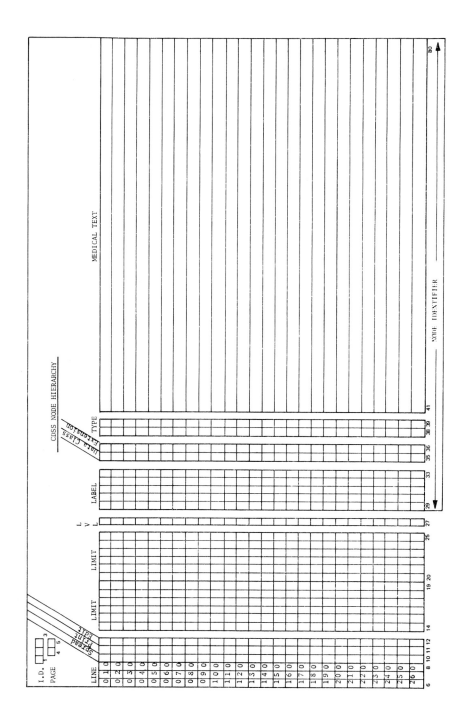

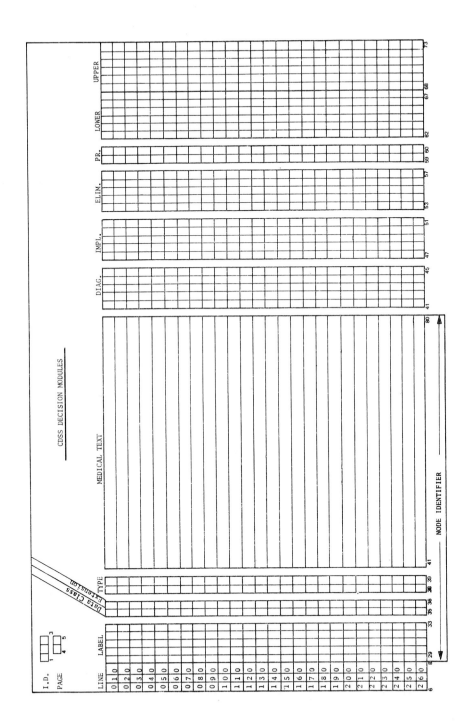

*In what sequence are they asked?*

Questions can be answered only one at a time. An important task in structuring a questioning process is to transform the questions from the disease-related orientation in which the physician thinks of the data to a sequence of questions to be answered one at a time.

*How do you translate the answers to standard medical terminology?*

The question is phrased so that it will be meaningful to the patient. To the physician, the question is equivalent to a specifically defined term which will be used in making decisions, in making his records, or in communicating with other medical practitioners.

*How to specify the questions?*

The physician must specify his questions onto the CDSS Questionnaire Specification Form (M61-0194). The I.D., PAGE, LINE and NODE IDENTIFIER are described in detail in part II. Each of the remaining fields are described below:

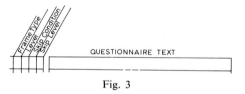

Fig. 3

*Questionnaire text*

The question will be formulated for display to the person answering the question (e.g., DYSPHAGIA? or DO YOU HAVE DIFFICULTY IN SWALLOWING?).

*Level—1 Column*

Enter one letter A to Z, which represents its relative position to other questions (see example).

*Skip condition—1 Column*

Enter Y (yes) or N (no): the answer under which questions of greater depth are to be skipped.

*Skip level—1 Column*

Enter one letter A to Z, which represents the level of the question to be answered where the questions of greater depth are skipped.

*Example*

In Form IV there is a set of questions designed to identify men between 45 and 65

CDSS- QUESTIONNAIRE SPECIFICATION FORM

I.D. JFK
PAGE 02

MEDICAL TEXT — NODE IDENTIFIER — TYPE — Data Class / Extension — LABEL — QUESTIONNAIRE TEXT

| LINE | Frame Type / Level Type / Skip Condition / Skip Level | QUESTIONNAIRE TEXT | LABEL |
|------|------|------|------|
| 010 | EAN | ARE YOU MALE ? | 3(4)01 |
| 020 | BYA | ARE YOU OVER 65? | M302 |
| 030 | BYA | ARE YOU UNDER 45? | M303 |
| 040 | SJNA | ARE YOU (BETWEEN 45 & 65? | M304 |
| 050 | MC | INDICATE WHICH CHILDHOOD | |
| 060 | D | DISEASES YOU HAVE HAD: | CD1 |
| 070 | D | MUMPS | CD2 |
| 080 | D | MEASLES | CD3 |
| 090 | D | WHOOPING COUGH | AD1 |
| 100 | C | HAVE YOU HAD TUBERCULOSIS, | |
| 110 | | PNEUMONIA, OR BRONCHITIS? | |
| 120 | CJ | HAVE YOU HAD MALARIA, | AD2 |
| 130 | | HEPATITIS, OR DIPTHERIA? | |
| 140 | | | |
| 150 | | | |
| 160 | | | |
| 170 | | | |
| 180 | | | |
| 190 | | | |
| 200 | | | |
| 210 | | | |
| 220 | | | |
| 230 | | | |
| 240 | | | |
| 250 | | | |
| 260 | | | |

with a history of certain infectious disorders. The top level question is to identify males. At the next level of depth, the age range is determined. For individuals within the range, the disease history is asked.

Individuals who are not males are given the instruction to skip the subquestions when they answer "no" to the first question. An answer of "yes" to "age over 65" of "age under 45" also causes a skip. For question one, the skip level is not specified and is, therefore, assumed to be the level of the question asked, that is, level A. For question two, the skip level must be specified, since the writer wishes the person answering questions to skip to an A level question.

### Frame type—1 Column

E, S, or M is entered. This establishes the rules for asking the questions which are at one level greater depth.

E, (exclusive). The E frame type associated with question one states that only one yes is to be accepted for the age questions at the next level.

S, (safe). The S frame type associated with question four states that an answer of yes or no is to be obtained for each of the questions at the next lower level.

M, (multiple option). The M frame type states that choices at the next level are to be answered "yes" if appropriate, and are otherwise not to be answered.

### Node identifier (See part II for details)

The standard medical term which the data base writer regards as equivalent to the question asked is stated in the field provided. In order to avoid unnecessary writing, this text may be identified by a label, which serves as a cross reference to the standard text defined in the hierarchy form. If a node identifier is not specified, the question text is treated as an instruction to the question answerer, which is not to receive an answer.

## IV. HOW TO WRITE HIERARCHY

As we have discussed in part II, "the computer has no medical knowledge". It needs a language. CDSS requires an all inclusive list of terms, and an organization or classification scheme for the terms. This organized list is called a "hierarchy".

The hierarchy establishes the format of the patient record summary and is used to enter the medical terms and their relationships between each other. Four concepts should be kept in mind while writing the hierarchy.

### Consistent language

The terms should be as close to standard medical nomenclature as practical. This enables other physicians to use the system, and to interpret the patient record summary in a standard method.

### Classification and grouping

The hierarchy promotes the classification and grouping of terms. This is a familiar concept to the physician. It allows him to lean heavily on his formal medical background. Also it allows him to easily add new terms in their proper position. One use for the hierarchy is to provide a format for the patient record summary. This allows the physician to present groups of medical findings in a systematic manner.

### Inference

The grouping allows for "inference" to other members of the group. If a man is male, it can be inferred he is not female. If a member of a class is present, the name of the class can be inferred to be the title for a section of the report. The value of inference will become more apparent as you create the decision criteria in part V.

### Meaningful data

Medical terms should be those useful to the physician in his data acquisition or decision criteria. This should not be an attempt at a thesaurus of equivalent terms, or a list of all possible laboratory tests, etc. The more pertinent the data, the more efficient and accurate the system.

### How to specify the hierarchy

You specify the hierarchy in order to enter the medical terms and their relationships into the computer. The terms are entered in three parts. The first part is the medical terms in the sequence in which they will be displayed in the patient record summary. The second part is all terms formerly used but not still required. This is for retrieving old records. The third part contains the names of any decisions that may be required (see part V).

The physician must order the terms in the hierarchy on the "CDSS NODE HIERARCHY" (form M61-0195). The I.D., PAGE, LINE, and NODE IDENTIFIER have been described in detail in part II. Specific information required for inference, printing and editing are required in the remaining six fields.

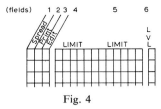

Fig. 4

### Spread—1 Column (field 1)

This column indicates what can be inferred from the hierarchy term. A blank ( ) or V or E may be used. We will use the expression of "father" and "sons" to refer to the class identification and the group members, respectively. Example: the class (COUGH) may have a son (COUGH, CHRONIC).

Blank or V : This is the normal type of inference. When the son is answered *yes,* the father is inferred to be *yes.*

Example: V COUGH

      COUGH, SEVERE

      COUGH, CHRONIC

      COUGH, PRODUCTIVE

An answer of *yes* to DOES HE HAVE A CHRONIC COUGH?, or the others, infers a *yes* to COUGH.

E           : exclusive inference: when a son is answered *yes*, the other sons (in this case daughter) are inferred to be *no*.

Example: E SEX

      MALE

      FEMALE

An answer of *yes* to IS HE MALE? infers *no* to FEMALE and *yes* to SEX. SEX may now be used as a part of your patient record summary.

*Print—1 Column (field 2)*

One letter is used to indicate under what conditions the item will be printed or displayed. All possible combinations are possible. The most frequently used are listed first.

Y Print only if answer is *yes*.

A Print under all conditions irrespective of answer.

X Do not print under any conditions.

N Print only if answer is *no*.

B Print if answer is either *yes* or unanswered.

C Print if answer is either *no* or unanswered.

D Print if answer is either *yes* or *no*.

U Print only if unanswered.

Example: (PRINT) (MEDICAL TERM)      (how used?)

      A    PATIENT RECORD SUMMARY  title of report

      X    ADMINISTRATIVE DATA    title of group of terms

      Y    MALE               answer to questionnaire

In the above example, PATIENT RECORD SUMMARY would be printed every time, followed by MALE if it was answered *yes*.

Example:

      A    PATIENT SUMMARY RECORD

      B    ADMINISTRATIVE DATA

      C    NAME

      C    SEX

      D    MALE

      D    FEMALE

      C    AGE

Levels can be thought of conceptually as a "tree". You probably would have found it convenient to construct that portion of the hierarchy with the following pattern in mind.

Example:

A (PATIENT RECORD SUMMARY)

B (ADMINISTRATIVE DATA)

C (NAME)  C (SEX)  C (AGE)

D (MALE)  D (FEMALE)

All previous examples in part IV are incorporated in the sample form V.

## V. HOW TO WRITE DECISION MODULES

### Decisions

The distinctive ability of the Clinical Decision Support System (CDSS) is to calculate decisions. The task of the data base writer is to define the decisions and to identify the criteria for making them. The criteria must be formulated prior to the system's use in a clinical environment.

### Decision modules

The basic unit of the system is a "decision module". This module consists of a label or name and its list of medical findings. This list resembles a set of diagnostic criteria. The label is the name of the "decision". Thus, the medical findings and their decision define a "decision module". One module represents one decision process.

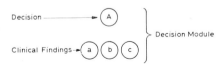

Fig. 5

### Weight relationships

The decision module also includes the "weight relationships" between the decision and its medical findings. Weights (numerical values) are assigned by the writer to each medical finding. The required decision is made when the combined weights of any of the medical findings add to 100 or more.

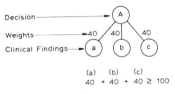

Fig. 6

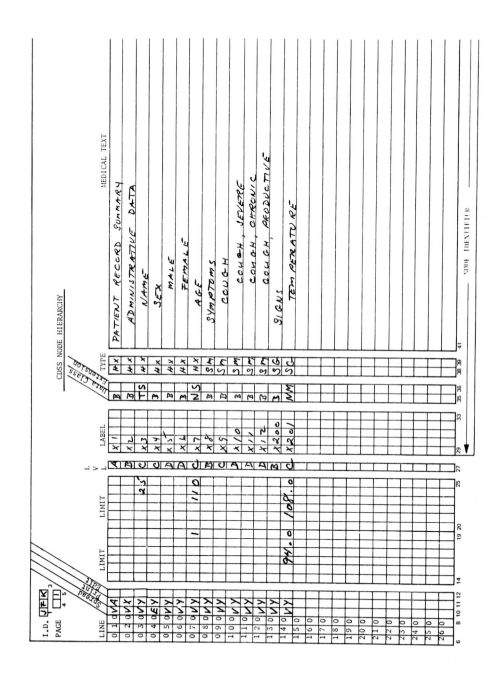

The example in Fig. 6 shows a physician's desire to require all three medical findings (a, b, c) to be present. Any one or two do not qualify because the sum is less than 100. Another variation would be where he desired to require a major finding plus at least one more to make a decision. Each of the other medical findings alone is not enough. He would then write the module as in Fig. 7.

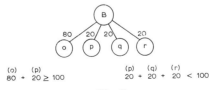

$$\begin{array}{cc} \text{(o)} & \text{(p)} \\ 80 + 20 \geq 100 \end{array} \qquad \begin{array}{ccc} \text{(p)} & \text{(q)} & \text{(r)} \\ 20 + 20 + 20 < 100 \end{array}$$

Fig. 7

*Complex decisions*

Simple decisions are written in the above manner. The physician will probably discover, on the other hand, some complex decisions depend on other decisions and then additional findings. Thus, two or more decision modules may be required to evoke this decision. Combining the two previous modules in Figs. 6 and 7 illustrates this case.

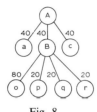

Fig. 8

In Fig. 8, a decision A is evoked by decision B and other findings (a and c). This technique can be especially useful when the decisions are of two different types. Decision B might be a disease and decision A might be the treatment.

*Sample decision module*

An actual example (Fig. 9) demonstrates a one-level decision module. The physician states that any of the first three findings would be sufficient to order a hematocrit. Weakness or fatigue alone are not sufficient. Together they are sufficient to order the hematocrit.

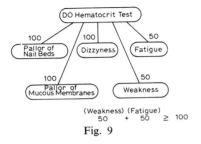

$$\begin{array}{cc} \text{(Weakness)} & \text{(Fatigue)} \\ 50 + 50 \geq 100 \end{array}$$

Fig. 9

*Notation*

With the introduction of the medical nomenclature, the writing of the decision modules becomes cumbersome. For ease in handling, we write the above module in the following manner.

| Name | Condition ( Y, N)* | Weight |
|------|--------------------|--------|
| DO Hematocrit Test | | |
| Pallor of Nail Beds | Y | 100 |
| Pallor of Mucous Membranes | Y | 100 |
| Dizzyness | Y | 100 |
| Weakness | Y | 50 |
| Fatigue | Y | 50 |

*Intermediate decisions*

Decisions are of several types. Two letters are used to designate each type:
DS  Disease
DO  Doctor's Order
RX  Treatment
Other types may be designated as required by the physician, such as:
IN  Intermediate Decision
An "Intermediate Decision" is a general grouping of more elementary decisions for ease of reference. Syndromes would be an intermediate decision. A group of findings or a pattern may, for convenience, be classified "Intermediate Decision". Large groups, however, become unwieldy and logically incorrect. Complex decisions are greatly simplified by breaking them into smaller intermediate decision groups. When writing decisions, it is prudent to make the groupings as small as practical.

The following module shows the use of IN's in a diagnostic process:
DO BARIUM SWALLOW
IN  TRACHEO-ESOPHAGEAL FISTULA, CLUES TO  Y    100
IN  HIATUS HERNIA, SUSPECTED                    Y    100
IN  etc... ... ...
The decision module in Form VI is used to coordinate several pertinent groups of medical findings. The intermediate decisions are independently defined for convenience and clarity.

*How to fill out the form*

The physician must transcribe the desired modules onto the CDSS Decision Modules

---

* YES (Y) and NO (N) conditions are both used. Both positive and negative findings may be used in a decision module.

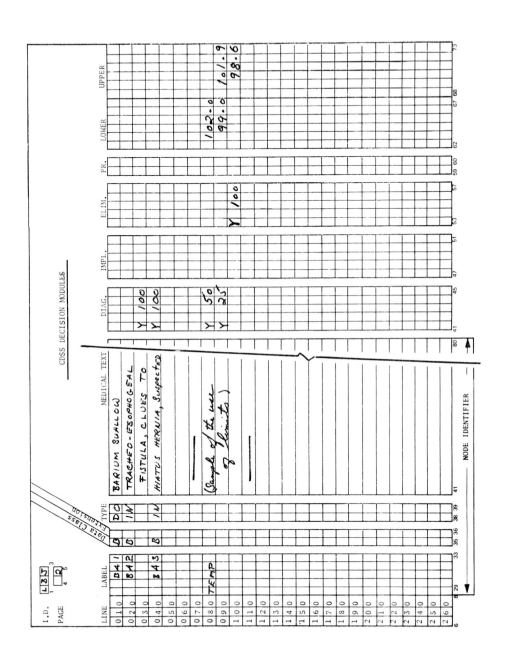

(form M61-0196). The I.D., PAGE, LINE, and NODE IDENTIFIER are described in detail in part II. Each of the remaining fields is described below.

The remaining six fields describe the weight relationships in our decision modules. At least one field must be completed; however, more may be required to describe the criteria.

### *Diagnostic (Diag.)—5 Columns (field 1)*

The "diagnostic" field contains the numerical weight required to help diagnose a decision and the condition (Yes or No) and the weight required to evoke the use of this weight (e.g., HIATUS HERNIA, SUSPECTED Y 100).

The conditions may be either yes, Y, or no, N, and the weights may range from 1 to 100. Samples: Y 100, N 50.

### *Implication (Impl.)—5 Columns (field 2)*

The "implication" field contains the numerical weight and condition required to implicate (e.g., consider but not diagnose) a decision. Special workups, expensive tests, serious medical conditions may be "implicated" but not necessarily diagnosed from the information available. This field is optional. In a final version of the data base, these will become diagnostic decisions.

Again, the conditions may be either yes, Y, or no, N, and the weights may range from 1 to 100. Samples: Y 100, N 50.

### *Elimination (Elim.)—5 Columns (field 3)*

The "elimination" decisions are used to specifically rule out a particular disease. For example, if the patient is male, pregnancy is ruled out. This is different from "failure to diagnose". That is where the remaining medical findings were all answered YES, and there is still not enough possible weight to diagnose "pregnancy".

Again, the conditions may be either yes, Y, or no, N, and the weights may range from 1 to 100. Samples: Y 100, N 50.

### *Priority (Pr.)—2 Columns*

This field is reserved for future expansion of the system. Please do not write in this field.

### *Lower/Upper—Two 6-column fields (5 and 6)*

All of the discussion has been of yes or no type findings. Other medical findings, however, such as temperature, solicit a numeric answer (e.g., 98.6 degrees).

With these findings, we have three possible actions:
1. Add weights (if patient's temperature is) above lower limit.
2. Add weights (if patient's temperature is) below upper limit.
3. Add weights (if patient's temperature falls) between given limits.

These limits are paired with their appropriate entry in the DIAGNOSTIC, IMPLICATION, or ELIMINATE fields. Each set requires a separate line on the form. For example:

| (Field 1) Diag. | (2) Impl. | (3) Elim. | (4) Pr. | (5) Lower | (6) Upper |
|---|---|---|---|---|---|
| Y 50 | | | | 102.0 | — |
| | | Y 100 | | — | 98.6 |
| Y 25 | | | | 99.0 | 101.9 |

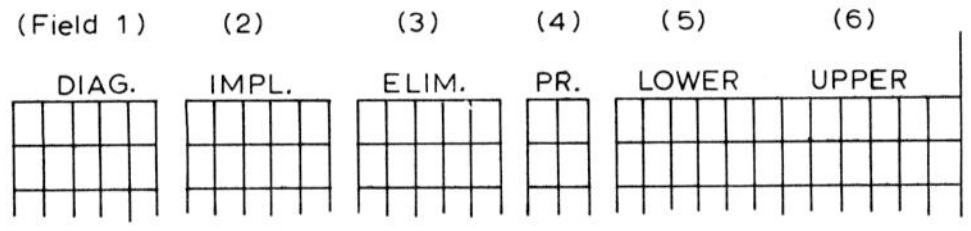

Fig. 10

*Sample form*

Form II is an example of some of the above examples entered on a CDSS Decision Module form.

## SUMMARY

The Clinical Decision Support System (CDSS) consists of computer programs to aid in the acquisition of patient data, and to suggest appropriate decisions on the basis of the data thus acquired. The decisions may be concerned with further data needed, procedures required, diagnoses, and treatments.

To guide the system in the data acquisition and display functions and in the decision making function, it is necessary to specify the data to be acquired and the decision criteria. This paper presents rules and formats that enable a physician to specify the medical concepts for implementation by the system.

# General Principles of Simulation Techniques

E. A. KOLDENHOF

*IBM—Netherlands Amsterdam (The Netherlands)*

This review does not assume much foreknowledge about brain research and related subjects, because its objective is to introduce the reader that part of the computer science which is probably not too well known in this area of science. The knowledge of many users about computer systems is mostly restricted to the hardware of the system and terms such as interphase and processor–controller are more or less well known. But it is a mistake to think that merely by writing a computer program, the computer will do whatever people would like to do with it. Following such a procedure will lead to disappointments, and two things will be discovered very soon. First of all, writing a program is much more difficult than people think it is and, secondly, connecting experiments to the computer system will lead to complications in the program if the results have to be calculated in what is called "real time". This mainly because the computer has a processor–controller which controls the flow of data within the computer, whereas the experiment has its own time scale and the synchronization between experiment and computer system has to be supported by program.

This review will deal mainly with those cases in which the real time aspect is not present. It is assumed that the data to be processed by the computer are somewhere in the core, and become available to the processor at the time they are needed. This is a very important point for the programming system—as will be explained in greater detail at the end of this review—for, in studying problems through the simulation of physical phenomena with a computer system, the most interesting thing is to compare the results with those obtained in real time with real experiments.

For simplicity, we start from the assumption that the experiment and the simulated model are separate. There is a data bank in the memory of the computer system, and we want to do something with the information stored in that data bank.

In simulation, certain phenomena are studied as a function of time. This aspect will always be dominant in simulation. There will always be some kind of model, and in one way or another the behaviour of this model as a function of time has to be studied. But again, it must be emphasized: it is *not* real time. The time axis corresponds to time "made" by the computer, hence it is possible to transform the time axis. The computer can run for several hours to simulate a process which happens in real time in a few seconds. In such cases no comparison can be made between the results of simulation by the computer and the results of the real time experiment, because too little work can be done with the computer system in the time available for the calculations. If such a comparison is necessary, either the model has to be simplified or the computer system has to be extended, e.g. with an analog computer, to a hybrid system.

The main portion of this review will deal with the software (i.e. "program") used for simulation in digital computer systems. Why is the word "software" used here? Because the organization of the programs used to simulate a model representing a problem is the main subject in this review. The basic of programming in general shall therefore be first explained, as far as needed for the understanding of simulation.

First of all, modern digital computers are constructed in words with bits which can be either a **1** or a **0**. Basically, there are three types of information stored in such words. The first type is an *instruction* for the machine, the second is an *address* (or a number to calculate an address), whereas the third one is *data* that is temporarily loaded into the accumulator and used for calculations.

Programming a computer means that every instruction and every address has to be defined. The most direct way to do this is writing a program in ASSEMBLER language, which is very inconvenient for a user because it requires the study of the entire data flow within the computer system. A more sophisticated step is to write programs not in ASSEMBLER language but in FORTRAN. In this language the user can express what he wants in an easily understandable form. The computer has a program which is called "compiler", and this program translates such a FORTRAN program into bits (in words) and defines the data flow within the computer system. An even more sophisticated step is the use of simulation languages. These languages have a so-called translator. The procedure is then extremely simple for the users: a computer program translates the user's program into FORTRAN, whereafter the compiler is used to get the bits in the words. Why all these steps in a programming system? Because this type of programming enables the user to write in a very short time a program which can easily be altered. The first example shown in this review was written and debugged in a few hours after defining the problem. It would have taken considerably longer time for the computer to produce reliable results that could be used for comparison with the experimental measurements, had the problem been programmed directly into FORTRAN or ALGOL.

Moreover, there are many features available in the translator which can be used in debugging the program, and many of these features cannot easily be programmed. This is particularly true for the *integration methods* to be used. In this simulation language one out of seven integration methods can be specified by a data card*. It will, therefore, only be necessary to study the specifications of the integration methods, and to decide which is the best one to solve the problem under investigation.

No real programming is needed to use such a simulation language, so the user need not be a programmer or a mathematician. Such a type of language enables the user to keep much closer to the problem than when a detailed program has to be written. Still, the gap between problem and its mathematical representation has to be bridged and this is already difficult enough. As these simulation languages are very young—they exist only a few years—and not much school training is provided for modeling, the gap between problem and the simulated model is a wide one. However, it is to be expected that with the frequent use of simulation languages, more successful work will be done in the future in this area.

---

* This is valid for the computer system IBM 360.

For a good understanding of simulation languages it is not necessary to give a detailed description of a complicated but powerful simulation tool, as CSMP-360 (Brennan, 1969). Neither is it useful to give an historical review of simulation languages here because this has been done elsewhere in the literature (Brennan, 1967). It is preferable to study in greater detail one simulation language that can very simply be used on a small computer system: the IBM 1130. (IBM, 1967). This simulation language and the examples given can demonstrate all important points, and the use of the language as such. The simulation language is called "Continuous Systems Modeling Program" and it is often abbreviated to CSMP-1130. The program follows the same principles as in an analog computer. The problem has to be represented in block form. For this purpose the user has a number of blocks with standard functions available (See Table 1).

A maximum of 75 blocks can be used in the model, apart from the simulated time which has to be defined as block number 76. Some of the blocks are very simple. An example is the adder, which is used when the user wants to have the sum of two inputs. Another one is the integration block, which applies a standard integration method. The entire model is merely a combination of such blocks which have to be numbered to define the direction of the calculations. In data cards the inputs of these blocks are specified and the necessary parameters are given. An example is given in Fig. 1.

The integration used needs an initial condition, which is specified as a parameter (see Table 1). The whole program consists then of data cards specifying the connections between the blocks. In the case given in Fig. 1, block 2, which is an integration, receives its input from 1. The method of integration is standard, pre-programmed in the computer once and for all, and does not need to be specified in CSMP-1130.

Studying simulation problems there is always one important fact that needs special attention. In one way or another, in at least one part of the block diagram, outputs of blocks return to other inputs. Or, in other words, each simulation model must contain at least one closed loop. This is demonstrated also in Fig. 1 in which the block diagram for solving the differential equation is given. This block diagram is the same as used for the computation on an analog computer. It is clearly shown that there is a closed loop within this block diagram consisting of the blocks 1, 2, 3 and 4.

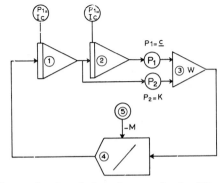

Fig. 1. Block diagram for the solution of a second order differential equation.

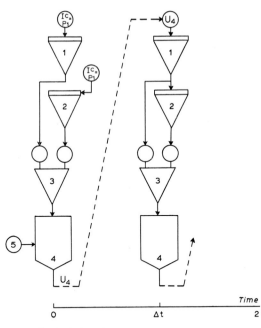

Fig. 2. Sequence of calculation due to the sorting mechanism in CSMP-1130.

What is the difference between digital simulation and analog simulation? In digital simulation a block can be a table containing experimental data. It is not really necessary to have the mathematical expression for that part of the problem. Any experimental univalent relation between two quantities is valid to be used as block.

In a problem like the one given in Fig. 1—this is a very simple one—the program basically consists first of the data cards specifying the connection and function of the blocks, and second, the cards specifying the constants and parameters. These cards are put into the computer, which immediately translates them into a program. But in order to translate them, the computer has to sort them. Why? The digital computer computes all results for a certain value of the time, and then it takes a time step in order to compute them for the next value of the time. But in order to be able to do this, it has to decide which data—output of a block—should be transferred from one cycle of calculation to the next one. This is necessary because when we calculate, e.g., for time zero the closed loop of Fig. 1, a decision must be made which input to start with. All outputs, including the one from which we have started, will be calculated from the first mentioned input. Normally the input value will not be exactly the same as the output value, calculated later and representing the same quantity. (Fig. 2, $U_4 \neq JC$). During sorting block 1 (integration) was chosen as a "transferring" block. The calculated value $U_4$, the output for $t = 0$, was used as the input value for the next cycle. This is shown in Fig. 2. Therefore the sorting program distinguishes two different types of blocks: a normal block and a block with so called "memory": the integration block is such a memory block. The sorting program also checks whether every closed loop in a simulation model has at least one such memory block. If this is not so, the program is not accepted and the closed loop has to be considered as an implicit loop for which a special iteration procedure is available. Why is this feature so important and why does it contribute so much in finding reliable results? Because building a model for a problem, usually many loops are to be connected, and it is often very difficult to ascertain whether the criterion that all closed loops have at least one memory block has been fulfilled.

Therefore, the program check for memory blocks is very helpful. If the computer finds that the model is not consistent in that respect, a message is generated, specifiying the block that has been improperly defined. Again: the whole program will check all statements to avoid improper results during the stimulation later on.

The CSMP-1130 is a program very simple to use and much can be done with it, but it should be investigated whether it is worth while to simulate a problem with CSMP-1130. Once the user has defined how the model looks and has ascertained that the results are more or less according to expectation, more refinement in the simulation is needed. This can be done with the other simulation program: the CSMP-360. This language is basically the same but the user does not need to write his program in block form, it can be written in "FORTRAN-like" statements. The output and input will have names and the program describing the model of Fig. 2 now reads:

$$X = (K \times XXX + C \times XX) \, M$$
$$XXX = INTGRL \, (XXX0, \, XX)$$
$$XX = INTGRL \, (XX0, \, X)$$

Again, a sorting program will sort all these statements and will generate a message if the closed loop program has not been properly defined. In this simulation language, programming is closer to normal programming than in CSMP-1130. This computer program is not so closely related to the analog computer, but still, there are many similarities in the principles. It only resembles a normal computer program.

The following example is derived from work carried out by Dr. de Valois from the Brain Research Institute of Amsterdam (1966). The model describes the diffusion of oxygen in the human brain. The values of the constants are probably incorrect because they are not known yet. For our purpose this is, however, not so important because the main point to be demonstrated is: how can such a simulation program be used to study and improve the knowledge of a problem. First of all, only physical properties are considered and not the human factors. There is a capillary containing a fluid with a certain content of oxygen (Fig. 3), and the diffusion problem, that means the concentration of oxygen as a function of time and place are the subject of study. The first assumption is that there is a certain consumption of oxygen in the brain, in other words, oxygen decreases as a function of distance from the capillary.

It is indifferent whether the absorption is due to a chemical reaction or to some other phenomenon, but there must be some consumption of oxygen, otherwise oxygen concentration would be the same over the whole brain. Several other assumptions are made to describe the problem by a differential equation. One of them is that within the capillary, the fluid has the same concentration of oxygen throughout the

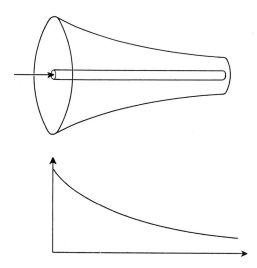

Fig. 3. Diffusion of oxygen from a capillary into an oxygen-absorbing medium.

entire cross section. With all assumptions the differential equation is still a difficult one, which is shown below. Not for the sake of mathematical presentation, but to show a very important feature of simulation on a digital computer: the improvement of the study by adding some experimental results in the model.

Basically the differential equation reads:

$$\frac{1}{D} \cdot \frac{\partial C}{\partial t} = \frac{1}{r} \cdot \left\{ \frac{\partial}{\partial r} \left( r \frac{\partial C}{\partial r} \right) + \frac{\partial}{\partial z} \left( r \frac{\partial C}{\partial z} \right) \right\} - \frac{K}{D} \cdot C \qquad [1]$$

In words: the time dependency of oxygen in a cylinder with symmetrical coordinates $r$ and $z$, is a function of the concentration gradient in the $r$-direction and in $z$-direction. The last term represents the consumption of oxygen at the point in the brain having the coordinates $(r, a)$. To solve this equation without a computer, usually the assumption is made that the gradient in $z$-direction is very small compared to that in the $r$-direction. Therefore it will be ignored in our case. After this simplification the analytical solution can be obtained by separating the variables $t$ and $r$.

To shorten a highly complex explanation which has been described elsewhere for a similar case (Koldenhof, 1963), the solution can be written as a power series. More important for practical purposes is that the differential equation is only valid in a small region close to the capillary. The greater $r$, the stronger is the influence of the neglected terms and the greater the difference between the solution and reality will be. From this equation, a simple 1130 program is made for constant $t$, taking $r$ as the only independent variable "time". The block diagram describing the diffusion around one capillary is given in Fig. 4.

Obviously, it is easy to simulate the first part of the curve. But unfortunately the model becomes unstable after a certain point, which can be characterized by $dc/dr$ crossing zero and, obviously, this is wrong because in reality $c$ and $dc/dr$ have to become zero when $r$ is infinite. Playing around with the coefficients a solution can be

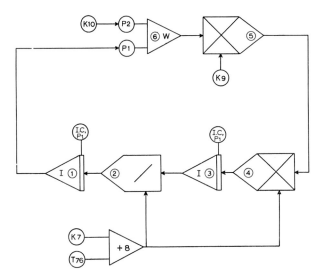

Fig. 4. Block diagram of the model representing the radial diffusion of oxygen for one capillary.

found in which $c = 0$ and $dc/dr = 0$ are almost fulfilled for a certain value of $r$. In the projected study this is not the solution that is really wanted, because we are not so much interested in the contribution of one capillary, but rather in the contribution of many. The real contents of oxygen is the sum of the contributions from all capillaries. This problem was also studied and one of the results was that the solution of [1] gives a satisfactory curve only when a wrong coefficient is used. Therefore it was necessary to change the model to give a better representation of reality for high values of $r$. In the digital computer this can easily be done in many ways, because there is a block which is called a relay. Using this it is easy to switch to another function under certain conditions. This new function must represent the mere two-dimensional diffusion problem for high values of $r$. Thus, the unsatisfactory part of the curve can easily be avoided. This type of simulation can be done with CSMP-1130 and the program is always short. In the model described here it consists of not more than about 20 cards.

The next step in the problem study can be the simulation of a model of two capillaries at a certain distance from each other. The concentration gradient between the two capillaries as function of the distance has to be found. Now another problem arises. In simulation the independent axis is always time, therefore we had to replace $r$ here by the time in the first model.

For two capillaries there are two $r$-axes possible, one of which has to be chosen as the time axis. An assumption has to be made about the distance between the capillaries. The whole problem can then be defined (Fig. 5) and solved.

The choice, however, will be influenced by the existence of an unstable region in the simplified model. Therefore, the distance $r = r_0$ must be so small that the unstable region should be beyond it in the simulation. The block diagram is shown in Fig. 6. Another problem is that the simulation starts for one capillary far from its axis. This

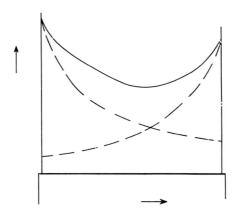

Fig. 5. Radial diffusion of oxygen into a medium between two capillaries.

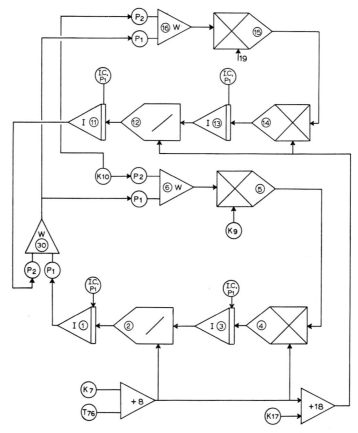

Fig. 6. Block diagram for a model, representing the diffusion of oxygen from two capillaries at a certain distance.

introduces a new problem with the same starting values. In short, we must use some kind of iterative procedure to find all these initial values. The problem becomes no longer suitable for the CSMP-1130. In such cases a program is needed to incorporate an iterative procedure into the simulated model. At this stage of the game it is preferable to change to CSMP-360 for the programming language to be used. But now the model is already well known, the problem has been defined when we introduce this more difficult simulation, so that the program can be directly written in a better form far more easily.

One other point has to be mentioned when we are dealing with differential equations. People generally endeavour to reduce equations to the first degree, for it is more convenient to solve linear equations. Analytical solution of other equations is very complicated and really difficult. In simulation, this would be a waste of effort. In digital simulation it is not important whether there is an $r^2$ instead of an $r$ in the formula, even an experimental curve can easily be incorporated in the model.

Once the model has been defined, programming is only a matter of minutes. The computer will give further instructions what has to be done, it knows exactly what to do. New principles can be applied easily. No matter how difficult a mathematical expression is, an experimental initial guess must be made, whereupon the results of a simulation can be studied. This leads to new ways of improving the model step by step. Using the computer with CSMP-1130 and studying the results and the remarks about the model, the user can work out a valid model within a reasonable time. If more refined calculations are required, then one can change over to a real computer program, such as CSMP-360, and very often additional programs have to be introduced. Again, in accordance with the organization of this simulation program, the problem can be coded in a simple, straightforward way, omitting the programming of problems that have been solved before at the time CSMP was developed.

Basically, two different types of problems can be studied with the aid of simulation languages. The first one is solving differential equations. Our model was complemented with assumptions and experimental data, but the main part of the problem was still a differential equation, in which the time factor was taken as the independent variable. The other type deals with the simulation of behaviour of a physical phenomenon against time. In this case it is really time that is the independent variable, but it is not necessarily on a real time scale. This means that through a transformation this time can be extended according to what is feasible in the computer system.

In the literature, a model consisting of 4 experimental parts, which represents the blood circulation in the human body was described (Guyton, 1966). As usual with this type of problems, the model has 3 tables of experimental data and one block that is partly a differential equation and partly an experimental equation (see Fig. 7). The CSMP-1130 program can easily be constructed from this model, and is given in Fig. 8. Trying to simulate this model on a 1130, the initial conditions caused a problem. Studying a phenomenon, it is advantageous to start from a steady state, because otherwise simulation— and computer time—are wasted before reaching the steady state. In this particular case, some problems were encountered in obtaining the proper constants for the steady state. It took several computer runs to find the proper con-

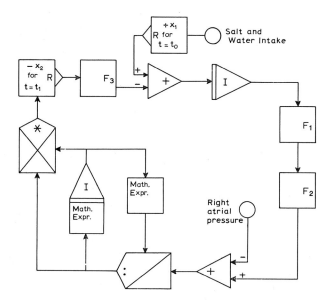

Fig. 7. Block diagram for a model representing the blood circulation in a human body.

stants. Starting from the steady state at time $t$, two changes were introduced: first the water intake was changed after a certain time. This can be explained, assuming that the model represents a patient in a hospital. At a certain moment the doctor orders him to drink a little bit more—change in water intake. What is the reaction on the factors defining the blood circulation, such as blood flow and blood pressure? As a second change it was assumed that after a certain time one of the kidneys was removed. This could be done easily because one of the experimental graphs represents the resistance of a kidney and this can be changed by a relay. The results are shown in Fig. 8. The coefficients are not quite correct, but it is at least interesting to see the dynamic reaction of the human body on such changes (see Fig. 8). In the beginning we have exactly the steady state, with an accuracy of 4 digits; it is a perfect steady state. Beginning at $t = 0.5$ the patient had to drink a little bit more (continuous water intake). The total blood volume increased slightly but after some time it went down slightly again. The removal of the kidney was much more spectacular: first there was a large increase but some time after the change at $t = 2.0$ steady state was reached again. That was the result of removing the kidney and the entire reaction can be studied in quantities. It was a shock which upset the whole body, but again the body recovered and the steady state returned to almost the starting value, the difference being only half a percent.

With this example we only showed what can be done in such cases, if somebody makes the effort to find the real coefficients. Experience shows that the actual data are also meaningful. Some results of the computer simulation will be unexpected.

Many people think that they understand the problems, and that these problems can be represented in a certain way, but often some of their ideas and theories have never been checked. This holds even more when the methods to measure quantities are poor.

CONTINUOUS SYSTEM MODELING PROGRAM

A DIGITAL ANALOG SIMULATOR PROGRAM FOR THE IBM 1130

INSTRUCTIONAL COMMENTS MAY BE SUPPRESSED AT ANY TIME BY TURNING ON SWITCH 10;

TURN ON SWITCH 1 TO ENTER OR MODIFY CONFIGURATION STATEMENTS VIA THE KEYBOARD;

TURN ON SWITCH 2 TO ENTER OR MODIFY INITIAL CONDITIONS OR ELEMENT PARAMETERS VIA;

TURNS ON SWITCH 3 TO ENTER OR MODIFY FUNCTION GENERATOR INTERCEPTS VIA THE KEYBOARD

CONFIGURATION SPECIFICATION

| OUTPUT NAME | BLOCK | TYPE | INPUT 1 | INPUT 2 | INPUT 3 |
|---|---|---|---|---|---|
| | 1 | F | 23 | 0 | 0 |
| | 2 | + | − 1 | 28 | 0 |
| | 3 | K | 0 | 0 | 0 |
| | 4 | I | 2 | 0 | 0 |
| | 5 | F | 4 | 0 | 0 |
| | 6 | F | 5 | 0 | 0 |
| | 7 | + | 6 | − 8 | 0 |
| | 8 | K | 0 | 0 | 0 |
| | 9 | / | 7 | 16 | 0 |
| | 10 | X | 9 | 11 | 0 |
| | 11 | I | 20 | 13 | 0 |
| | 13 | K | 0 | 0 | 0 |
| | 14 | / | 11 | 15 | 0 |
| | 15 | K | 0 | 0 | 0 |
| | 16 | G | 18 | 0 | 0 |
| | 17 | K | 0 | 0 | 0 |
| | 18 | + | 14 | 17 | 0 |
| | 19 | I | 0 | 0 | 0 |
| | 20 | X | 9 | 13 | 0 |
| | 21 | K | 0 | 0 | 0 |
| | 22 | + | −21 | 76 | 0 |
| | 23 | R | 22 | 24 | 10 |
| | 24 | + | −25 | 10 | 0 |
| | 25 | K | 0 | 0 | 0 |
| | 26 | K | 0 | 0 | 0 |
| | 27 | + | −26 | 76 | 0 |
| | 28 | R | 27 | 40 | 3 |
| | 29 | G | 10 | 0 | 0 |
| | 40 | K | 0 | 0 | 0 |

Fig. 8. The CSMP-1130 program for the blood circulation in a human body.

## INITIAL CONDITIONS AND PARAMETERS

| | | | |
|---|---|---|---|
| 1 | 125.0000 | 75.0000 | 0.0000 |
| 3 | 1.30001 | 0.0000 | 0.0000 |
| 4 | 15.0000 | 0.0000 | 0.0000 |
| 5 | 22.0000 | 12.0000 | 0.0000 |
| 6 | 6.6000 | 3.3000 | 0.0000 |
| 8 | 6.0302 | 0.0000 | 0.0000 |
| 11 | 20.0000 | −5.0000 | 0.0000 |
| 13 | 50.0000 | 0.0000 | 0.0000 |
| 15 | 18.0000 | 0.0000 | 0.0000 |
| 16 | 0.0500 | 0.0000 | 0.0000 |
| 17 | 2.8889 | 0.0000 | 0.0000 |
| 19 | 20.0000 | 0.0000 | 0.0000 |
| 21 | 2.0000 | 0.0000 | 0.0000 |
| 25 | 60.0000 | 0.0000 | 0.0000 |
| 26 | 0.5000 | 0.0000 | 0.0000 |
| 29 | 0.3333 | 0.0000 | 0.0000 |
| 40 | 2.4000 | 0.0000 | 0.0000 |

## FUNCTION GENERATOR SPECIFICATIONS

| | | | | |
|---|---|---|---|---|
| 1 | 0.2000 | 0.3000 | 0.5000 | 0.7000 |
| | 0.9000 | 1.3000 | 1.9000 | 2.4000 |
| | 2.9000 | 3.5000 | 4.1000 | |
| 5 | 3.4000 | 3.7000 | 4.0000 | 4.3000 |
| | 4.6000 | 4.9000 | 5.2000 | 5.5000 |
| | 5.8000 | 6.1000 | 6.4000 | |
| 6 | 4.0000 | 5.0000 | 6.0000 | 7.0000 |
| | 8.0000 | 9.0000 | 10.0000 | 11.0000 |
| | 12.0000 | 13.0000 | 14.0000 | |

.01 ) INTEGRATION INTERVAL

3.0 ) TOTAL TIME

0.1 ) PRINT INTERVAL

Fig. 9. The results of a simulation of a change in water intake and of removal of a kidney on the blood circulation.

In such cases even the interpretation of measurements is somewhat uncertain. Making a model and testing the theories with simulation runs, the computer will show exactly what would happen if this model were true. It acts as a highly objective test method.

During the last few years quite a number of models have been simulated, and every model is a new surprise in one way or another. If the research worker is open for such a check he can make good use of the computer system, which is one of the best means of testing ideas and theories. My opinon is that the simulation languages will enable the user to program problems easily, without spending much time on programming, and that they will contribute significantly to the future progress in many research areas

## REFERENCES

BRENNAN, R. (1969) *Continuous Systems Modeling Programs. State-of-the-Art and Prospectus for Development.*

GUYTON, A. C., MILHORN HR., H. T. AND COLEMAN, T. G. (1967) *Simulation of Physical Mechanisms, Part II, Simulation,* p. 73.

*IBM* (1967) *Application Program Manual H20-0209. System/1130 Continuous Systems Modeling Program. Application Description.*

*IBM* (1968) *Application Program Manual H20-0367. System/360 Continuous Modeling Program User's Manual.*

KOLDENHOF, E. A. (1963) Laminar boundary layers on continuous cylinders. *Thesis, Eindhoven.*

DE VALOIS, J. C. (1966) An electrophysiological study of cerebral anoxia. *Thesis, Amsterdam.*

# Examples of the Application of Computer Programs to Neurophysiological Projects

# Computer Programming for Parameter Analysis of the Electroencephalogram

J. SMITH AND J. P. SCHADÉ

*Central Institute for Brain Research, Amsterdam (The Netherlands)*

## INTRODUCTION

Five aspects are of primary importance in obtaining the optimal information from a particular signal:

1. *sensing*: pick-up, conversion etc.;
2. *transmission* to recorder or to computer;
3. *recording*, including play-back and time-sampling;
4. *computation*: formulas, computing circuit performance etc.;
5. *interpretation*.

In each of these stages the quality of performance, e.g. noise, level, and distortion, will be of significance. The present account deals with the computational and interpretation aspects of signal analysis.

The quantitative analysis of a continuous random signal in time would either require the exact measurement of an infinitely long piece of the random signal, or a collection of pieces of infinite total length. From these data an infinitely detailed computation should then be made.

Since these two requirements are rather impractical, other means have to be employed. Approximation of signals raises numerous questions, such as how many data of a given accuracy are required, which computation approach should be used, and how reliable are the results.

## TIME-DOMAIN

We will first consider a continuous random signal in time (Fig. 1) which may be an electroencephalogram, electromyogram or some other bioelectric phenomenon. A number of parameters such as amplitude, frequency and phase may be determined over time. We can define the phase over time as the accumulated number of cycles starting from an initial time.

However, during consecutive intervals, the frequency, amplitude and phase change in time. For a simple sine wave the mathematical formulation is as follows:

$$x(t) = X \sin(2\pi f t + \theta_0) \tag{1}$$

in which $\qquad\qquad$ $X$ is the amplitude

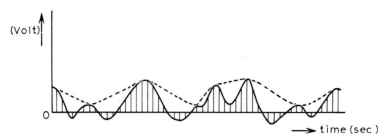

Fig. 1. Continuous random function $x(t)$ in the time-domain.

$f$ is the frequency

$\theta_0$ is the phase at the initial time.

For a continuous random signal in time—EEG—in which the amplitude, frequency and phase change in time, we can write the equation:

$$x(t) = X(t) \sin [2\pi f(t) \cdot t + \theta_0(t)] \tag{2}$$

in which $\quad X(t)$ means the amplitude is a function of time

$f(t)$ means the frequency is a function of time

$\theta_0(t)$ means the phase is a function of time.

Although this procedure will give an analytical tool for continuous random signals in the time-domain, the frequency-domain is often of more help in the interpretation of physiological and pathological phenomena.

### FREQUENCY-DOMAIN

The relation between the time-domain and the frequency-domain is given by the Fourier transformation. Generally, several formulations of Fourier transformations are being used according to custom, convenience, or taste. The formulation noted here is used by Campbell and Foster (1942). Given a function of time $x(t)$, its Fourier transform is a function of frequency and is given by the equation:

$$X(f) = \int_{-\infty}^{\infty} x(t) \exp(-j2\pi ft) \, dt \tag{3}$$

Conversely, given a function of frequency $X(f)$, its Fourier transform is a function of time, and is given by the equation:

$$x(t) = \int_{-\infty}^{\infty} X(f) \exp(+j2\pi ft) \, dt \tag{4}$$

A continuous random signal in time as in Fig. 1 will give in the frequency-domain a pattern as illustrated in Fig. 2.

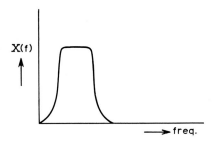

Fig. 2. Spectrum of the continuous random signal $x(t)$ in the frequency-domain.

## SAMPLING PROCEDURE

We will consider a continuous record $x(t)$ over time of a narrow band. By "narrow band" we mean a signal with a relatively narrow spectral width—$B$—distributed around a relatively high center frequency $f_0$. The signal spectrum $X(f)$ defined according to (3) has the condition that

$$X(f) = 0 \text{ if } f_0 - \frac{B}{2} < f < f_0 + \frac{B}{2}$$

where $f_0 \geqslant 1.5\ B$.

The Shannon "sampling theorem" states that any signal $x(t)$ can be represented by a series of samples, taken at a *minimum* rate equalling twice the highest frequency present in the signal spectrum $X(f)$. This method is primarily used for wide-band signals, particularly if $X(f)$ ranges from direct current up to a maximum frequency $f_H$.

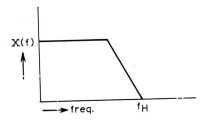

Fig. 3. Frequency spectrum of a wide-band signal.

Shannon's theorem, however, is very inefficient when applied to a narrow-band signal as it prescribes a sampling rate:

$$F = 2 f_H = 2 \left( f_0 + \frac{B}{2} \right)$$

Depending on the value of $f_0$, the sampling rate may be very high compared to $2 f_H$ samples/sec.

A solution was given by the sampling theorem of Woodward (1953) stating that a narrow-band signal can be represented by a series of samples, taken at miminum rate, equalling twice the bandwidth of the signal spectrum $X(f)$. The maximum time $\Delta t$ between two samples is thus:

$$\Delta t = \frac{1}{2f_H} \, .$$

### Choice of the sampling time $\Delta t$

Depending on the resolution one can choose another $\Delta t$, according the equation:

$$t_{j+1} - t_j = \Delta t = \frac{1}{2f_H K} \text{ where } K \text{ is an integer constant.} \qquad (5)$$

Let us consider a pure sinusoid:

$$x(t) = \sin(2\pi f_H t + \theta_0) \text{ and let } \Delta t = \frac{1}{2f_H K} \, . \qquad (6)$$

In this way the phase increment $\Delta\theta$ for various values of the constant $K$ may be obtained. Thus:

$$(\Delta\theta)_j = 2\pi f_H t_j + \theta_0 - \theta_0 = \theta_{j+1} - \theta_j. \qquad (7)$$

In table form:

| $K$ | $\Delta\theta = 2\pi f_H \dfrac{1}{2f_H \cdot K}$ (degrees) |
|---|---|
| 2 | 90° |
| 3 | 60° |
| 4 | 45° |

etc.

In practice a value of $K$ equalling 3 or 4 will suffice. To determine the amplitude, frequency and phase of a continuous record over time, the record is sampled with a sampling time $\Delta t$, (5). The continuous record is thus transformed in a time sequence of numbers, representing the equally spaced values of $\Delta t$ units of time, apart from the continuous record, $x_j$.

Therefore a proper choice of $\Delta t$ is important. If $\Delta t$ is too large the time sequence of numbers $x_j$ fails to adequately reflect the properties of the continuous record $x(t)$. However, if $\Delta t$ is too small the time sequence of numbers $x_j$ becomes too large and the number of computations required to determine amplitude, frequency and phase becomes unnecessarily large. There are certain advantages in choosing a small $\Delta t$, because rapidly varying changes in amplitude are discernable.

### Narrow-band stationary signal contaminated with additive wide-band stationary noise

It is known that stationary signals with a narrow-band spectral density function approximate the appearance of a sine wave if rather short time intervals are being considered. The frequency of the sine wave is located near the mid-band frequency of the spectrum density. A typical appearance of a stationary signal, possessing a spectral density function is shown in Fig. 4.

### Narrow-band spectral density function

The frequency and amplitude of a sine wave changes in the course of various time intervals. If the band is sufficiently narrow, the changes over time in frequency and

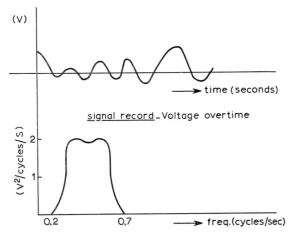

Fig. 4. Narrow-band spectral density function of the continuous signal in time.

amplitude are rather slow. The phase over time may be defined as the accumulated number of cycles starting from the initial time.

The narrow-band stationary signal is often contaminated with wide-band stationary noise. In that case the frequency, amplitude and phase of the narrow-band stationary signal is not discernable of the contaminated record. It is therefore necessary to define frequency, amplitude and phase for wide-band stationary noise and also to establish a mathematical method for measuring the frequency, amplitude and phase of wide-band stationary noise when such a noise is contaminated by additive extraneous wide-band stationary noise.

With the theory mentioned above, it is possible to choose the proper $\Delta t$ for the normal case. When additive wide-band noise is contaminated in the process, a smaller $\Delta t$ is required. If $f_{Hn}$ denotes the highest effective frequency of the spectral density of the additive extraneous wide-band noise, and $f > f_{Hn}$ spectral density is zero, then the following statements are true:

$$\text{if } f_{Hn} \leqslant (2K-1)f_H, \text{ then } \Delta t = \frac{1}{2f_H \cdot K}$$

$$\text{if } f_{Hn} > (2K-1)f_H, \text{ then } \Delta t = \frac{1}{f_H + f_{Hn}}$$

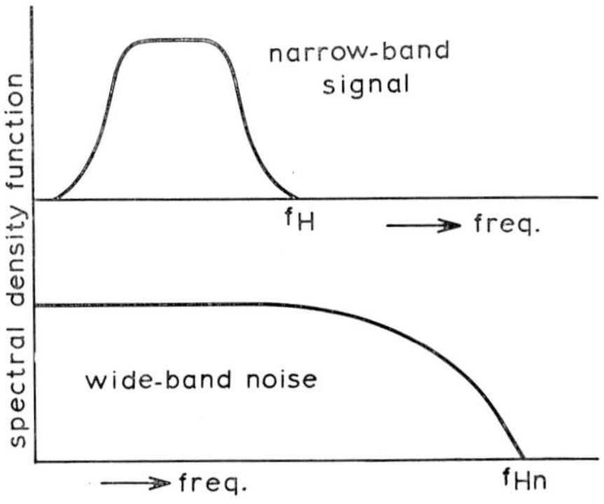

Fig. 5. Narrow-band and wide-band signal.

*Moving averages*

The continuous record $x(t)$ may be described in a sequence of numbers $X_j = X(j\Delta t)$, where $j = -j_f, ..., -2, -1, 0, 1, 2, ... j_l$. The next step is the calculation of the moving averages for each $j$.

$$\tilde{X}_j = \sum_{l=-m}^{m} b_l X_{j+l}$$

$$\tilde{Y}_j = \sum_{l=-m}^{m} a_l X_{j+l} \tag{8}$$

The constants $(a_l, b_l)$, $l = -m, ..., +m ...$, are the same for each $l$, and are determined by the filter used. From equation (8) one can compute for each $j$ the amplitude $\tilde{A}_j$ and phase $\overset{\circ}{\theta}_j$ by the equation:

$$\tilde{A}_j \, e^{i\,\theta_j} = \tilde{X}_j + i\tilde{Y}_j \tag{9}$$

The corresponding frequency is then:

$$\tilde{\omega}_j = \frac{\theta_j - \theta_{j-1}}{\Delta t} \quad \text{where} \quad -\pi \leqslant \theta_j - \theta_{j-1} \leqslant \pi \tag{10}$$

In fact $\tilde{\omega}_j$ is the average frequency of $x(t)$ over the time interval $(k-1)\, t \leqslant \Delta t \leqslant k\,\Delta t$.

In determining the constants $(a_l, b_l)$ we take into account that there is a one to one correspondence between averages (equation 8) and trigonomic polynomials (filters in the frequency domain). The filters corresponding to the parameters in equation (8) are shown in Figs. 6 and 7.

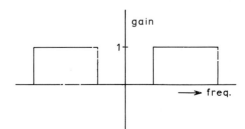

Fig. 6. Ideal in-phase filter.

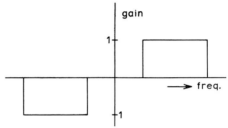

Fig. 7. Ideal in-quadrature filter.

The computer program may be composed in such a way as to compute trapezoidal filters. By combining a suitable number of properly located and overlapping triangular filters, the trapezoidal filters of desired bandwidth and frequency will be obtained. (See Fig. 8).

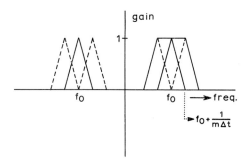

Fig. 8. Trapezoidal filters formed by a combination of triangular filters.

*Transformation of trapezoidal filters from triangular filters*

It may be noted that the bandwidth of a triangular filter amounts to $\dfrac{2}{m\Delta t}$ . One has only to specify $m$, the frequency location $fo$ and the number of triangular form filter $N$, in order to obtain the trapezoidal filter desired. These data allow the computation of the constants $(a_l, b_l)$ $l = -m, \ldots m$ (equation (8)), and in this way the frequency, amplitude and phase will be determined.

*Filters*

The data input series $X_j$ smoothed by the filter $C_{m, N, \omega_0}(\omega)$ is symbolized by $\tilde{X}_j$. The relation between these two sets of data is:

$$\tilde{X}_j = \sum_{l=-m}^{m} b_l \, X_{j+l} \text{ where } b_{-j} = b_1.$$

The data input series $X_j$ smoothed by the filter $S_{m, N, \omega_0}(\omega)$ is symbolized by $\tilde{Y}_j$, with the relation

$$\tilde{Y}_j = \sum_{l=m}^{m} a_j \, X_{j+1} \text{ where } a_{-j} = a_1.$$

The filter is given by

$$T_m(\omega) = \frac{1}{m} + \frac{2}{m} \sum_{l=1}^{m-1} \left[ 0.54 + 0.46 \cos\left(\frac{l\pi}{m}\right) \right] \cos(l\omega)$$

$$+ \frac{1}{m} \left[ 0.54 + 0.46 \cos(\pi) \right] \cos(m\omega)$$

Depending of the number of triangles ($N$) which can be even or odd, the generalized Tukey filters $C_{m, N, \omega_0}(\omega)$ and $S_{m, N, \omega_0}(\omega)$ can be expressed in the following polynomials:

*When N is even*

$$C_{m, N, \omega_0}(\omega) = \frac{2N}{m} + \frac{4}{m} \sum_{l=1}^{m=1} \left[ 0.54 + 0.46 \cos\left(\frac{l\pi}{m}\right) \right] \cos(l\omega_0)$$

$$\left[ \frac{\sin(Nl\pi/m)}{\sin(l\pi/m)} \right] \cos(l\omega) - \frac{2N}{m} \left[ 0.54\, 0.46 \cos(\pi) \right] \cos(m\omega_0) \cos(m\omega)$$

*and*:

$$S_{m, N, \omega_0}(\omega) = \frac{4}{m} \sum_{l=1}^{m-1} \left[ 0.54 + 0.46 \cos\left(\frac{l\pi}{m}\right) \right] \sin(l\omega_0)$$

$$\left[ \frac{\sin(Nl\pi/m)}{\sin(l\pi/m)} \right] \sin(l\omega) - \frac{2N}{m} \left[ 0.54 + 0.46 \cos(\pi) \right] \sin(m\omega_0)\ \sin(m\omega)$$

*When N is odd*

$$C_{m, N, \omega_0}(\omega) = \frac{2N}{m} + \frac{4}{m} \sum_{l=1}^{m-1} \left[ 0.54 + 0.46 \cos\left(\frac{l\pi}{m}\right) \right] \cos(l\omega_0)$$

$$\left[ \frac{\sin(Nl\pi/m)}{\sin(l\pi/m)} \right] \cos(l\omega) + \frac{2N}{m} \left[ 0.54 + 0.46 \cos(\pi) \right] \cos(m\omega_0) \cos(\omega m)$$

*and*:

$$S_{m, N, \omega_0}(\omega) = \frac{4}{m} \sum_{l-1}^{m-1} \left[ 0.54 + 0.46 \cos\left(\frac{l\pi}{m}\right) \right] \sin(l\omega_0)$$

$$\left[ -\frac{\sin(Nl\pi/m)}{\sin(l\pi/m)} \right] \sin(l\omega) + \frac{2N}{m} \left[ 0.54 + 0.46 \cos(\pi) \right] \sin(m\omega_0) \sin(m\omega)$$

A simplification is obtained by introducing the following coefficients:

$$C_{m, N, \omega_0}(\omega) = b_0 + \sum_{l=1}^{m-1} b_l \cdot \cos(l\omega) + b_m$$

$$S_{m, N, \omega_0}(\omega) = \sum_{l=1}^{m-1} a_l \sin(l\omega) + a_m$$

$$b_0 = \frac{2N}{m}$$

$$b_1 = \frac{4}{m} \left[ 0.54 + 0.46 \cos\left(\frac{l\pi}{m}\right) \right] \left[ \frac{\sin(Nl\pi/m)}{\sin(l\pi/m)} \right] \cos(l\omega_0)$$

with $l = 1, 2 \ldots, m - 1$

$$b_m = \frac{2N}{m} \left[ 0.54 + 0.46 \cos(\pi) \right] \cos(m\omega_0) \text{ if } N \text{ is odd}$$

$$= -\frac{2N}{m}\left[0.54 + 0.46\cos(\pi)\right]\cos(m\omega_0)\ \text{if } N \text{ is even}$$

$$a_0 = 0$$

$$a_1 = \frac{-4}{m}\left[0.54 + 0.46\cos(l\pi/m)\right]\left[\frac{\sin(Nl\pi/m)}{\sin(l\pi/m)}\right]\sin(l\omega_0)$$

with $l = 1, 2, \ldots, m-1$

$$a_m = -\frac{2N}{m}\left[0.54 + 0.46\cos(\pi)\right]\sin(m\omega_0)\ \text{if } N \text{ is odd}$$

$$= \frac{2N}{m}\left[0.54 + 0.46\cos(\pi)\right]\sin(m\omega_0)\ \text{if } N \text{ is even.}$$

### COMPUTATION OF FREQUENCY, AMPLITUDE AND PHASE

Knowing the coefficients $(a_l, b_l)$, one can compute the corresponding finite moving averages

$$\widetilde{X}_j,\ \widetilde{Y}_j\ \text{for each } j\ (\text{equation (8)}).$$

The frequency, amplitude and phase are then computed according the following equations:

$$j^e\text{-frequency} = (\theta_j - \theta_{j-1})/\Delta t$$

$$j^e\text{-amplitude} = \sqrt{\widetilde{X}_j^2 + \widetilde{Y}_j^2}$$

$$j^e\text{-phase} = \text{Arg}(\widetilde{X}_j + i\widetilde{Y}_j) = \theta_j$$

### SUMMARY

The analysis of a continuous random signal in time, e.g. an electroencephalogram, can be achieved in a number of ways. The method described here deals with the determination of the frequency, amplitude and phase of an electroencephalogram (EEG), with the aid of a computer program.

As the EEG is a continuous signal in time the data are first sampled, according to the well-known "sampling theorem" stated by Shannon, combined with Woodward's "sampling theorem" for narrow-band signals.

So the continuous record is transformed into a time sequence of numbers, representing the equally spaced values of the continous record $X(j\Delta t)$. This sequence of numbers forms the input data of the program. As a basis for the computation a 7094-IBM program has been used, developed by Dixon (1968).

### REFERENCES

BLACKMAN, R. B. AND TUKEY, J. W. (1958) *The Measurement of Power Spectra from the Point of View of Communications Engineering*, Dover, New York.

CAMPBELL, G. A. AND FOSTER, R. M. (1942) *Fourier Integrals for Practical Applications*, Van Nostrand, New York.

DIXON, W. J. (1968) *Biomedical Computer Programs*, Univ. of California Press.

SHANNON, C. E. (1949) Communication in the presence of noise. *Proc. I.R.E.*, **37**.

WOODWARD, P. M. (1953) *Probability and Information Theory with Applications to Radar*, Pergamon, London.

```
*ID              FREQUENCY, AMPLITUDE AND PHASE                      BMD 0010
*     MAP                                                            BMD 0020
*     XEQ                                                            BMD 0030
*     LABEL                                                          BMD 0040
*     FORTRAN                                                        BMD 0050
CBMD01T              FREQUENCY, AMPLITUDE AND PHASE                  BMD 0060
        DIMENSION X(5000),FMT(120),YSQ(500),Y(1500),SYM(15),YP(15),  BMD 0070
     1A(1000),B(1000),XX(5000),YY(5000)                              BMD 0080
        COMMON X,FMT,YSQ,Y,SYM,YP,A,B,XX,YY,AMPL,PHASE,TG,FILTER,KPROB, BMD 0090
     1NDATA,FTRI,NTRI,M,FM,NPOINT,POINT,WO,ANS,PI,H                  BMD 0100
        EQUIVALENCE (YES,IYES)                                       BMD 0110
C                                                                    BMD 0120
  304   FORMAT(45H0CONTROL CARDS INCORRECTLY ORDERED OR PUNCHED)     BMD 0130
  305   FORMAT (43H COMPUTATIONAL ANALYSIS OF, 1.THE FREQUENCY/      BMD 0140
     151H                                    2.THE AMPLITUDE/        BMD 0150
     251H                                    3.AND THE PHASE/        BMD 0160
     314H PROBLEM CODE A6,/                                          BMD 0170
     423H NUMBER OF DATA POINTS I5,///)                              BMD 0180
 1000 FORMAT(1H1)                                                    BMD 0190
 1002 FORMAT(10X,38HVALUE OF INTEGRAL OF F(X) SQUARE FROM F10.5,     BMD 0200
     14H TO F10.5,3H = F10.5//)                                      BMD 0210
 1003 FORMAT(1H1,9X47HB IS THE COEFFICIENT OF COS J.OMEGA IN C(OMEGA)/ BMD 0220
     1 10X,75HAND A IS THE COEFFICIENT OF SIN J.OMEGA IN S(OMEGA) IN SECBMD 0230
     2TION FOUR STEP 2 ///)                                          BMD 0240
 1004 FORMAT (10X,2HA(I4,4H) = F10.5,20X,2HB(I4,4H) = F10.5)         BMD 0250
 1005 FORMAT(1H0,9X,34HTHESE ARE THE VALUE OF THE FILTER//)          BMD 0260
 1006 FORMAT(1H0,9X,10HRESOLUTION7X,16HNO. OF TRIANGLES9X,11HCENTERED ATBMD 0270
     18X,9HBANDWIDTH,10X,19HLEAKAGE IN PER CENT//)                   BMD 0280
 1007 FORMAT(7F12.6)                                                 BMD 0290
 1008 FORMAT(13X,I3,18X,I3,15X,F11.8,8X,F10.7,12X,F12.8)             BMD 0300
 1009 FORMAT(10X16HA(  0) =    0.024X9HB(  0) =F11.5)                BMD 0310
 1010 FORMAT(1H1,20X,19HGRAPH OF THE FILTER//)                       BMD 0320
 1011 FORMAT(10X,5H* * */10X,28HBANDWIDTH CHOSEN IN PROBLEM I3,      BMD 0330
     1 50H LARGER THAN PI, PROGRAM GOES TO NEXT PROBLEM CARD/10X,5H* * *BMD 0340
     2)                                                              BMD 0350
 1017 FORMAT(10X,25HORIGINAL DATA OF PROBLEM I3//)                   BMD 0360
 1018 FORMAT(10F12.6)                                                BMD 0370
 1019 FORMAT(10X,49H*****THE MAIN LOBE OF THE FILTER OF THIS PROBLEM(I3,BMD 0380
     166H) IS NOT BETWEEN 0 AND PI,PROGRAM GOES TO NEXT PROBLEM, IF  BMD 0390
     2ANY)                                                           BMD 0400
 1020 FORMAT (1H1,31X,56HGRAPH OF THE FILTERED INPUT AT THE INDICATED DABMD 0410
     XA POINT//)                                                     BMD 0420
 1023 FORMAT(1H1,20X,72HAVERAGE FREQUENCY, AMPLITUDE, PHASE AND FINITE MBMD 0430
     XOVING AVERAGES OF SERIES I4/32X,53H(FREQUENCY IN RADIANS/UNIT TIMEBMD 0440
     X AND PHASE IN RADIANS)//)                                      BMD 0450
 1024 FORMAT(1H I5,4XF12.6,4(8X,F12.6))                              BMD 0460
 1025 FORMAT(2X,4HDATA,7X,9HFREQUENCY,11X,9HAMPLITUDE,13X,5HPHASE,7X,38HBMD 0470
     XFINITE MOVING AVERAGES USING CONSTANTS/1X,5HPOINT,68X,4HB(J),16X, BMD 0480
     X4HA(J)//)                                                      BMD 0490
 2000 FORMAT(1H0)                                                    BMD 0500
 5001 FORMAT(2A6,4A3,I3,I4,I3,I4,I3,F5.0,22X,2I2)                    BMD 0510
 5003 FORMAT(12A6)                                                   BMD 0520
C                                                                    BMD 0530
      A123=(+6HFINISH)                                               BMD 0540
      B123=(+6HPROBLM)                                               BMD 0550
      YES =(+3HYES)                                                  BMD 0560
      NTAPE=5                                                        BMD 0570
C        READ INPUT TAPE                                            BMD 0580
  500 READ INPUT TAPE 5,5001,TODE,CODE,KG,KDATA,ILTER,KOOL,KPROB,NDATA BMD 0590
```

```
     1,NTRI,M,NPOINT,WO,INFORM,KVR                                   BMD 0600
B        IF(B123*(-TODE)+TODE*(-B123)) 300,20,300                    BMD 0610
B 300    IF(A123*(-TODE)+TODE*(-A123)) 302,303,302                   BMD 0620
  302 WRITE OUTPUT TAPE 6,304                                        BMD 0630
  303 IF(NTAPE-5)372,372,371                                         BMD 0640
  371 CALL REMOVE(NTAPE)                                             BMD 0650
  372 CALL EXIT                                                      BMD 0660
   20 CALL TPWD(INFORM,NTAPE)                                        BMD 0670
      WRITE OUTPUT TAPE 6,305,CODE,NDATA                             BMD 0680
C         CHECK NR. OF TRIANGLES, MUST BE POSITIVE                   BMD 0690
      IF(-NTRI)25,302,302                                            BMD 0700
   25 FTRI=NTRI                                                      BMD 0710
C         CHECK NR.OF RESOLUTIONS, MUST BE SMALLER THAN OR EQUAL 4000 BMD 0720
      IF(M-4000)255,255,302                                          BMD 0730
  255 FM=M                                                           BMD 0740
      PI=3.14159265                                                  BMD 0750
C         CHECK HALF(THE NUMBER OF RESOLUTIONS-2) MUST BE BIGGER THAN THEBMD 0760
C         NR.OF TRIANGLES                                            BMD 0770
      CRIT=(FM-2.0)/2.0                                              BMD 0780
      IF(CRIT-FTRI)  11,11,12                                        BMD 0790
   11 DO 90 I=1,6                                                    BMD 0800
   90 WRITE OUTPUT TAPE 6,2000                                       BMD 0810
      WRITE OUTPUT TAPE 6,1011,KPROB                                 BMD 0820
      PI=-4000                                                       BMD 0830
C         TEST KVR, IF KVR SMALLER OR EQUAL 0, OR BIGGER 10 THAN KVR=1, BMD 0840
C         ELSE KVR IS RIGHT.                                         BMD 0850
   12    CALL VFCHCK(KVR)                                            BMD 0860
  210 KVR=KVR*12                                                     BMD 0870
      READ INPUT TAPE 5,5003,(FMT(I),I=1,KVR)                        BMD 0880
C         TEST NR.OF DATAS, MUST BE BIGGER THAN 49 AND SMALLER THAN 5001,BMD 0890
C         CONTINUED THE PROCESS WITH STATEMENT 215.                  BMD 0900
      IF((NDATA-49)*(NDATA-5001))215,302,302                         BMD 0910
  215 MISTAK=0                                                       BMD 0920
      READ INPUT TAPE NTAPE,FMT,(X(I),I=1,NDATA)                     BMD 0930
      IF(-PI)40,500,500                                              BMD 0940
   40 IF(KG-IYES)30,45,30                                            BMD 0950
   45 CALL TRANS( MISTAK)                                            BMD 0960
      IF( MISTAK) 500,30,500                                         BMD 0970
   30 IF(KDATA-IYES)60,65,60                                         BMD 0980
   65 WRITE OUTPUT TAPE 6,2000                                       BMD 0990
      WRITE OUTPUT TAPE 6,1017,KPROB                                 BMD 1000
      WRITE OUTPUT TAPE 6,1018,(X(I),I=1,NDATA)                      BMD 1010
   60 IF(ILTER-IYES)126,95,126                                       BMD 1020
C         TEST NR.OF POINTS FOR FILTER EVALUATION, MUST BE BIGGER THAN BMD 1030
C         49, CONTINUE STAT.NR.951, AND CHECK WO MUST BE BIGGER THAN 0 BMD 1040
C         AND SMALLER THAN PI                                        BMD 1050
   95 POINT=NPOINT                                                   BMD 1060
      IF(50-NPOINT)951,951,302                                       BMD 1070
  951 IF(WO*(WO-PI))1955,955,96                                      BMD 1080
C         H A REAL CONSTANT BETWEEN 0.0628 AND 0.00314.              BMD 1090
C         G A REAL CONSTANT, DEFINING THE BANDWIDTH B OF THE FILTER USED.BMD 1100
C         WO A REAL CONSTANT,DEFINING THE CENTER FREQUENTIE OF THE FILTERBMD 1110
  955 H=PI/POINT                                                     BMD 1120
      G=(FTRI+1.0)*2.0*PI/FM                                         BMD 1130
      BONE=WO-.5*G                                                   BMD 1140
      IF(BONE) 96,96,97                                              BMD 1150
   96 WRITE OUTPUT TAPE 6,1019,KPROB                                 BMD 1160
      GO TO 500                                                      BMD 1170
C         COMPUTE THE INTEGRAL OF C**2 ,LOWER BOUND=0, UPPER BOUND=WO-B/2BMD 1180
```

```
C           NONE INTEGER CONST., DEFINING THE NR.OF STEPS FOR INTEGRAL CAL-BMD 1190
C           CULATION, BETWEEN THE L.B.AND U.B., IDEM NTWO, NTHREE        BMD 1200
   97 NONE=(BONE/H)+0.5                                                  BMD 1210
      WRITE OUTPUT TAPE 6,1000                                          BMD 1220
      CALL LANAI (NONE,0.0,0)                                           BMD 1230
      AA=ANS                                                            BMD 1240
  100 WRITE OUTPUT TAPE 6,2000                                          BMD 1250
      ZERO=0.0                                                          BMD 1260
      WRITE OUTPUT TAPE 6,1002,ZERO,BONE,AA                             BMD 1270
C           COMPUTE THE INTEGRAL OF C**2, LOWER BOUND=WO-B/2,           BMD 1280
C                                    UPPER BOUND=WO+B/2                  BMD 1290
      BTWO=WO+.5*G                                                      BMD 1300
      IF(BTWO-PI) 101,101,102                                           BMD 1310
  102 WRITE OUTPUT TAPE 6,1019,KPROB                                    BMD 1320
      GO TO 500                                                         BMD 1330
  101 NTWO=(G/H)+0.5                                                    BMD 1340
      CALL LANAI (NTWO,BONE,NONE)                                       BMD 1350
      BB=ANS                                                            BMD 1360
  105 WRITE OUTPUT TAPE 6,2000                                          BMD 1370
      WRITE OUTPUT TAPE 6,1002,BONE,BTWO,BB                             BMD 1380
C           COMPUTE THE INTEGRAL OF C**2, LOWER BOUND=WO+B/2,           BMD 1390
C                                    UPPER BOUND=3.1415                  BMD 1400
      NTHREE=((PI-BTWO)/H)+0.5                                          BMD 1410
      KK=NONE+NTWO                                                      BMD 1420
      CALL LANAI(NTHREE,BTWO,KK)                                        BMD 1430
      CC=ANS                                                            BMD 1440
  110  WRITE OUTPUT TAPE 6,2000                                         BMD 1450
      WRITE OUTPUT TAPE 6,1002,BTWO,PI,CC                               BMD 1460
C           COMPUTE THE LEAKAGE OF THE FILTER.                          BMD 1470
      PC=(AA+CC)*100.0/(AA+BB+CC)                                       BMD 1480
      WRITE OUTPUT TAPE 6,1006                                          BMD 1490
      WRITE OUTPUT TAPE 6,1008,M,NTRI,WO,G,PC                           BMD 1500
  115 WRITE OUTPUT TAPE 6,2000                                          BMD 1510
      WRITE OUTPUT TAPE 6,1005                                          BMD 1520
C           NPOINT IS THE TOTAL NR.OF POINTS BETWEEN O-PI, EVALUATING   BMD 1530
C           THE FILTER                                                  BMD 1540
      NPOINT=NONE+NTWO+NTHREE                                           BMD 1550
      POINT=NPOINT-1                                                    BMD 1560
      WRITE OUTPUT TAPE 6,1007,(Y(I),I=1,NPOINT)                        BMD 1570
      WRITEOUTPUT TAPE 6,1010                                           BMD 1580
C           PLOTTING THE FILTER-GRAPH, AFTER CALCULATING THE YMAX AND YMIN BMD 1590
      YMAX=-10**10                                                      BMD 1600
      YMIN=10**10                                                       BMD 1610
      DO 120 I=1,NPOINT                                                 BMD 1620
      YMAX=MAX1F(Y(I),YMAX)                                             BMD 1630
  120 YMIN=MIN1F(Y(I),YMIN)                                             BMD 1640
      SYM=(+6H*00000)                                                   BMD 1650
      DO 125 I=1,NPOINT                                                 BMD 1660
      FI=I-1                                                            BMD 1670
      XX=FI*PI/POINT                                                    BMD 1680
      YP(1)=Y(I)                                                        BMD 1690
  125 CALL PLOTR (XX,0.0,PI,YP,SYM,YMIN,YMAX,1,-1)                      BMD 1700
      CALL PLOTR (XX,0.0,PI,YP,SYM,YMIN,YMAX,-1,-1)                     BMD 1710
  126 IF(KOOL-IYES)131,127,131                                          BMD 1720
C           CALLING THE SUBR. COEVV. FOR CALCULATING THE COEFF.A AND B  BMD 1730
C           AND LISTING OF THIS COEFF                                   BMD 1740
  127 CALL COEVV(A,B)                                                   BMD 1750
      BZERO=2.0*FTRI/FM                                                 BMD 1760
      WRITE OUTPUT TAPE 6,1003                                          BMD 1770
```

```
        WRITE OUTPUT TAPE 6,1009,BZERO                              BMD 1780
        DO 130 I=1,M                                                BMD 1790
   130 WRITE OUTPUT TAPE 6,1004,I,A(I),I,B(I)                       BMD 1800
C          COMPUTE THE DATA-INPUT SERIES SMOOTHED BY THE FILTER     BMD 1810
   131 DO 140 K=1,NDATA                                             BMD 1820
        XX(K)=0.0                                                   BMD 1830
        YY(K)=0.0                                                   BMD 1840
        DO 155 J=1,M                                                BMD 1850
        JS=K+M+J                                                    BMD 1860
        KS=K+M-J+1                                                  BMD 1870
        IF((JS+1)-NDATA) 145,145,150                                BMD 1880
   145 YY(K)=YY(K)+A(J)*(X(JS)-X(KS))                               BMD 1890
   155 XX(K)=XX(K)+B(J)*(X(JS+1)+X(KS-1))                           BMD 1900
        IS=M+K+1                                                    BMD 1910
        XX(K)=BZERO*(X(IS)+X(IS-1))+XX(K)                           BMD 1920
   140 CONTINUE                                                     BMD 1930
   150 WRITE OUTPUT TAPE 6,1020                                     BMD 1940
        K=K-1                                                       BMD 1950
        YMAX=-10.0**10                                              BMD 1960
        YMIN= 10.0**10                                              BMD 1970
C          CHOOSE THE BIGGEST AND SMALLEST VALUE OF XX(I)           BMD 1980
        DO 157 I=1,K                                                BMD 1990
        YMAX=MAX1F(XX(I),YMAX)                                      BMD 2000
   157 YMIN=MIN1F(XX(I),YMIN)                                       BMD 2010
        IF(YMAX-YMIN-1.0)1575,1575,158                              BMD 2020
  1575 DIV=(YMAX-YMIN)/3.0                                          BMD 2030
        YMAX=YMAX+DIV                                               BMD 2040
        YMIN=YMIN-DIV                                               BMD 2050
   158 FK=M                                                         BMD 2060
        FMAX=NDATA-M                                                BMD 2070
        DO 159 I=1,K                                                BMD 2080
        FK=FK+1.0                                                   BMD 2090
        YP(1)=XX(I)                                                 BMD 2100
   159 CALL PLOTR(FK,FM,FMAX,YP,SYM,YMIN,YMAX, 1,-1)                BMD 2110
        CALL PLOTR(FK,FM,FMAX,YP,SYM,YMIN,YMAX,-1,-1)               BMD 2120
        WRITE OUTPUT TAPE 6,1023,KPROB                              BMD 2130
        WRITE OUTPUT TAPE 6,1025                                    BMD 2140
C          CALLING SUBROUTINE FOR COMPUTING THE PHASE Z             BMD 2150
        CALL PHAZE(XX(1),YY(1),Z1)                                  BMD 2160
        J=M+1                                                       BMD 2170
C          COMPUTING FOR EACH J THE FREQUENTIE,AMPLITUDE AND PHASE  BMD 2180
        DO 165 I=2,K                                                BMD 2190
        J=J+1                                                       BMD 2200
        AMPL    =SQRTF(XX(I)**2+YY(I)**2)                           BMD 2210
        CALL PHAZE(XX(I),YY(I),Z2)                                  BMD 2220
        FREQ=Z2-Z1                                                  BMD 2230
        IF(FREQ)160,164,164                                         BMD 2240
   160 DIV= FREQ+(2.0*PI)                                           BMD 2250
        FREQ=-FREQ                                                  BMD 2260
        FREQ=MIN1F(DIV,FREQ)                                        BMD 2270
        IF(FREQ-DIV)163,164,164                                     BMD 2280
   163 FREQ=-FREQ                                                   BMD 2290
   164 WRITE OUTPUT TAPE 6,1024,J,FREQ,AMPL,Z2,XX(I),YY(I)          BMD 2300
   165 Z1=Z2                                                        BMD 2310
        GO TO 500                                                   BMD 2320
        END                                                         BMD 2330
                                                                    BMD 2340
C                                                                   BMD 2350
  *     LABEL                                                       BMD 2350
  *     FORTRAN                                                     BMD 2360
```

```
CCOEVV          SUBROUTINE COEVV FOR BMD01T                          BMD 2370
        SUBROUTINE COEVV (A,B)                                       BMD 2380
        DIMENSION X(5000),FMT(120),YSQ(500),Y(1500),SYM(15),YP(15),  BMD 2390
       1A(1000),B(1000),XX(5000),YY(5000)                            BMD 2400
        DIMENSION S(1000)                                            BMD 2410
        COMMON X,FMT,YSQ,Y,SYM,YP,A,B,XX,YY,AMPL,PHASE,TG,FILTER,KPROB, BMD 2420
       1NDATA,FTRI,NTRI,M,FM,NPOINT,POINT,WO,ANS,PI,H                BMD 2430
C          M INTEGER CONST., DEFINING NR.OF RESOLUTIONS=FM           BMD 2440
C          COMPUTING THE COEFF. A AND B                             BMD 2450
        MMO=M-1                                                      BMD 2460
        ARG=FM*WO                                                    BMD 2470
        AA=2.0*FTRI*(.54+.46*COSF(PI))*SINF(ARG)/FM                  BMD 2480
        BB=2.0*FTRI*(.54+.46*COSF(PI))*COSF(ARG)/FM                  BMD 2490
C          TEST NR.OF TRIANGLES EVEN-CONT.STAT.NR.10, ODD-CONT.STAT.NR.20 BMD 2500
        KT=NTRI/2                                                    BMD 2510
        IF(NTRI-KT*2)20,10,20                                        BMD 2520
C          NTRI IS ODD                                              BMD 2530
   20 A(M)=-AA                                                       BMD 2540
        B(M)=BB                                                      BMD 2550
C          NTRI IS EVEN                                             BMD 2560
        GO TO 30                                                     BMD 2570
   10 A(M)=AA                                                        BMD 2580
        B(M)=-BB                                                     BMD 2590
C          COMPUTING THE A AND B COEFF.FOR J IS 1 UNTILL (M-1)      BMD 2600
   30 DO 105 J=1,MMO                                                 BMD 2610
        FJ=J                                                         BMD 2620
        ARGA=FJ*PI/FM                                                BMD 2630
        ARGB=FJ*FTRI*PI/FM                                           BMD 2640
  105 S(J)=4.0*(.54+.46*COSF(ARGA))*SINF(ARGB)/(FM*SINF(ARGA))       BMD 2650
        DO 120 J=1,MMO                                               BMD 2660
        FJ=J                                                         BMD 2670
        ARG=FJ*WO                                                    BMD 2680
        A(J)=-S(J)*SINF(ARG)                                         BMD 2690
  120 B(J)=S(J)*COSF(ARG)                                            BMD 2700
        RETURN                                                       BMD 2710
        END                                                          BMD 2720
C                                                                    BMD 2730
*     LABEL                                                          BMD 2740
*     FORTRAN                                                        BMD 2750
CDINT    SUBROUTINE DINT FOR BMD01T                                  BMD 2760
        SUBROUTINE DINT(YSQ,NN,H,ANS)                                BMD 2770
        DIMENSION YSQ(500),CONS(4)                                   BMD 2780
C          YSQ A REAL VAR. EQUAL TO C**2                            BMD 2790
        CONS(1)=0.34861111                                           BMD 2800
        CONS(2)=1.24583333                                           BMD 2810
        CONS(3)=0.87916667                                           BMD 2820
        CONS(4)=1.02638889                                           BMD 2830
        X=0.0                                                        BMD 2840
        J=NN                                                         BMD 2850
        DO 10 I=1,4                                                  BMD 2860
        X=X+(YSQ(I)+YSQ(J))*CONS(I)                                  BMD 2870
        J=J-1                                                        BMD 2880
   10 CONTINUE                                                       BMD 2890
        DO 20 I=5,J                                                  BMD 2900
        X=X+YSQ(I)                                                   BMD 2910
   20 CONTINUE                                                       BMD 2920
        ANS=X*H                                                      BMD 2930
        RETURN                                                       BMD 2940
        END                                                          BMD 2950
```

```
C                                                                        BMD 2960
*        FAP                                                             BMD 2970
         COUNT    50                                                     BMD 2980
*        SUBROUTINE FORM2 OF PLOTR                                       BMD 2990
         LBL      FORM2                                                  BMD 3030
*                                                                        BMD 3040
*        CALLING SEQUENCE   CALL FORM2(T,M,SYMB)                         BMD 3050
*                                                                        BMD 3060
         ENTRY    FORM2                                                  BMD 3070
FORM2    CLA*     2,4                                                    BMD 3080
         ARS      18                 SET SHIFT ADDRESSES                 BMD 3090
         STA      TT                                                     BMD 3100
         STA      COM                                                    BMD 3110
         CAL*     1,4                 GET T                              BMD 3120
TT       ALS      **                  SHIFT                              BMD 3130
         LAS      SMASK               PERFORM COMPARISONS TO FIND RANGE OF BMD 3140
         REM                              ORIGINAL CHARACTER IN POSITION  M  BMD 3150
         REM                              OF  T                          BMD 3160
         TRA      PT                  GREATER THAN /  --SUBSTITUTE 2     BMD 3170
         TRA      4,4                 /  --LEAVE ALONE                   BMD 3180
         LAS      BLANK               COMPARE WITH BLANK                 BMD 3190
IMASK    OCT      310000000000        (CAN NEVER COME HERE, SO PLACE CONSTANT BMD 3200
         REM                              IN THIS LOCATION)              BMD 3210
         TRA      FIX                 BLANK--SET TO SYMB                 BMD 3220
         LAS      NINE                COMPARE WITH 9                     BMD 3230
         TRA      TTT                 GREATER--CONTINUE COMPARISON       BMD 3240
         CAL      AMASK               9  --SET TO A                      BMD 3250
ADD1     ADD      ONE                 LESS THAN 9 --ADD 1                BMD 3260
         TRA      COM                                                    BMD 3270
TTT      LAS      IMASK               COMPARE WITH   I                   BMD 3280
         TRA      PT                  GREATER THAN I  --SET TO 2         BMD 3290
         CAL      BLANK               I  --SET TO SLASH                  BMD 3300
         LAS      AMASK               COMPARE WITH 1 LESS THAN A         BMD 3310
         TRA      ADD1                A-H  --ADD 1                       BMD 3320
         TRA      PT                  +  --SET TO 2                      BMD 3330
PT       CAL      TWO                 OTHER--SET TO 2                    BMD 3340
         TRA      COM                                                    BMD 3350
FIX      CAL*     3,4                 GET SYMB                           BMD 3360
         ANA      MASK                REMOVE REST OF CHARACTERS FROM SYMB BMD 3370
COM      ARS      **                  SHIFT TO PROPER POSITION IN WORD   BMD 3380
         SLW*     1,4                 STORE AS NEW T                     BMD 3390
         TRA      4,4                 RETURN                             BMD 3400
*        CONSTANTS                                                       BMD 3410
BLANK    OCT      600000000000                                          BMD 3420
AMASK    OCT      200000000000                                          BMD 3430
SMASK    OCT      610000000000                                          BMD 3440
ONE      OCT      010000000000                                          BMD 3450
TWO      OCT      020000000000                                          BMD 3460
NINE     OCT      110000000000                                          BMD 3470
MASK     OCT      770000000000                                          BMD 3480
         END                                                            BMD 3490
C                                                                        BMD 3500
*        LABEL                                                           BMD 3510
*        FORTRAN                                                         BMD 3520
CLANAI           SUBROUTINE LANAI FOR BMD01T                            BMD 3530
         SUBROUTINE LANAI (NN,BASE,KIT)                                 BMD 3540
         DIMENSION X(5000),FMT(120),YSQ(500),Y(1500),SYM(15),YP(15),    BMD 3550
        1A(1000),B(1000),XX(5000),YY(5000)                              BMD 3560
         COMMON X,FMT,YSQ,Y,SYM,YP,A,B,XX,YY,AMPL,PHASE,TG,FILTER,KPROB, BMD 3570
```

```
      1NDATA,FTRI,NTRI,M,FM,NPOINT,POINT,WO,ANS,PI,H            BMD 3580
C                                                               BMD 3590
 1000 FORMAT(1H0,21HVALUES OF F(X) SQUARE//)                    BMD 3600
 1001 FORMAT(7F12.6)                                            BMD 3610
C                                                               BMD 3620
C         NN INTEGER CONST.DEFINING THE NR.OF STEPS FOR THE INYEGRAL CALCBMD 3630
C         BASE REAL CONST.DEFINING THE LOWER BOUND OF THE INTEGRAL  BMD 3640
C         KIT INTEGER CONST.DEFINING THE NR.OF PRECEDING STEPS.  BMD 3650
      DO 100 I=1,NN                                             BMD 3660
      FI=I                                                      BMD 3670
      OMEGA=FI*H+BASE                                           BMD 3680
      CALL TABBY (OMEGA,YY)                                     BMD 3690
C         COMPUTING AND STORING THE C(M,N,WO)(OMEGA)-VALUES AND THEIR  BMD 3700
C         SQUARES.                                              BMD 3710
      L=I+KIT                                                   BMD 3720
      Y(L)=YY                                                   BMD 3730
  100 YSQ(I)=YY**2                                              BMD 3740
      WRITE OUTPUT TAPE 6,1000                                  BMD 3750
      WRITE OUTPUT TAPE 6,1001,(YSQ(I),I=1,NN)                  BMD 3760
      CALL DINT (YSQ,NN,H,ANS)                                  BMD 3770
      RETURN                                                    BMD 3780
      END                                                       BMD 3790
C                                                               BMD 3800
*     LABEL                                                     BMD 3810
*     FORTRAN                                                   BMD 3820
CPLOTR           SUBROUTINE PLOTR                               BMD 3830
      SUBROUTINE PLOTR(X,ZMIN,ZMAX,Y,SYM,WMIN,WMAX,NC,NP)       BMD 3840
C     PLOTR WAS MODIFIED THIS DATE TO GIVE BETTER SCALES.       BMD 3850
      DIMENSION XY(51,17),Y(15),CLAB(12),XM(16),SYM(15),GF(10),FMT(10)  BMD 3860
C                                                               BMD 3870
  100 FORMAT(1H 6X5(F12.3,8X),F12.3/17X,5(F12.3,8X))            BMD 3880
  101 FORMAT(1H F12.3,1X,A1,16A6,A5,A1,F12.3)                   BMD 3890
  102 FORMAT(1H 13X,A1,16A6,A5,A1)                              BMD 3900
 1000 FORMAT(1H   14X,101A1)                                    BMD 3910
 1001 FORMAT(15X,20(5H+....),1H+)                               BMD 3920
C                                                               BMD 3930
      BLANKS=(+6H        )                                      BMD 3940
      IF(NCC)48,50,48                                           BMD 3950
   50 KL=0                                                      BMD 3960
C         DEFINE THE REAL VAR. XM(I),GF(I),FMT(I),TC AND TP.    BMD 3970
B     XM(1)=770000000000                                       BMD 3980
B      XM(2)=007700000000                                      BMD 3990
B      XM(3)=000077000000                                      BMD 4000
B       XM(4)=000000770000                                     BMD 4010
B       XM(5)=000000007700                                     BMD 4020
B       XM(6)=000000000077                                     BMD 4030
      GF(1)=(+6H1X      )                                       BMD 4040
      GF(2)=(+6H2X      )                                       BMD 4050
      GF(3)=(+6H3X      )                                       BMD 4060
      GF(4)=(+6H4X      )                                       BMD 4070
      GF(5)=(+6H5X      )                                       BMD 4080
      GF(6)=(+6H6X      )                                       BMD 4090
      GF(8)=(+6H8X      )                                       BMD 4100
      GF(9)=(+6H9X      )                                       BMD 4110
      GF(10)=(+6H10X     )                                      BMD 4120
      FMT(1)=(+6H(17X    )                                      BMD 4130
      FMT(2)=BLANKS                                             BMD 4140
      FMT(3)=BLANKS                                             BMD 4150
      FMT(4)=(+6H5(F12.)                                        BMD 4160
```

```
      FMT(5)=(+6H3,8X)/)                                        BMD 4170
      FMT(6)=(+6H7X,    )                                        BMD 4180
      FMT(8)=(+6H4(F12.)                                        BMD 4190
      FMT(9)=(+6H3,8X),)                                        BMD 4200
      FMT(10)=(+6HF12.3))                                       BMD 4210
      TC=(+1H.)                                                 BMD 4220
      TP=(+1H+)                                                 BMD 4230
      CALL SCALE(WMIN,WMAX,100.0,JY,YMIN,YMAX,YIJ)              BMD 4240
      YR=YMAX-YMIN                                              BMD 4250
C         TEST JY, FOR JY EQUAL 0, 10 OR BIGGER 10,TEST KL FOR CALC.CLAB BMD 4260
C         TEST JY, FOR JY SMALLER 0 OR 1 UNTILL 9, COMPUTE CLAB(I)  BMD 4270
  230 J=JY                                                      BMD 4280
      IF(J*(J-10))204,201,201                                   BMD 4290
  201 IF(KL)220,220,231                                         BMD 4300
  231 WRITE OUTPUT TAPE 6,1001                                  BMD 4310
      IF(KL)250,250,220                                         BMD 4320
  220 CLAB(1)=YMIN                                              BMD 4330
      DO 222 I=2,11                                             BMD 4340
  222 CLAB(I)=CLAB(I-1)+YIJ                                     BMD 4350
      WRITE OUPUT TAPE 6,100,(CLAB(I),I=1,11,2),(CLAB(J),J=2,10,2  BMD 4360
      IF(KL)231,231,14                                          BMD 4370
  204 IF(J-5)205,221,207                                        BMD 4380
  207 J=J-5                                                     BMD 4390
  205 JYT=5-J                                                   BMD 4400
  221 CONTINUE                                                  BMD 4410
      IF(KL)226,226,227                                         BMD 4420
  226 FMT(3)=GF(JY)                                             BMD 4430
  225 FMT(7)=GF(JY)                                             BMD 4440
      TT=JY                                                     BMD 4450
      TT=TT*YIJ/10.                                             BMD 4460
      CLAB(1)= YMIN+TT                                          BMD 4470
      DO 223 I=2,10                                             BMD 4480
  223 CLAB(I)=CLAB(I-1) +YIJ                                    BMD 4490
      WRITE OUTPUT TAPE 6,FMT,(CLAB(I),I=2,10,2),(CLAB(J),J=1,9   ,2)  BMD 4500
      IF(KL)227,227,14                                          BMD 4510
  227 IF(JY-5)208,209,208                                       BMD 4520
  209 WRITE OUTPUT TAPE 6,1001                                  BMD 4530
      IF(KL)250,250,226                                         BMD 4540
  208 WRITE OUTPUT TAPE 6,1000,(TC,I=1,J ),((TP,(TC,I=1,4)),K=1,19),TP,(BMD 4550
     1 TC,I=1,JYT)                                              BMD 4560
      IF(KL)250,250,226                                         BMD 4570
  250 CONTINUE                                                  BMD 4580
      NCC=1                                                     BMD 4590
      IC=0                                                      BMD 4600
C         TEST INTEGER VARIABLE NP                              BMD 4610
      IF(NP)80,11,11                                            BMD 4620
C         COMPUTE K,L AND XY(I,J)                               BMD 4630
   11 DO 1 I=1,51                                               BMD 4640
      DO 1 J=1,17                                               BMD 4650
    1 XY(I,J)=BLANKS                                            BMD 4660
      CALL SCALE (ZMIN,ZMAX,50.,JX,XMIN,XMAX,XIJ)               BMD 4670
      XR=XMAX-XMIN                                              BMD 4680
C         TEST INTEGER VARIABLE NC, NC=0 COMPUTE RLAB           BMD 4690
   48 IF(NC)52,13,49                                            BMD 4700
   49 IF(NP)80,10,10                                            BMD 4710
   10 DO 9 N=1,NC                                               BMD 4720
      SYMB=SYM(N)                                               BMD 4730
      XDIFFR=XMAX-X                                             BMD 4740
      IF(XDIFFR)105,106,106                                     BMD 4750
```

```
    105 XDIFFR=0.0                                                      BMD 4760
    106 YDIFFR=YMAX-Y(N)                                                BMD 4770
        IF(YDIFFR)107,108,108                                           BMD 4780
    107 YDIFFR=0.0                                                      BMD 4790
    108 L=51.-(50.*XDIFFR)/XR+.5                                        BMD 4800
        K=101.-(100.*YDIFFR)/YR+.5                                      BMD 4810
        M=XMODF(K,6)                                                    BMD 4820
        K=(K-1)/6+1                                                     BMD 4830
        IF(M)21,16,21                                                   BMD 4840
     16 M=6                                                             BMD 4850
     21 LL=M                                                            BMD 4860
        M=(M-1)*6                                                       BMD 4870
B   19 T=XY(L,K)*XM(LL)                                                 BMD 4880
        CALL FORM2(T,M,SYMB)                                            BMD 4890
B       XY(L,K)=(XY(L,K)*(-XM(LL)))+T                                   BMD 4900
  9     CONTINUE                                                        BMD 4910
        GO TO 15                                                        BMD 4920
C          COMPUTE K AND XY(I,J)                                        BMD 4930
     80 DO 86 I=1,17                                                    BMD 4940
     86 XY(1,I)=BLANKS                                                  BMD 4950
        L=1                                                             BMD 4960
        DO 95 N=1,NC                                                    BMD 4970
        SYMB=SYM(N)                                                     BMD 4980
        YDIFFR=YMAX-Y(N)                                                BMD 4990
        IF(YDIFFR)860,865,865                                           BMD 5000
    860 YDIFFR=0.0                                                      BMD 5010
    865 K=101.-(100.*YDIFFR)/YR+.5                                      BMD 5020
        M=XMODF(K,6)                                                    BMD 5030
        IF(M)90,91,90                                                   BMD 5040
     91 M=6                                                             BMD 5050
     90 LL=M                                                            BMD 5060
        K=(K-1)/6+1                                                     BMD 5070
        M=(M-1)*6                                                       BMD 5080
B       T=XY(L,K)*XM(LL)                                                BMD 5090
        CALL FORM2(T,M,SYMB)                                            BMD 5100
B    95 XY(L,K)=(XY(L,K)*(-XM(LL)))+T                                   BMD 5110
        IF(XMODF(IC,5))97,96,97                                         BMD 5120
     96 W=TP                                                            BMD 5130
        GO TO 98                                                        BMD 5140
     97 W=TC                                                            BMD 5150
     98 WRITE OUTPUT TAPE 6,101,X,W,(XY(1,N),N=1,17),W,X                BMD 5160
        IC=IC+1                                                         BMD 5170
        GO TO 15                                                        BMD 5180
C          COMPUTE RLAB                                                 BMD 5190
     13 M=6-JX                                                          BMD 5200
        LL=50+M                                                         BMD 5210
        T=JX                                                            BMD 5220
        IF(5-JX)131,131,135                                             BMD 5230
    131 T=0.0                                                           BMD 5240
    135 RLAB=XMAX-(T*XIJ)/5.0                                           BMD 5250
        W=TC                                                            BMD 5260
        K=52                                                            BMD 5270
        DO 31 L=M,LL                                                    BMD 5280
        K=K-1                                                           BMD 5290
        I=XMODF(L,5)                                                    BMD 5300
        IF(I-1)2,3,2                                                    BMD 5310
      3 W=TP                                                            BMD 5320
        WRITE OUTPUT TAPE 6,101,RLAB,W,(XY(K,N),N=1,17),W,RLAB         BMD 5330
        RLAB=RLAB-XIJ                                                   BMD 5340
```

```
       W=TC                                                         BMD 5350
       GO TO 31                                                     BMD 5360
    2 WRITE OUTPUT TAPE 6,102,W,(XY(K,N),N=1,17),W                  BMD 5370
   31 CONTINUE                                                      BMD 5380
   52 KL=1                                                          BMD 5390
       GO TO 230                                                    BMD 5400
   14 NCC=0                                                         BMD 5410
   15 RETURN                                                        BMD 5420
          END                                                       BMD 5430
C                                                                   BMD 5440
*      FAP                                                          BMD 5450
       COUNT    20                                                  BMD 5460
       TTL      SUBROUTINE REMOVE FOR BMD01T                        BMD 5470
       LBL      REMOVE,X                                            BMD 5480
*               ENTRY--    CALL REMOVE(I)                           BMD 5490
       ENTRY    REMOVE                                              BMD 5500
REMOVE CLA*     1,4              GET LOCAL TAPE NUMBER              BMD 5510
       SXA      SAVX4,4          SAVE I.R. 4                        BMD 5520
       ADD      =020                                                BMD 5530
       TSX      $(IOS),4         SET UP TAPE ADDRESSES              BMD 5540
       CLA*     $(REW)           GENERATE UNLOAD ADDRESS            BMD 5550
       STA      RUN                                                 BMD 5560
       STA      SDN                                                 BMD 5570
  SDN  SDN      **               WAIT TO FINISH REWINDING           BMD 5580
RUN    RUN      **               REWIND AND UNLOAD                  BMD 5590
SAVX4  AXT      **,4             RESTORE I.R. 4                     BMD 5600
       TRA      2,4              RETURN                             BMD 5610
       END                                                         BMD 5620
C                                                                   BMD 5630
*      LABEL                                                        BMD 5640
*      FORTRAN                                                      BMD 5650
CTABBY    SUBROUTINE TABBY FOR BMD01T                              BMD 5660
       SUBROUTINE TABBY (OMEGA,YY)                                  BMD 5670
       DIMENSION X(5000),FMT(120),YSQ(500),Y(1500),SYM(15),YP(15),  BMD 5680
      1A(1000),B(1000),XX(5000),YY(5000)                            BMD 5690
       COMMON X,FMT,YSQ,Y,SYM,YP,A,B,XX,YY,AMPL,PHASE,TG,FILTER,KPROB, BMD 5700
      1NDATA,FTRI,NTRI,M,FM,NPOINT,POINT,WO,ANS,PI,H                BMD 5710
C         M,FM= NR OF RESOLUTIONS, NTRI,FTRI= NR.OF TRIANGLES MAKING THE BMD 5720
C         FILTER, WO= FREQ.AT WHICH THE FILTER IS CENTERED, P1=3.14159265BMD 5730
       SUM=0.0                                                      BMD 5740
       MMO=M-1                                                      BMD 5750
C         COMPUTING THE SUBEQUATION OF C(M,N,WO)(OMEGA), THE SECOND TERM BMD 5760
       DO 100 J=1,MMO                                               BMD 5770
       FJ=J                                                         BMD 5780
       P=FJ*PI/FM                                                   BMD 5790
       Q=FJ*WO                                                      BMD 5800
       R=FTRI*FJ*PI/FM                                              BMD 5810
       ARG=FJ*OMEGA                                                 BMD 5820
  100 SUM=SUM+(.54+.46*COSF(P))*COSF(Q)*SINF(R)*COSF(ARG)/SINF(P)   BMD 5830
       SUM=4.0*SUM/FM                                               BMD 5840
       S=FM*WO                                                      BMD 5850
       T=FM*OMEGA                                                   BMD 5860
C         TEST FOR THE NR OF TRIANGLES N=NTRI=EVEN -STAT.NR.300, ODD-STATBMD 5870
C         NR.200                                                    BMD 5880
       NIT=NTRI/2                                                   BMD 5890
       IF(NTRI-NIT*2) 200,300,200                                   BMD 5900
C         COMPUTING THE TOTAL EQUATION OF C(M,N,WO)(OMEGA), DEPENDING N BMD 5910
C         IS EVEN OR ODD                                            BMD 5920
  200 YY= (2.0*FTRI/FM)+SUM+2.0*FTRI*(.54+.46*COSF(PI))*COSF(S)*COSF(T)/BMD 5930
```

```
      1FM                                                            BMD 5940
        GO TO 400                                                    BMD 5950
  300 YY= (2.0*FTRI/FM)+SUM-2.0*FTRI*(.54+.46*COSF(PI))*COSF(S)*COSF(T)/BMD 5960
      1FM                                                            BMD 5970
  400 RETURN                                                         BMD 5980
        END                                                          BMD 5990
C                                                                    BMD 6000
*       LABEL                                                        BMD 6010
*       FORTRAN                                                      BMD 6020
CTPWD       SUBROUTINE TPWD FOR BMD01T                               BMD 6030
        SUBROUTINE TPWD(NT1,NT2)                                     BMD 6040
        IF(NT1)40,10,12                                              BMD 6050
 10     NT1=5                                                        BMD 6060
 12     IF(NT1-NT2)14,19,14                                          BMD 6070
 14     IF(NT2-5)15,19,17                                            BMD 6080
   15 REWIND NT2                                                     BMD 6090
        GO TO 19                                                     BMD 6100
   17 CALL REMOVE(NT2)                                               BMD 6110
   19 IF(NT1-5)18,24,18                                              BMD 6120
 18     IF(NT1-6)22,40,22                                            BMD 6130
 22     REWIND NT1                                                   BMD 6140
 24     NT2=NT1                                                      BMD 6150
 28     RETURN                                                       BMD 6160
 40     WRITE OUTPUT TAPE 6,49                                       BMD 6170
        CALL EXIT                                                    BMD 6180
 49     FORMAT(25H ERROR ON TAPE ASSIGNMENT)                        BMD 6190
        END                                                          BMD 6200
C                                                                    BMD 6210
*       LABEL                                                        BMD 6220
*       FORTRAN                                                      BMD 6230
CTRANS          SUBROUTINE TRANS FOR BMD01T                          BMD 6240
        SUBROUTINE TRANS (MISTAK)                                    BMD 6250
        DIMENSION X(5000),FMT(120),YSQ(500),Y(1500),SYM(15),YP(15), BMD 6260
      1A(1000),B(1000),XX(5000),YY(5000)                            BMD 6270
        DIMENSION IBIN (10),CON(10)                                  BMD 6280
        COMMON X,FMT,YSQ,Y,SYM,YP,A,B,XX,YY,AMPL,PHASE,TG,FILTER,KPROB, BMD 6290
      1NDATA,FTRI,NTRI,M,FM,NPOINT,POINT,WO,ANS,PI,H                BMD 6300
        EQUIVALENCE(ITG,SPECTG)                                      BMD 6310
C                                                                    BMD 6320
 1001 FORMAT(11H0DATA POINT I5,57H VIOLATES THE RESTRICTION FOR TRANSGENBMD 6330
      XERATION OF THE TYPEI3,52H. THE PROGRAM CONTINUES LEAVING THE VALUEBMD 6340
      X UNCHANGED.)                                                  BMD 6350
 1002 FORMAT(A6,I1,8(I2,F6.0))                                       BMD 6360
 1003 FORMAT(58H0CONTROL CARD ERROR. PROGRAM EXPECTED A SPECTG CARD BUT BMD 6370
      XA A6,16H CARD WAS FOUND.)                                    BMD 6380
 1004 FORMAT(42H0PROGRAM WILL GO TO NEXT PROBLEM CARD.)             BMD 6390
 1005 FORMAT(40H0ILLEGAL TRANSGENERATION CODE SPECIFIED.)           BMD 6400
C                                                                    BMD 6410
        ASNF(V)=ATANF(V)/SQRTF(1.0-V**2)                            BMD 6420
        SPECTG=(+6HSPECTG)                                          BMD 6430
        READ INPUT TAPE5,1002,KODE,NTRAN,(IBIN(I),CON(I),I=1,NTRAN) BMD 6440
C         FOR KODE EQUAL TO ITG, COMPUTE JESUS.                     BMD 6450
        IF(KODE-ITG)900,400,900                                     BMD 6460
  400 DO 500 I=1,NTRAN                                               BMD 6470
        IF(IBIN(I)-17) 605,600,605                                  BMD 6480
  605 JESUS=IBIN(I)                                                  BMD 6490
C         JESUS MUST BE NOT BE EQUAL 6 FOR THIS ROUTE.              BMD 6500
        IF(JESUS-6)610,905,610                                      BMD 6510
  600 JESUS=6                                                        BMD 6520
```

```
   610 CC=CON(I)                                                     BMD 6530
C          TEST JESUS, MUST BE 1. UNTILL 10.                         BMD 6540
       IF(JESUS*(JESUS-11)) 620,905,905                              BMD 6550
C          COMPUTE FOR JESUS BETWEEN 1.UNTILL 10.THE REAL VARIABLE X(K)  BMD 6560
   620 DO 150 K=1,NPOINT                                             BMD 6570
       GO TO (10,20,30,40,50,60,70,80,90,100)   ,JESUS              BMD 6580
    10 IF(X(K))200,150,14                                            BMD 6590
    14 X(K)=SQRTF(X(K))                                              BMD 6600
       GO TO 150                                                     BMD 6610
    20 IF(X(K))200,22,23                                             BMD 6620
    22 X(K)=1.0                                                      BMD 6630
       GO TO 150                                                     BMD 6640
    23  X(K)=SQRTF(X(K))+SQRTF(X(K)+1.0)                             BMD 6650
       GO TO 150                                                     BMD 6660
    30 IF(X(K))200,200,31                                            BMD 6670
    31 X(K)=0.4342944819*LOGF(X(K))                                  BMD 6680
       GO TO 150                                                     BMD 6690
    40 X(K)=EXPF(X(K))                                               BMD 6700
       GO TO 150                                                     BMD 6710
    50 IF(X(K))200,150,53                                            BMD 6720
    53 IF (X(K)-1.0) 54,55,200                                       BMD 6730
    54  ARG =SQRTF(X(K))                                             BMD 6740
       X(K)=ASNF(ARG)                                                BMD 6750
       GO TO 150                                                     BMD 6760
    55 X(K)=PI/2.0                                                   BMD 6770
       GO TO 150                                                     BMD 6780
    60 IF(X(K))200,200,61                                            BMD 6790
    61 X(K)=LOGF(X(K))                                               BMD 6800
       GO TO 150                                                     BMD 6810
    70 IF(X(K))71,200,71                                             BMD 6820
    71 X(K)=1.0/X(K)                                                 BMD 6830
       GO TO 150                                                     BMD 6840
    80 X(K)=X(K)+CC                                                  BMD 6850
       GO TO 150                                                     BMD 6860
    90 X(K)=X(K)*CC                                                  BMD 6870
       GO TO 150                                                     BMD 6880
   100 IF(X(K))200,200,101                                           BMD 6890
   101 X(K)=X(K)**CC                                                 BMD 6900
       GO TO 150                                                     BMD 6910
   200 WRITE OUTPUT TAPE 6,1001,K,IBIN(I)                            BMD 6920
   150 CONTINUE                                                      BMD 6930
   500 CONTINUE                                                      BMD 6940
   300 RETURN                                                        BMD 6950
   900 WRITE OUTPUT TAPE 6,1003,KODE                                 BMD 6960
   901 WRITE OUTPUT TAPE 6,1004                                      BMD 6970
       MISTAK=17                                                     BMD 6980
       GO TO 300                                                     BMD 6990
   905 WRITE OUTPUT TAPE 6,1005                                      BMD 7000
       GO TO 901                                                     BMD 7010
       END                                                           BMD 7020
C                                                                    BMD 7030
*      LABEL                                                         BMD 7040
*      FORTRAN                                                       BMD 7050
CVFCHCK     SUBROUTINE TO CHECK FOR PROPER NUMBER OF VARIABLE FORMAT CRDSBMD 7060
       SUBROUTINE VFCHCK(NVF)                                        BMD 7070
       IF(NVF)10,10,20                                               BMD 7080
    10 WRITE OUTPUT TAPE 6,4000                                      BMD 7090
       NVF=1                                                         BMD 7100
    50 RETURN                                                        BMD 7110
```

```
C                                                                    BMD 7120
 20     IF(NVF-10)50,50,10                                           BMD 7130
C                                                                    BMD 7140
 4000 FORMAT(1H023X71HNUMBER OF VARIABLE FORMAT CARDS INCORRECTLY SPECIFBMD 7150
     XIED, ASSUMED TO BE 1.)                                         BMD 7160
      END                                                            BMD 7170
C                                                                    BMD 7180
*       LABEL                                                        BMD 7190
*       FORTRAN                                                      BMD 7200
CSCALE          SUBROUTINE SCALE FOR SUB PLOTR                       BMD 7210
      SUBROUTINE SCALE(YMIN,YMAX,YINT,JY,TYMIN,TYMAX,YIJ)            BMD 7220
      DIMENSION C(10)                                                BMD 7230
      C(1)=1.0                                                       BMD 7240
      C(2)=1.5                                                       BMD 7250
      C(3)=2.0                                                       BMD 7260
      C(4)=3.0                                                       BMD 7270
      C(5)=4.0                                                       BMD 7280
      C(6)=5.0                                                       BMD 7290
      C(7)=7.5                                                       BMD 7300
      C(8)=10.0                                                      BMD 7310
B     TEST=154400000000                                              BMD 7320
C        TEST FOR (YMAX-YMIN)/YINT IS A POWER OF 10 OR NOT.          BMD 7330
 50   YR=YMAX-YMIN                                                   BMD 7340
      TT=YR/YINT                                                     BMD 7350
      J=LOG10F(TT)                                                   BMD 7360
      E=10.0**J                                                      BMD 7370
C        WHEN'OLD'-TT IS A POWER OF 10, THEN 'NEW'-TT IS 1.          BMD 7380
      TT=TT/E                                                        BMD 7390
      I=0                                                            BMD 7400
      IF(TT-1.0)205,201,201                                          BMD 7410
 205  TT=TT*10.0                                                     BMD 7420
      E=E/10.0                                                       BMD 7430
 201  I=I+1                                                          BMD 7440
      IF(8-I)1,2,2                                                   BMD 7450
 1    E=E*10.0                                                       BMD 7460
      I=1                                                            BMD 7470
C        TEST (TT-C(I)) VALUE 1.BIGGER ZERO, INCREASE I AND TEST AGAIN BMD 7480
C                             2.EQUAL ZERO,COMPUTE YMIN/C(I) TO CALC.YIJBMD 7490
C                             3.SMALLER ZERO, COMPUTE YIJ             BMD 7500
 2    IF(TT-C(I))233,202,201                                         BMD 7510
C        COMPUTE TYMIN,TYMAX,JY, AND YIJ AS A OUTPUT OF THIS SUBROUTINE.BMD 7520
 233  YIJ=C(I)*E                                                     BMD 7530
      GO TO 203                                                      BMD 7540
 202  Y=YMIN/C(I)                                                    BMD 7550
      J=Y                                                            BMD 7560
      T=J                                                            BMD 7570
      IF(0.0001-ABSF(T-Y)204,233,233                                BMD 7580
 204  YIJ=C(I+1)*E                                                   BMD 7590
 203  X=((YMAX+YMIN)/YIJ-YINT )/2.0+.0001                            BMD 7600
      K=X                                                            BMD 7610
      IF(K)235,240,240                                               BMD 7620
 235  Y=K                                                            BMD 7630
      IF(X-Y)236,240,236                                             BMD 7640
 236  K=K-1                                                          BMD 7650
 240  TYMIN=K                                                        BMD 7660
      TYMIN=YIJ*TYMIN                                                BMD 7670
      TYMAX=TYMIN+YINT*YIJ                                           BMD 7680
C        TEST (YMAX-TYMAX) MUST BE SMALLER OR EQUAL TEST-VALUE.      BMD 7690
      IF(YMAX-TYMAX-TEST)10,10,201                                   BMD 7700
```

```
      10 TT=YINT/10.                                              BMD 7710
         JY=TT+.000001                                            BMD 7720
         YIJ=YINT*(YIJ/10.0)                                      BMD 7730
         J=TYMIN/ YIJ                                             BMD 7740
         IF (K)242,241,241                                        BMD 7750
     242 J=J-1                                                    BMD 7760
     241 J=J*JY+JY-K                                              BMD 7770
         JY=J                                                     BMD 7780
         RETURN                                                   BMD 7790
         END                                                      BMD 7800
C                                                                 BMD 7810
*     LABEL                                                       BMD 7820
*     FORTRAN                                                     BMD 7830
CPHAZE          SUBROUTINE PHAZE FOR BMD01T                       BMD 7840
         SUBROUTINE PHAZE(X,Y,Z)                                  BMD 7850
C        DEFINE CONSTANTS PI AND PI2                              BMD 7860
         PI=3.14159265                                            BMD 7870
         PI2=2.0*PI                                               BMD 7880
C        COMPUTE THE PHAZE Z, DEPENDING ON THE X AND Y VALUES, FOR THE   BMD 7890
C        CALCULATION OF THE ARGUMENT PHI=ARCTG(Y/X)              BMD 7900
C        X=NEG    Y=NEG    PHI=POS    PHAZE Z=PI+PHI             BMD 7910
C        X=NEG    Y=0      PHI=0      PHAZE Z=PI                 BMD 7920
C        X=NEG    Y=POS    PHI=NEG    PHAZE Z=PI-PHI             BMD 7930
         AB=ABSF(Y/X)                                            BMD 7940
         PHI=ATANF(AB)                                           BMD 7950
         IF(X.)11,12,13                                          BMD 7960
      11 IF(Y)17,30,18                                           BMD 7970
      17 Z=PI+PHI                                                BMD 7980
         GO TO 50                                                BMD 7990
      30 Z=PI                                                    BMD 8000
         GO TO 50                                                BMD 8010
      18 Z=PI-PHI                                                BMD 8020
         GO TO 50                                                BMD 8030
C        X=0      Y=NEG    PHI=-INFINITY    PHAZE Z=270          BMD 8040
C        X=0      Y=0      PHI=0            PHAZE Z=0            BMD 8050
C        X=0      Y=POS    PHI=+INFINITY    PHAZE Z=90          BMD 8060
      12 IF(Y)35,15,40                                           BMD 8070
      35 Z=0.75*PI2                                              BMD 8080
         GO TO 50                                                BMD 8090
      15 Z=0.0                                                   BMD 8100
         GO TO 50                                                BMD 8110
      40 Z=PI/2.0                                                BMD 8120
         GO TO 50                                                BMD 8130
C        X=POS    Y=NEG    PHI=NEG    PHAZE Z=PI2-PHI            BMD 8140
C        X=POS    Y=0      PHI=0      PHAZE Z=0                  BMD 8150
C        X=POS    Y=POS    PHI=POS    PHAZE Z=PHI               BMD 8160
      13 IF(Y)14,15,16                                           BMD 8170
      14 Z=PI2-PHI                                               BMD 8180
         GO TO 50                                                BMD 8190
      16 Z=PHI                                                   BMD 8200
      50 RETURN                                                  BMD 8210
         END                                                     BMD 8220
*     DATA                                                       BMD 8230
*STORE                                                           BMD 8240
```

# Estimation of the Parameters of a Truncated Gamma Distribution in the Case of Neuronal Spike Data

J. L. BLOM*, J. OOSTERHOFF AND R. WIGGERS

*Netherlands Central Institute for Brain Research and Mathematical Center, Amsterdam (The Netherlands)*

## INTRODUCTION

Since the publication of Brink *et al.* (1946) which concerned the interspike-interval histogram of a chemically excited nerve fiber, quantitative analysis of neuronal activity has used a variety of statistical procedures.

In a review article Moore *et al.* (1966) distinguished two different kinds of approach, one dealing with methods describing the observed activity in terms of statistical functions, the other one describing the spike generating process with theoretically derived models (e.g. Gerstein and Mandelbrot, 1964; Stein, 1965; Gluss, 1967; Enright, 1967).

In the description in terms of statistical functions of the observed spike data, the serial aspect can be dealt with by auto- and serial correlation functions and its derivatives (Cox *et al.*, 1966). With this method the stability of the firing pattern and the interdependency of the spike intervals can be analysed (Werner *et al.*, 1963).

The interspike-interval histogram of neuronal activity is a sample of grouped observations taken during a definite period of time. With this method the time sequence of the observed activity is lost.

In analysing this distribution many authors find a resemblance of the empirical distribution to a gamma- or exponential distribution (Kuffler *et al.*, 1957; Rodieck *et al.*, 1962; Hyvärinen, 1966). However, the right hand tails of the empirical distributions tend to be much heavier than predicted by a gamma distribution. Since these deviations have a relatively high influence on the estimation of the scale and shape parameters of the distribution, we investigated the question whether a truncated gamma distribution could be fitted to the major part of the observations, discarding the large interspike intervals.

We describe here our procedure for estimating the origin, scale, and shape parameters of a truncated gamma distribution which is based on a paper by Chapman (1956). The text of an ALGOL-60 program which was run on the EL X-8 computer of the Mathematical Center (Amsterdam) to analyse the data recorded by one of us (J.L.B.) is also presented.

---

* Present address: Laboratory of Ergonomic Psychology TNO, Zuiderzeeweg 10, Amsterdam (The Netherlands).

*References p. 229*

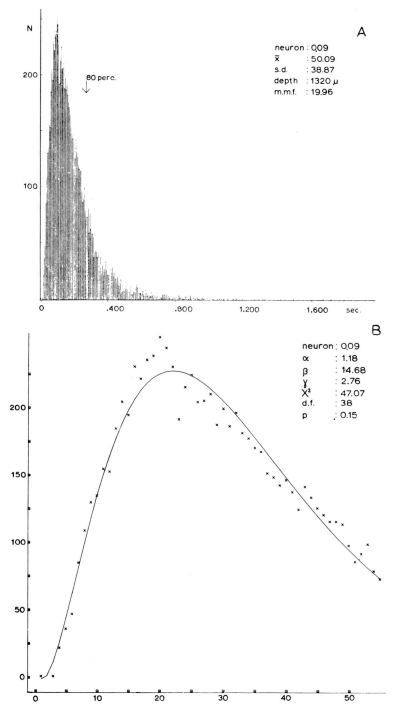

Fig. 1. Untruncated (A) and truncated (B) interval histogram of neuron nr. 009. In this neuron 8.146 intervals were used, covering 55 classes. A good fit was found to the truncated gamma-distribution. Its S-value was 0.006.

The input for this program is derived from interval histograms generated with a Data Retrieval Computer (DRC, Nuclear Chicago). Herewith the number of classes is restricted to 400. Different epochs—an epoch being the span of time of the longest measurable interval—were used to cover more than 98% of all recorded intervals. By means of a conversion (see program description) based on the different epochs all times were expressed in milliseconds.

A graphical display of the in- and output of the program was made with special plot procedures in ALGOL-60 on the EL X-1 computer of the Mathematical Center (Amsterdam). (Fig. 1A, B)

### MATHEMATICAL DESCRIPTION

Let the random variable $t$ be distributed according to a truncated gamma distribution with density function

$$p(t; \alpha, \beta, \gamma) = \begin{cases} \dfrac{1}{K} \, e^{-\beta(t-\alpha)} (t-\alpha)^{\gamma-1} & \alpha < t < M \\ 0 & \text{elsewhere} \end{cases} \quad (1)$$

where

$$K = K(\alpha, \beta, \gamma) = \int_{\alpha}^{M} e^{-\beta(t-\alpha)} (t-\alpha)^{\gamma-1} dt$$

In this formula, $M$ is a fixed point of truncation, $\alpha$ is the origin, $\beta$ the scale parameter and $\gamma$ the shape parameter of the distribution. If $\gamma = 1$, the distribution is a translated and truncated exponential distribution.

Let $n$ independent observations of $t$ be grouped into $m$ classes, where class $i$ extends from $1_i - h_i$ to $1_i + h_i$, $i = 1, 2, \ldots, m$, and $1_1 - h_1 = \alpha$,
$$1_i + h_i = 1_{i+1} \quad (i = 1, 2, \ldots, m-1), \quad 1_m + h_m = M.$$
Let $x_i$ denote the number of observations falling into class $i$ ($i = 1, 2, \ldots, m$). The basic approximation proposed by Chapman transforms the estimation problem to a least-squares problem. Define

$$p_i = \frac{1}{K} \int_{1_i - h_i}^{1_i + h_i} e^{-\beta(t-\alpha)} (t-\alpha)^{\gamma-1} dt \quad (i = 1, 2, \ldots, m) \quad (2)$$

and approximate the right-hand member by

$$2h_i \, \frac{1}{K} \, e^{-\beta \, (1_i - \alpha)} (1_i - \alpha)^{(\gamma-1)}$$

Then approximately

$$\ln(p_i/p_{i+1}) \simeq \beta(1_{i+1} - 1_i) + (\gamma - 1) \left[ (\ln(1_i - \alpha) - \ln(1_{i+1} - \alpha) \right] + \ln(h_i/h_{i+1}) \quad (3)$$

suggesting that for a given $\alpha$ the parameters $\beta$ and $\gamma$ can be estimated by a least-squares procedure, replacing $p_i$ by its estimate $x_i/n$. As the random variables $\ln(x_i/x_{i+1})$ are heteroscedastic, weights have to be introduced which must be estimated from the observations.

Let us assume for a moment that $\alpha$ is known. Define

$$y_i = \ln(x_i/x_{i+1}) - \ln (h_i/h_{i+1}), \ i = 1, 2, ..., m-1. \tag{4}$$

and let $y$ denote the corresponding column vector. Chapman has shown that $y_1, y_2,$ ..., $y_{m-1}$ have asymptotically for $n \to \infty$ a multivariate normal distribution with means

$$\beta (1_{i+1} - 1_i) + (\gamma - 1) [\ln(1_i - a) - \ln(1_{i+1} - a)] \ \ (i = 1, 2, ..., m-1)$$

and covariance matrix

$$C = \frac{1}{n} \begin{bmatrix} \left[\dfrac{1}{p_1} + \dfrac{1}{p_2}\right] & \left[-\dfrac{1}{p_2}\right] & 0 & & \cdots & 0 \\[2ex] \left[-\dfrac{1}{p_2}\right] & \left[\dfrac{1}{p_2} + \dfrac{1}{p_3}\right] & \left[-\dfrac{1}{p_3}\right] & & \cdots & 0 \\[2ex] [0] & \left[-\dfrac{1}{p_3}\right] & \left[\dfrac{1}{p_3} + \dfrac{1}{p_4}\right] & & \cdots & 0 \\[2ex] & \cdot & \cdot & \cdot & & \cdot \\ & \cdot & \cdot & \cdot & & \cdot \\ & \cdot & \cdot & \cdot & & \cdot \\ 0 & 0 & 0 & & \left[\cdots \ \dfrac{1}{p_{m-1}} + \dfrac{1}{p_m}\right] \end{bmatrix}$$

Hence, least-squares estimates of $\beta$ and $\gamma$ are found by minimizing the quadratic form

$$(y - Ey)^T \ C^{-1}(y - Ey) \tag{5}$$

where $y$ denotes a column vector, the superscript $^T$ denotes transposition, $C^{-1}$ is the inverse of the matrix $C$, and $E$ denotes expectation.

Since the true values of the $p_i$ are not known, it is necessary to replace the $p_i$ in $C$ by their estimates $x_i/n$. Let us denote the resulting matrix by $\hat{C}$.

Let

$$\begin{aligned} f_i &= 1_{i+1} - 1_i & (i = 1, 2, ..., m-1) \\ g_i &= \ln(1_i - a) - \ln(1_{i+1} - a) & (i = 1, 2, ..., m-1) \\ w_i &= y_i - \beta f_i - (\gamma - 1)g_i & (i = 1, 2, ..., m-1) \end{aligned}$$

and let $f$, $g$ and $w$ denote the corresponding column vectors. The quadratic form (5) transforms into

$$w^T \ \hat{C}^{-1}w$$

and this form is minimized by the least-squares estimates $\hat{\beta}$ and $\hat{\gamma}$ of $\beta$ and $\gamma$ defined by

$$\hat{\beta} = \hat{\varLambda}^{-1} \mid (g^T \ \hat{C}^{-1}g) \, (f^T \ \hat{C}^{-1}w) - (f^T \ \hat{C}^{-1}g) \, (g^T \ \hat{C}^{-1}w) \mid \tag{6}$$

$$\hat{\gamma} = \hat{\varLambda}^{-1} \mid (f^T \ \hat{C}^{-1}f) \, (g^T \ \hat{C}^{-1}w) - (f^T \ \hat{C}^{-1}g) \, (f^T \ \hat{C}^{-1}w) \mid \tag{7}$$

where

$$\hat{\varLambda} = (f^T \ \hat{C}^{-1}f) \, (g^T \ \hat{C}^{-1}g) - (f^T \ \hat{C}^{-1}g)^2. \tag{8}$$

The computation of $\hat{\beta}$ and $\hat{\gamma}$ from these quotations is facilitated by the tridiagonal form of the matrix $\hat{C}$.

Having obtained the estimates $\hat{\beta}$ and $\hat{\alpha}$, the probabilities $p_i$ ($i = 1, 2, \ldots, m$) are estimated from (2), replacing $\beta$ and $\gamma$ by $\hat{\beta}$ and $\hat{\gamma}$, with the aid of a procedure for computing the incomplete gamma function. This leads to a new estimate $\hat{\hat{C}}$, of the matrix $C$, and we repeat the same process to obtain better estimates $\hat{\hat{\beta}}$ and $\hat{\hat{\gamma}}$ of $\beta$ and $\gamma$, replacing $\hat{C}$ by $\hat{\hat{C}}$ in (6), (7) and (8).

An asymptotic estimate of the covariance matrix of the ultimate estimators $\hat{\hat{\beta}}$ and $\hat{\hat{\gamma}}$ is

$$\hat{\hat{A}}^{-1} \begin{bmatrix} f^T \hat{C}^{-1} f & -f^T \hat{C}^{-1} g \\ -f^T \hat{C}^{-1} g & g^T \hat{C}^{-1} g \end{bmatrix}$$

If the origin $\alpha$ is unknown we also have to estimate $\alpha$. The method of linearization as proposed in the paper by Chapman (1956) cannot be applied since the restriction introduced by Chapman for this case is not satisfied in the present problem. However, we can obtain an approximate least-squares estimate $\hat{\alpha}$ (or $\hat{\hat{\alpha}}$ respectively) in such a way that the quadratic form

$$w^T \hat{C}^{-1} w \text{ (or } w^T \hat{\hat{C}}^{-1} w \text{ respectively)}$$

is approximately minimized. To this end, a number of trial values for $\alpha$ is investigated and the value that is best in this sense is chosen as an estimate for $\alpha$. This estimation process may be expected to produce reasonable results if the class frequencies $x_i$ are not too small and the width of the classes not too great. If the frequencies $x_i$ are smaller than some predetermined number $Q$, depending on the total number of observations $n$, adjacent classes are pooled.

The definition of $\beta$ and $\gamma$ implies that both parameters are positive. However, the estimation procedure does not necessarily produce positive estimates. In those cases in which one of both estimates turned out to be negative, a coarser grouping was tried. The program contains a transformation of the scale and the origin to reduce the time span to msec. An example of the results is presented. The details are dealt with elsewhere by one of us (J. L. B., 1969). (Table I).

As was pointed out at the start, the point of truncation M should be fixed. In the present problem truncation of the gamma distribution was introduced because Blom (1969) found that the right-hand tails of the empirical distributions were too heavy to give a reasonable fit to an untruncated gamma distribution. As a point of truncation the 80% sample percentile was chosen rather arbitrarily. Since this point of truncation depends on the observations, the foregoing analysis is not quite correct. However, when the samples are large, the 80% sample percentile has a small variance and one may expect that the estimation procedure is satisfactory in this case. We note that the more sophisticated estimation procedure discussed by Wilk *et al.* (1962), which is based on the $n$ smallest from a total of $N$ observations, cannot be applied to this problem since the 80% points of the empirical distribution is not the 80% point of a sample from a gamma distribution, due to the heavy tails of the samples.

To judge the fit of observations to a theoretical distribution one should always inspect the fit by eye. This is especially important if one does not expect that the observations follow the hypothetical distribution exactly (in this case the truncated gamma distribution) aiming only at a reasonable description of the observations. To obtain a

# TABLE 1

NEURON NR. 911. DURING 70 MINUTES REGISTRATION 1508 INTERVALS WERE RECORDED FROM WHICH 1206, BEING 80 PERCENT OF THE TOTAL, ARE ANALYZED IN THE PROGRAM. EPOCH TIME WAS 4000 MSEC. GIVING A CLASS WIDTH OF 10 MSEC.

Neuron = 911
Sum of observations = 1206
Estimated parameters first step:

| Alpha | Beta | Gamma | Sum of sq |
|---|---|---|---|
| +1.700000 | +.058361 | +1.168485 | +18.863530 |
| +1.650000 | +.059066 | +1.182517 | +18.697640 |
| +1.600000 | +.059756 | +1.196382 | +18.606058 |
| +1.550000 | +.060432 | +1.210093 | +18.581785 |
| +1.500000 | +.061095 | +1.223662 | +18.618583 |
| +1.450000 | +.061746 | +1.237102 | +18.710874 |
| +1.400000 | +.062385 | +1.250421 | +18.853657 |
| +1.350000 | +.063013 | +1.263629 | +19.042431 |
| +1.300000 | +.063631 | +1.276734 | +19.273142 |
| +1.250000 | +.064239 | +1.289745 | +19.542121 |

Estimated parameters second step

| | | | |
|---|---|---|---|
| +1.700000 | +.059219 | +1.172729 | +17.909893 |
| +1.650000 | +.059914 | +1.186075 | +17.687146 |
| +1.600000 | +.060601 | +1.199422 | +17.541154 |
| +1.550000 | +.061281 | +1.212775 | +17.464628 |
| +1.500000 | +.061954 | +1.226133 | +17.451088 |
| +1.450000 | +.062622 | +1.239501 | +17.494753 |
| +1.400000 | +.063284 | +1.252879 | +17.590445 |
| +1.350000 | +.063941 | +1.266268 | +17.733514 |
| +1.300000 | +.064592 | +1.279669 | +17.919769 |
| +1.250000 | +.065238 | +1.293085 | +18.145423 |

Best estimations: Alfastar  = + 15.000000
Betastar  = +161.408907
Gammastar = +1.226133

Estimated beta and gamma covariance matrix:  +.000020    +.000225
+.000225    +.003303

| Classes | Expected freq. | Observed freq. | Chi-sq. diff. |
|---|---|---|---|
| 2 – 3 | +58.561994 | +61 | +.101497 |
| 4 – 4 | +47.380051 | +44 | +.241130 |
| 5 – 5 | +48.870325 | +46 | +.168584 |
| 6 – 6 | +49.044325 | +45 | +.333506 |
| 7 – 7 | +48.494526 | +54 | +.625024 |
| 8 – 8 | +47.505750 | +49 | +.047000 |
| 9 – 9 | +46.239461 | +50 | +.305835 |
| 10 – 10 | +44.796415 | +43 | +.072039 |
| 11 – 11 | +43.243473 | +47 | +.326327 |
| 12 – 12 | +41.626872 | +48 | +.975734 |
| 13 – 13 | +39.979493 | +48 | +1.609038 |
| 14 – 14 | +38.325162 | +30 | +1.808429 |
| 15 – 16 | +71.742198 | +70 | +.042308 |
| 17 – 18 | +65.398410 | +60 | +.445620 |
| 19 – 20 | +59.388454 | +66 | +.736044 |
| 21 – 22 | +53.770018 | +47 | +.852392 |
| 23 – 24 | +48.566420 | +48 | +.006606 |
| 25 – 26 | +43.780008 | +47 | +.236828 |
| 27 – 28 | +39.400306 | +32 | +1.389952 |
| 29 – 31 | +51.732401 | +56 | +.352050 |
| 32 – 34 | +43.961088 | +41 | +.199450 |
| 35 – 38 | +48.387261 | +48 | +.003099 |
| 39 – 42 | +38.718180 | +35 | +.357064 |
| 43 – 48 | +43.915226 | +39 | +.550138 |
| 49 – 57 | +43.172184 | +52 | +1.805105 |

→

Chi-square = +13.590802
D.F. = +22
P = +.915364

numerical measure of the fit to the truncated gamma distribution, a chi-square test of goodness of fit was performed, comparing the estimated class frequencies $n\hat{p}_i$ (based on $\hat{\hat{\beta}}, \hat{\hat{\gamma}}$ and $\hat{\hat{\alpha}}$) and the observed class frequencies, where classes with small expectations were pooled again. The tail probability of this test may then serve as a measure of the fit. Since small deviations from the hypothetical distribution may lead to extremely small tail probabilities if the number of observations is large, these tail probabilities should be interpreted with sufficient care. For a lucid exposition of the chi-square test we refer to a paper by Cochran (1952).

## INPUT–OUTPUT DESCRIPTION

### Control numbers

1. integer number indicating the number of problems to be calculated (nprob).
2. number of classes constituting the interval histogram, equal for all problems (classes).
3. sample percentile of truncation, no truncation is 1 (truncation).
4. nprob times the specific numbers code and scale, the last being a power of two, for converting the class value to milliseconds.
   For scale = 0 the epoch time of the DRC is 125 milliseconds.
5. nprob times a set of observations.

### Used input- and output procedures

| | |
|---|---|
| READ: | reads the next number from tape. |
| CARRIAGE(n): | printer steps up n lines. |
| PRINTTEXT(s): | prints a string of characters s, given in the program. |
| FIXT(n,m,x): | prints the numeric value of number x with n characters before and m characters after the dec. point, adding a sign and the dec. point. |
| ABSFIXT(n,m,x): | analogon of FIXT(n,m,x) except that no sign is printed. |
| NEW PAGE: | printing continues on top of new page. |
| PRSYM(n): | prints the character internally represented in the decimal value n. |
| NLCR: | printing continues on new line, carriage returns. |
| SPACE(n): | advances the printing position n spaces. |
| FIXP(n,m,x): | punching analogon of FIXT(n,m,x). |
| ABSFIXP(n,m,x): | punching analogon of ABSFIXT(n,m,x). |
| PUNLCR: | punching analogon of NLCR. |
| PUHEP(n): | punches the binary representation of n as one heptad. |
| RUNOUT: | provides tapefeed. |

←━━

The estimated parameters together with the least square estimate for different $\alpha$ from first and second step are given, the best $\alpha$, the best $\alpha$, $\beta$ and $\gamma$ and covariance matrix of $\beta$ and $\gamma$, and thereafter the expected and observed frequency distributions are printed together with the class number comprised for calculations of the chi-square differences. At the end the chi-square value, the degree of freedom and the tail probability according to the chi-square test for goodness of fit are given

*References p. 229*

```
begin integer n, i, i0, q, q1, q2, aantal, j, j1, som, k1, k2, s, s0, prob, nprob, m,
  code, scale, classes;
  real v1, v2, v3, v4, v5, var1, var2, var3, tau, det, c1, c2, c3, c4, c5, func1, func2,
  som2, chi, Pchi, KK, min, truncation;
  boolean b;
  real array alfa, beta, betaster, gamma, gammaster, Kster, K, V1, V2, V4[1:40];
  boolean array Kgrof, Kstergrof, stap1[1:40];

  procedure FIX(l, m, n);
  begin ABSFIXT(l, m, n); ABSFIXP(l, m, n);  end;


  real procedure DETSOLTRI(n, a, b, c, d); value n, a, b, c; integer n; array a, b, c, d;
  comment a,d[1:n],b,c[1:n-1];
  begin comment DETSOLTRI calculates the determinant of a tridiagonal matrix;
    integer i;
    real det, s, m;
    det:= 1;
    for i:= 1 step 1 until n - 1 do
    begin if abs(a[i]) > abs(c[i]) then
        begin m:= - c[i] / a[i]; a[i + 1]:= m × b[i] + a[i + 1];
          d[i + 1]:= m × d[i] + d[i + 1]; c[i]:= 0
        end
        else
        begin m:= a[i] / c[i]; a[i]:= c[i]; s:= b[i]; b[i]:= a[i + 1];
          a[i + 1]:= m × b[i] - s; s:= d[i]; d[i]:= d[i + 1]; d[i + 1]:= m × d[i] - s;
          if i < n - 1 then
          begin c[i]:= b[i + 1]; b[i + 1]:= m × c[i] end
        end;
        det:= a[i] × det
    end UPPER;
    DETSOLTRI:= a[n] × det; d[n]:= d[n] / a[n];
    d[n - 1]:= (d[n - 1] - b[n - 1] × d[n]) / a[n - 1];
    for i:= n - 2 step - 1 until 1 do d[i]:= (d[i] - b[i] × d[i + 1] - c[i] × d[i + 2])
    / a[i]
  end DETSOLTRI;


  real procedure lika(x); value x; real x;
  begin real y;
    boolean alfa;
    if x < 0 then
    begin alfa:= true; x:= abs(x);  end
    else alfa:= false; x:= x / sqrt(2); y:= 1 / (1 + 0.3275911 × x);
    y:= ((((0.94064607 × y - 1.28782245) × y + 1.25969513) × y - 0.252128668) × y +
    0.225836846) × y × 1.12837917 × exp( - x × x);
    lika:= if alfa then y / 2 else 1 - y / 2;
  end lika;


  real procedure GAM(q); value q; real q;
  begin comment GAM calculates the function value of the complete gammafunction, 0<q<200;
    real t, s;
    s:= 1.0;
GG: if q < 4 then
    begin s:= s × q; q:= q + 1; goto GG;  end;
    t:= 1 / q;
    GAM:= exp( - q) × q ∧ (q - 0.5) × 2.506628275 × (1.0 + (.8333333333₁₀ - 1 +
    (.34722222₁₀ - 2 - .2681327₁₀ - 2 × t) × t) × t) / s;
```

```
end GAM;


real procedure incgam(x, p); value x, p; real x, p;
begin comment incgam calculates the function value of the incomplete gammafuntion;
    real a, b, A, Z;
    a:= x ∧ (p − 1); b:= 1; A:= 0;
incga: if p < 5 then
    begin b:= b × p; a:= x × a / p; A:= A + a; p:= p + 1; goto incga;  end;
    a:= p − 0.3333333 + (0.0197531 + 0.0072114 / p) / p; a:= ln(x / a);
    a:= sqrt(p − 0.2777778 + 0.0270576 / p) × a × (1 + a × (0.1666667 − (0.0098765 +
    0.0036057 / p) / p + a × (0.0277778 − 0.0009774 / p + a × (0.0037037 − 0.0000184
    / p + a × (0.0004244 + a × (0.0000312 + a × 0.0000020))))))); Z:= lika(a);
    if A > + 0.1₁₀ − 20 then Z:= Z + exp( − x) × b × A / GAM(p); incgam:= Z;
end incgam;


real procedure vecvec(l, u, shift, a, b); value l, u, shift; integer l, u, shift;
array a, b;
begin integer k;
    real s;
    s:= 0;
    for k:= 1 step 1 until u do s:= a[k] × b[shift + k] + s; vecvec:= s
end vecvec;


real procedure SUM(i, a, b, x); value b; integer i, a, b; real x;
begin real s;
    s:= 0;
    for i:= a step 1 until b do s:= s + x; SUM:= s
end;

nprob:= READ; classes:= READ; truncation:= READ;
begin integer array x, z, z1, k, L, Z[1:classes], cel[1:nprob,1:2];
    real array h, h1, l, l1, pster, P, chichi[1:classes];
    for i:= 1 step 1 until nprob do
    for j:= 1, 2 do cel[i,j]:= READ;
    for prob:= 1 step 1 until nprob do
    begin code:= cel[prob,1]; scale:= cel[prob,2]; n:= s:= 0; b:= true;
        for i:= 1 step 1 until 40 do Kgrof[i]:= Kstergrof[i]:= stap1[i]:= false;
        for i:= 1 step 1 until classes do
        begin x[i]:= READ; n:= n + x[i]; if b ∧ x[i] > 0 then
            begin i0:= i; b:= false end
        end;
        for i:= 1 step 1 until classes do
        begin s:= s + x[i]; if s / n ≥ truncation then
            begin m:= i; n:= s; i:= classes end
        end;
        q2:= q:= if n ≤ 60 then 5 else entier((n ∧ (2 / 3)) / 3) + 1;
        q1:= if n ≤ 60 then 5 else entier((n ∧ (2 / 3)) / 5) + 1;
        for s:= 1 step 1 until 20 do alfa[s]:= i0 − s / 20; aantal:= 20; if i0 > 1 then
        begin for s:= 21 step 1 until 30 do alfa[s]:= i0 + 1 − s / 10; aantal:= 30;
            if i0 > 2 then
            begin aantal:= 30 + 4 × (i0 − 2); if aantal > 40 then aantal:= 40;
                for s:= 31 step 1 until aantal do alfa[s]:= i0 + 5.5 − s / 4
            end
        end;
        som:= 0; j:= 1; i:= i0; k1:= − 1;
CYC1:   z[j]:= 0;
        for i:= i, i + 1 while z[j] < q1 do
```

```
begin z[j]:= z[j] + x[i]; k2:= i end;
k2:= k2 - i0; som:= som + z[j]; if som ≤ n - q1 then
begin l[j]:= i0 + .5 × (k1 + k2); h[j]:= .5 × (k2 - k1); k1:= k2; j:= j + 1;
     goto CYC1
end;
k2:= m - i0; z[j]:= n - SUM(i, 1, j - 1, z[i]); l[j]:= i0 + .5 × (k2 + k1);
h[j]:= .5 × (k2 - k1); c1:= l[1]; c2:= h[1];
tweeq: q2:= 2 × q2; som:= 0; j1:= 1; i:= i0; k1:= - 1;
cyc: z1[j1]:= 0;
     for i:= i, i + 1 while z1[j1] < q2 do
     begin z1[j1]:= z1[j1] + x[i]; k2:= i end;
     k2:= k2 - i0; som:= som + z1[j1]; if som ≤ n - q2 then
     begin l1[j1]:= i0 + .5 × (k1 + k2); h1[j1]:= .5 × (k2 - k1); k1:= k2;
          j1:= j1 + 1; goto cyc
     end;
     k2:= m - i0; z1[j1]:= n - SUM(i, 1, j1 - 1, z1[i]); l1[j1]:= i0 + .5 × (k2 + k1);
     h1[j1]:= .5 × (k2 - k1); c4:= l1[1]; c5:= h1[1]; if j1 = j then goto tweeq;
     begin array y, f, fhulp, a, b, g, ghulp, w, whulp[1:j - 1], p[1:j], y1, f1,
          fhulp1, a1, b1, g1, ghulp1[1:j1 - 1];
          for s:= 1 step 1 until aantal do
          begin l[1]:= c1 + .5 × (1 + alfa[s] - i0);
               h[1]:= c2 + .5 × (i0 - 1 - alfa[s]);
               for i:= 1 step 1 until j - 1 do
               begin y[i]:= ln(z[i] × h[i + 1] / (z[i + 1] × h[i]));
                    fhulp[i]:= f[i]:= l[i + 1] - l[i]; a[i]:= - 1 / z[i + 1];
                    b[i]:= 1 / z[i] + 1 / z[i + 1];
                    ghulp[i]:= g[i]:= ln((l[i] - alfa[s]) / (l[i + 1] - alfa[s]))
               end;
               l1[1]:= c4 + .5 × (1 + alfa[s] - i0); h1[1]:= c5 + .5 × (i0 - 1 - alfa[s]);
               for i:= 1 step 1 until j1 - 1 do
               begin y1[i]:= ln(z1[i] × h1[i + 1] / (z1[i + 1] × h1[i]));
                    fhulp1[i]:= f1[i]:= l1[i + 1] - l1[i]; a1[i]:= - 1 / z1[i + 1];
                    b1[i]:= 1 / z1[i] + 1 / z1[i + 1];
                    ghulp1[i]:= g1[i]:= ln((l1[i] - alfa[s]) / (l1[i + 1] - alfa[s]))
               end;
               DETSOLTRI(j - 1, b, a, a, fhulp); v1:= vecvec(1, j - 1, 0, f, fhulp);
               v3:= vecvec(1, j - 1, 0, y, fhulp);
               v2:= vecvec(1, j - 1, 0, fhulp, ghulp); DETSOLTRI(j - 1, b, a, a, ghulp);
               v4:= vecvec(1, j - 1, 0, ghulp, g); v5:= vecvec(1, j - 1, 0, ghulp, y);
               gamma[s]:= (v2 × v3 - v1 × v5) / (v2 × v2 - v1 × v4) + 1;
               beta[s]:= (v3 × v4 - v2 × v5) / (v1 × v4 - v2 × v2);
               if gamma[s] < .000001 ∨ beta[s] < .000001 then
               begin Kgrof[s]:= true; DETSOLTRI(j1 - 1, b1, a1, a1, fhulp1);
                    v1:= vecvec(1, j1 - 1, 0, f1, fhulp1);
                    v3:= vecvec(1, j1 - 1, 0, y1, fhulp1);
                    v2:= vecvec(1, j1 - 1, 0, fhulp1, ghulp1);
                    DETSOLTRI(j1 - 1, b1, a1, a1, ghulp1);
                    v4:= vecvec(1, j1 - 1, 0, ghulp1, g1);
                    v5:= vecvec(1, j1 - 1, 0, ghulp1, y1);
                    gamma[s]:= (v2 × v3 - v1 × v5) / (v2 × v2 - v1 × v4) + 1;
                    beta[s]:= (v3 × v4 - v2 × v5) / (v1 × v4 - v2 × v2);
                    if gamma[s] < .000001 ∨ beta[s] < .000001 then
                    begin Kster[s]:= ₙ6; goto out end
               end;
               for i:= 1 step 1 until j - 1 do
               begin whulp[i]:= w[i]:= y[i] - beta[s] × f[i] - (gamma[s] - 1) × g[i] end;
               DETSOLTRI(j - 1, b, a, a, whulp); K[s]:= vecvec(1, j - 1, 0, whulp, w);
               KK:= incgam(beta[s] × (m - alfa[s]), gamma[s]); func1:= 0;
               for i:= 1 step 1 until m do
               begin func2:= incgam(beta[s] × (l[i] + h[i] - alfa[s]), gamma[s]);
```

```
                p[i]:= KK / ((func2 - func1) × n); func1:= func2
        end;
        for i:= 1 step 1 until j - 1 do
        begin a[i]:= - p[i + 1]; b[i]:= p[i] + p[i + 1]; fhulp[i]:= f[i];
             ghulp[i]:= g[i]
        end;
        DETSOLTRI(j - 1, b, a, a, fhulp); V1[s]:= vecvec(1, j - 1, 0, fhulp, f);
        v3:= vecvec(1, j - 1, 0, fhulp, y); V2[s]:= vecvec(1, j - 1, 0, fhulp, g);
        DETSOLTRI(j - 1, b, a, a, ghulp); V4[s]:= vecvec(1, j - 1, 0, ghulp, g);
        v5:= vecvec(1, j - 1, 0, ghulp, y);
        gammaster[s]:= (V2[s] × v3 - V1[s] × v5) / (V2[s] × V2[s] - V1[s] ×
        V4[s]) + 1;
        betaster[s]:= (v3 × V4[s] - V2[s] × v5) / (V1[s] × V4[s] - V2[s] × V2[s]);
        if betaster[s] < .000001 ∨ gammaster[s] < .000001 then
        begin func1:= 0; Kstergrof[s]:= true;
            for i:= 1 step 1 until j1 do
            begin func2:= incgam(beta[s] × (l1[i] + h1[i] - alfa[s]), gamma[s]);
                p[i]:= KK / ((func2 - func1) × n); func1:= func2
            end;
            for i:= 1 step 1 until j1 - 1 do
            begin a[i]:= - p[i + 1]; b[i]:= p[i] + p[i + 1]; fhulp1[i]:= f1[i];
                ghulp1[i]:= g1[i]
            end;
            DETSOLTRI(j1 - 1, b1, a1, a1, fhulp1);
            V1[s]:= vecvec(1, j1 - 1, 0, fhulp1, f1);
            v3:= vecvec(1, j1 - 1, 0, fhulp1, y1);
            V2[s]:= vecvec(1, j1 - 1, 0, fhulp1, g1);
            DETSOLTRI(j1 - 1, b1, a1, a1, ghulp1);
            V4[s]:= vecvec(1, j1 - 1, 0, ghulp1, g1);
            v5:= vecvec(1, j1 - 1, 0, ghulp1, y1);
            gammaster[s]:= (V2[s] × v3 - V1[s] × v5) / (V2[s] × V2[s] - V1[s] ×
            V4[s]) + 1;
            betaster[s]:= (v3 × V4[s] - V2[s] × v5) / (V1[s] × V4[s] - V2[s] ×
            V2[s]); if betaster[s] < .000001 ∨ gammaster[s] < .000001 then
            begin stap1[s]:= true; betaster[s]:= beta[s]; gammaster[s]:= gamma[s];
                goto out
            end
        end;
        for i:= 1 step 1 until j - 1 do whulp[i]:= w[i]:= y[i] - betaster[s] ×
        f[i] - (gammaster[s] - 1) × g[i]; DETSOLTRI(j - 1, b, a, a, whulp);
        Kster[s]:= vecvec(1, j - 1, 0, w, whulp);
out:
end;
s0:= 1; min:= Kster[1];
for i:= 2 step 1 until aantal do if Kster[i] < min then
begin s0:= i; min:= Kster[i] end;
if min = ₁₀6 then
begin CARRIAGE(3); PRINTTEXT(⊲neuron:⊳); ABSFIXT(6, 0, code); CARRIAGE(3);
    PRINTTEXT(⊲sum of observations=⊳); ABSFIXT(6, 0, n); CARRIAGE(6);
    PRINTTEXT(⊲parameter estimation not possible⊳); NEW PAGE; goto einde
end;
var1:= alfa[s0]; var2:= betaster[s0]; var3:= gammaster[s0]; v1:= V1[s0];
v2:= V2[s0]; v4:= V4[s0]; det:= v1 × v4 - v2 × v2;
tau:= 125 × 2 ∧ scale / classes; c1:= v4 / det; c2:= - v2 / det;
c3:= v1 / det; KK:= incgam(var2 × (m - var1), var3); func1:= 0;
for i:= i0 step 1 until m do
begin func2:= incgam(var2 × (i - var1), var3);
    pster[i]:= (func2 - func1) / KK; func1:= func2
end;
j:= 1; i:= i0; som2:= 0;
```

```
CYC2: P[j]:= 0; Z[j]:= 0;
      for i:= i, i + 1 while P[j] < q / n do
      begin P[j]:= P[j] + pster[i]; Z[j]:= Z[j] + x[i]; L[j]:= i end;
      som2:= som2 + P[j]; if som2 ≤ 1 - q / n then
      begin j:= j + 1; goto CYC2 end;
      L[j]:= m; P[j]:= SUM(i, L[j - 1] + 1, m, pster[i]);
      Z[j]:= SUM(i, L[j - 1] + 1, m, x[i]); chi:= 0;
      for i:= 1 step 1 until j do
      begin real s;
          s:= (Z[i] - n × P[i]) ⋀ 2 / (n × P[i]); chi:= chi + s; chichi[i]:= s
      end;
      Pchi:= 1 - incgam(.5 × chi, .5 × (j - 3)); CARRIAGE(2); if prob = 1 then
      begin PRINTTEXT(◁number of problems :▷); FIX(6, 0, nprob); CARRIAGE(5) end;
      PRINTTEXT(◁neuron=▷); PUHEP(122); FIX(4, 0, code); CARRIAGE(3); PUNLCR;
      PRINTTEXT(◁sum of observations=▷); ABSFIXT(6, 0, n); CARRIAGE(3); PRINTTEXT(
      ◁estimated parameters first step:▷); PRINTTEXT(
      ◁         alpha          beta            gamma           sum of sq▷); NLCR;
      NLCR;
      for i:= 1 step 1 until aantal do
      begin SPACE(33); FIXT(6, 6, alfa[i]); FIXT(6, 6, beta[i]);
          FIXT(6, 6, gamma[i]); FIXT(10, 6, K[i]); if Kgrof[i] then PRINTTEXT(
          ◁    coarse grouping▷); NLCR
      end;
      NLCR; NLCR; PRINTTEXT(◁estimated parameters second step▷); NLCR; NLCR;
      for i:= 1 step 1 until aantal do
      begin SPACE(33); FIXT(6, 6, alfa[i]); FIXT(6, 6, betaster[i]);
          FIXT(6, 6, gammaster[i]); FIXT(10, 6, Kster[i]);
          if stap1[i] then PRINTTEXT(
          ◁    =first step▷) else if Kstergrof[i] then PRINTTEXT(
          ◁    coarse grouping▷); NLCR
      end;
      NLCR; PRINTTEXT(◁best estimations:    alfastar =▷); FIXT(3, 6, var1 × tau);
      NLCR; PRINTTEXT(◁                     betastar =▷); FIXT(3, 6, tau / var2);
      NLCR; PRINTTEXT(◁                    gammastar=▷); FIXT(3, 6, var3); NLCR;
      NLCR; PRINTTEXT(◁estimated beta and gamma covariance matrix:    ▷);
      FIXT(3, 6, c1); SPACE(3); FIXT(3, 6, c2); NLCR; NLCR; SPACE(50);
      FIXT(3, 6, c2); SPACE(3); FIXT(3, 6, c3); CARRIAGE(5); PRINTTEXT(
      ◁ classes    expected freq.   observed freq.    chi-sq. diff.▷); NLCR;
      NLCR; ABSFIXT(3, 0, i0); PRSYM(65); ABSFIXT(3, 0, L[1]);
      FIXT(6, 6, n × P[1]); FIXT(14, 0, Z[1]); FIXT(11, 6, chichi[1]); NLCR;
      for i:= 1 step 1 until j - 1 do
      begin ABSFIXT(3, 0, L[i] + 1); PRSYM(65); ABSFIXT(3, 0, L[i + 1]);
          FIXT(6, 6, n × P[i + 1]); FIXT(14, 0, Z[i + 1]);
          FIXT(11, 6, chichi[i + 1]); NLCR;
      end;
      CARRIAGE(3); PRINTTEXT(◁chi-square=▷); FIXT(3, 6, chi); NLCR; NLCR;
      PRINTTEXT(◁d.f.=▷); FIXT(3, 0, j - 3); NLCR; NLCR; PRINTTEXT(◁p=▷);
      FIXT(3, 6, Pchi); NEW PAGE;
      for i:= i0 step 1 until m do
      begin FIXP(3, 0, i); PUHEP(62); FIXP(4, 6, n × pster[i]); PUHEP(62);
          FIXP(4, 0, x[i]); PUNLCR;
      end;
      FIXP(1, 0, 0); PUNLCR; RUNOUT;
einde:
      end
   end
 end
end
```

## REFERENCES

BLOM, J. L. (1969) *Thesis, Amsterdam*.

BRINK, F. J. VAN, BRONK, D. W. AND RUDJORD, T. (1946) Chemical excitation of nerve. *Ann. N. Y. Acad. Sci.*, **47**: 457–485.

CHAPMAN, D. G. (1956) Estimating the parameters of a truncated gamma distribution. *Ann. Math. Statist.*, **27**, 498–506.

COCHRAN, W. G. (1952) The chi-square test of goodness of fit. *Ann. Math. Statist.*, **23**: 315–345.

COX, D. R. AND LEWIS, P. A. W. (1966) *The Statistical Analysis of Series of Events*, Methuen, London, Wiley & Sons, New York.

ENRIGHT, J. T. (1967) The spontaneous neuron subject to tonic stimulation. *J. Theor. Biol.*, **16**, 54–78.

GERSTEIN, G. L. AND MANDELBROT, B. (1964) Random walk models for the spike activity of a single neuron. *Biophys. J.*, **4**: 41–68.

GLUSS, B. (1967) A model for neuron firing with exponential decay of potential resulting in diffusion equations for probability density. *Bull. Math. Biophys.*, **29**, 233–242.

HYVÄRINEN, J. (1966) Analysis of spontaneous spike potential activity in the developing rabbit diencephalon. *Acta Physiol. Scand.*, **68**: suppl. 278.

KUFFLER, S. W., FITZHUGH, R. AND BARLOW, H. B., (1957) Maintained activity in the cat's retina in light and darkness. *J. Gen. Physiol.*, **40**: 685–702.

MOORE, G. P., PERKEL, O. H. AND SEGUNDO, J. P. (1966) Statistical analysis and functional interpretation of neuronal spike data. *Ann. Rev. Physiol.*, **28**: 495–522.

RODIECK, R. W., KIANG, N. Y. S. AND GERSTEIN, G. L. (1962) Some quantitative methods for the study of spontaneous activity of single neurons. *Biophys. J.*, **2**: 351–368.

STEIN, R. B. (1965) A theoretical analysis of neuronal variability. *Biophys. J.*, **5**: 175–195.

WERNER, G. AND MOUNTCASTLE, V. B. (1963) The variability of central neural activity in a sensory system and its implications for the central reflections of sensory events. *J. Neurophysiol.*, **26**: 958–977.

WILK. M. B., GNANADESIKAN, R. AND HUET, M. J. (1962) Estimation of parameters of the gamma distribution using order statistics. *Biometrika*, **49**: 525–545.

# A Computer Program for the Determination of Cerebral Blood Flow using the Kr-85 or Xe-133 Intra-arterial Injection Method

J. C. DE VALOIS, J. SMITH AND J. P. C. PEPERKAMP

*Central Institute for Brain Research, IJdijk 28, Amsterdam (The Netherlands)*

## INTRODUCTION

Cerebral blood flow can be determined in a number of ways. The present paper is based on the intra-arterial injection method as introduced by Lassen and Munck (1955). The theoretical basis is extensively discussed by Hoedt-Rasmussen (1967). The computer program is adapted from a program in Algol-60 developed by Sveinsdottir (1965).

After injection of a bolus of radioactive $^{85}$Kr or $^{133}$Xe (dissolved in saline) into one of the internal carotid arteries the clearance curves of the isotope are recorded externally. The general shape of this curve is a high order polynominal which can be described as the sum of two exponential curves. The program is written in Fortran IV and can be used on most IBM computers. The underlying version is adapted to be used on the IBM 1130 computer. It gives an analysis of the clearance curves into two mono-exponentials based on an iterative least-square method. The mean blood flow is also calculated on a non-compartmental basis.

## MATHEMATICAL PROCEDURES

The point of departure is a set of $n$ data points which are considered to belong to the function $f(t)$ (experimental curve). The function $g(t)$ is to be considered as a two-compartmental best fit to $f(t)$. The general shape of $g(t)$ is

$$g(t) = a\,\mathrm{e}^{-at} + b\,\mathrm{e}^{-\beta t} \quad . \quad . \quad . \quad . \quad . \quad . \quad . \quad . \quad . \quad . \quad . \quad (1)$$

$t$, $a$, $a$, $b$, and $\beta$ are the unknown parameters of this function.

### Initial guess procedure

The tail of the curve is characteristic of the slowly perfused parts of the brain, and *not* influenced by the first part of the curve after a certain time $t_{n_2}$ (see Fig. 1). The tail part of the curve is only dependent on $b$ and $\beta$:

$$g(t) = b\,\mathrm{e}^{-\beta t}$$

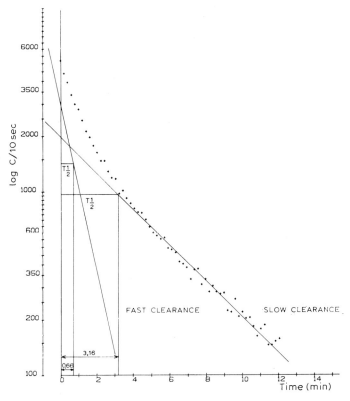

Fig. 1. Cerebral blood flow clearance curves. Graphical analysis. Flow fast = 96 ml/100 g/min. Flow slow = 27 ml/100 g/min. Flow mean = 52 ml/100 g/min.

After logarithmic conversion a linear expression can be formulated (expr. 2):

$$\ln g(t) = \ln b - \beta t$$

$$assume: \begin{cases} y = \ln g(t) \\ c = \ln b \\ ax = -\beta t \end{cases}$$

$$y = ax + c \quad \ldots \ldots \ldots \ldots \ldots \ldots (2)$$

A least square best fit can be obtained after *minimalization* of

$$\sum_{n_2}^{n} (y_i - y)^2$$

in which $y_i$ are $(n - n_2)$ data points.

This simple statistical problem results in the values of $a$ and $c$ (expr. 2) and the so called initial guess values for $b$ and $\beta$ (expr. 3 and 4):

$$\beta = -a = \frac{(n - n_2)\, \Sigma xy - \Sigma x \cdot \Sigma y}{(n - n_2)\, \Sigma x^2 - (\Sigma x)^2} \quad \ldots \ldots \ldots \ldots (3)$$

$$b = e^c = \exp. \frac{\Sigma x^2 \cdot \Sigma y - \Sigma x \cdot \Sigma xy}{(n - n_2) \ \Sigma x^2 - (\Sigma x)^2} \quad \cdots \cdots \cdots (4)$$

The same approach is used for the initial guess of $a$ and $\alpha$:

$$g\,(t) - b\,e^{-\beta t} = a\,e^{-\alpha t} \cdot \ldots \ldots \ldots \ldots 1$$

resulting in

$$g'\,(t) = ae^{-\alpha t}$$

$$a = \frac{n_1 \ \Sigma xy - \Sigma x \cdot \Sigma y}{n_1 \ \Sigma x^2 - (\Sigma x)^2} \quad \cdots \cdots \cdots \cdots (5)$$

$$a = \exp. \left\{ \frac{\Sigma x^2 \cdot \Sigma y - \Sigma x \cdot \Sigma xy}{n_1 \ \Sigma x^2 - (\Sigma x)^2} \right\} \quad \cdots \cdots \cdots (6)$$

The four initial guess values are indexed $a_0$, $\alpha_0$, $b_0$, and $\beta_0$, and used for the final iteration process.

### Iteration

The function $g\,(t) = a\,e^{-\alpha t} + b\,e^{-\beta t}$ can be developed in a Taylor series of the initial guess values:

$$g\,(t,\,a,\,\alpha,\,b,\,\beta) = g\,(t,\,a_0,\,\alpha_0,\,b_0,\,\beta_0) + (a_1 - a_0) \left(\frac{dg}{da}\right)_0 + (\alpha_1 - \alpha_0) \left(\frac{dg}{d\alpha}\right)_0 +$$

$$+ (b_1 - b_0) \left(\frac{dg}{db}\right)_0 + (\beta_1 - \beta_0) \left(\frac{dg}{d\beta}\right)_0 + \theta,$$

higher order terms, which are disregarded.

$$\left(\frac{dg}{da}\right)_0 = C_1 = e^{-a_0 t}$$

$$x_1 = a_1 - a_0$$

$$\left(\frac{dg}{d\alpha}\right)_0 = C_2 = -a_0\,t\,e^{-a_0 t}$$

$$x_2 = \alpha_1 - \alpha_0$$

$$\left(\frac{dg}{db}\right)_0 = C_3 = e^{-\beta_0 t}$$

$$x_3 = b_1 - b_0$$

$$\left(\frac{dg}{d\beta}\right)_0 = C_4 = -b_0\,t\,e^{-\beta_0 t}$$

$$x_4 = \beta_1 - \beta_0$$

Calculated over $n$ data points $n$ equations in four unknowns, $x_1$, $x_2$, $x_3$ and $x_4$, are obtained. The shape of any of these equations is (expr. 7):

$$g\,(t_i,\,a,\,\alpha,\,b,\,\beta) = g\,(t_i,\,a_0,\,\alpha_0,\,b_0,\,\beta_0) +$$
$$C_{i1}\,x_1 + C_{i2}\,x_2 + C_{i3}\,x_3 + C_{i4}\,x_4 \quad . . . . . . . . (7)$$
$$(i = 1,\,n).$$

Since this is a point to point fitting an error term $r\,(t_i)$ must be introduced. This error term is

$$r(t_i) = g(t_i) - f(t_i) . \quad . . . . . . . . . . . . (8)$$

This can be rearranged:

$$f(t_i) + r(t_i) = g(t_i) = g(t_i)_0 + C_{i1}\,x_1 + . . . . . . + C_{i4}\,x_4$$
$$g(t_i)_0 - f(t_i) = v(t_i)$$
$$r(t_i) = -v(t_i) + C_{i1}\,x_1 + . . . . . . . . + C_{i4}\,x_4 . \quad . . . . . . (9)$$

The final best fit is reached by minimalisation of the function $E$:

$$E = \sum_{i=1}^{n} r_i^2$$

Minimalization requires that the partial derivatives of $E$ in respect to $a$, $\alpha$, $b$, and $\beta$ be zero. This gives the four normal equations

$$\left.\begin{array}{l} \displaystyle\sum_{i=1}^{n}\,(-v_i + C_{i1}\,x_1 + . . . . . . . . + C_{i4}\,x_4)\,\dfrac{\mathrm{d}r_i}{\mathrm{d}a} = 0 \\[2em] \displaystyle\sum_{i=1}^{n}\,(-v_i + C_{i1}\,x_1 + . . . . . . . . + C_{i4}\,x_4)\,\dfrac{\mathrm{d}r_i}{\mathrm{d}\alpha} = 0 \end{array}\right\} \quad . . . . (10)$$

$$etc.$$

$$\left(\frac{\mathrm{d}r_i}{\mathrm{d}a}\right)_0 = \mathrm{e}^{-a_0 t_i} = C_{i1}; \quad \left(\frac{\mathrm{d}r_i}{\mathrm{d}\alpha}\right)_0 = -a t_i\,\mathrm{e}^{-a_0 t_i} = C_{i2};$$

$$\left(\frac{\mathrm{d}r_i}{\mathrm{d}b}\right)_0 = \mathrm{e}^{-\beta_0 t_i} = C_{i3}; \quad \left(\frac{\mathrm{d}r_i}{\mathrm{d}\beta}\right)_0 = -b_0 t_i\,\mathrm{e}^{-\beta_0 t_i} = C_{i4}.$$

Expr. (10) changes to expr. (11) after substitution and placement in matrix form:

$$\begin{bmatrix} \Sigma C_{i1}{}^2 & \Sigma C_{i1}C_{i2} & \Sigma C_{i1}C_{i3} & \Sigma C_{i1}C_{i4} \\ & \Sigma C_{i2}{}^2 & \Sigma C_{i2}C_{i3} & \Sigma C_{i2}C_{i4} \\ & & \Sigma C_{i3}{}^2 & \Sigma C_{i3}C_{i4} \\ & & & \Sigma C_{i4}{}^2 \end{bmatrix} \begin{bmatrix} x_1 \\ x_2 \\ x_3 \\ x_4 \end{bmatrix} = \begin{bmatrix} \Sigma C_{i1}v_i \\ \Sigma C_{i2}v_i \\ \Sigma C_{i3}v_i \\ \Sigma C_{i4}v_i \end{bmatrix}$$

The values of $x_1$ to $x_4$ can now easily be calculated by using determinants. This results in new values $a_1$, $\alpha_1$, $b_1$ and $\beta_1$ composed of $(a_0 + x_1)$, $(a_0 + x_2)$ etc. Iteration stops if:

$$\mid x_{1_n}/a_0\mid + \mid x_{2_n}\mid + \mid x_{3_n}/b_0\mid + \mid x_{4_n}\mid \leqslant 10^{-4}$$

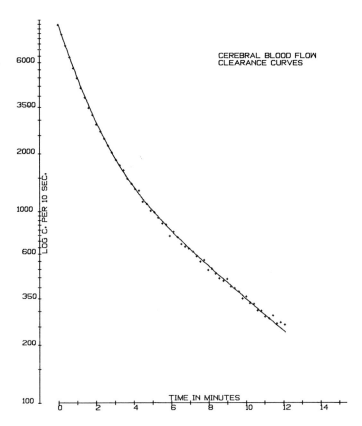

Fig. 2. Cerebral blood flow clearance curves. Computer analysis. Flow fast $=$ 92.3 ml/100 g/min. Flow slow $=$ 28.9 ml/100 g/min. Flow mean $=$ 52.5 ml/100 g/min.

## RESULTS

The present program has been used to evaluate clearance curves from the rabbit brain, in order to obtain blood flow data under normal conditions and under a variety of experimental conditions, *e.g.* hypo- and hypercarbia, hypo- and hypertension, drug studies, etc. The typical computer output obtained under normal conditions is shown. Besides the flow data, punch card output is produced to facilitate plotting of the clearance curves in equation form $(f(t) = a\,e^{-\alpha t} + b\,e^{-\beta t})$. In Fig. 2, the plot of the definite clearance curve is shown in relation to the original data points, after subtraction of the background. In a comparative study of 52 clearance curves in which flow values were obtained by three methods (graphical analysis, graphical analysis + least squares best fit, and the present method) the differences were significant ($P < 0.001$). The mean flow is underestimated by the former methods by 6%. The fast flow is even underestimated by at least 25%.

The graphical (hand-) analysis merely gives a rough approximation of the flow values to be expected.

```
// FOR
*LIST SOURCE PROGRAM                                                RCBF0010
*IOCS(CARD,TYPEWRITER,1132PRINTER)                                  RCBF0020
*ONE WORD INTEGERS                                                  RCBF0030
*EXTENDED PRECISION                                                 RCBF0040

C PROGRAM RCBF,TAYLOR DEVELOPMENT                                   RCBF0050

      DIMENSIONA(91) ,Y(91) ,SOM(4,4) ,HULP(4) ,SOMV(4) ,CUR(91) ,D(91) RCBF0060
    5 PAUSE5555                                                     RCBF0070
      L = 1                                                        RCBF0080
      CALL DATSW(10,LL)                                            RCBF0090
      GOTO(15,10),LL                                               RCBF0100
   10 L = L + 2                                                    RCBF0110

C     BACKGROUND,PARTIAL CO2 PRESSURE,TIME INTERVAL AND INJECTION SITE RCBF0120

   15 READ(2,195)BGND,PCO2,DT,PCORR,INJ                            RCBF0130
      WRITE(L,200)                                                 RCBF0140
      AREA = 0.                                                    RCBF0150

C     DATA POINTS A(I),N=1,91                                      RCBF0160

      DO 25 I=1,91                                                 RCBF0170
      READ(2,205)A(I)                                              RCBF0180
      IF (A(I)) 30,30,20                                           RCBF0190
   20 N = I                                                        RCBF0200
      A(I) = A(I) - BGND                                           RCBF0210
      AREA = AREA + A(I)                                           RCBF0220
   25 CONTINUE                                                     RCBF0230
   30 K = 28                                                       RCBF0240
      WRITE(L,210)                                                 RCBF0250
      WRITE(L,285)(A(I),I=1,N)                                     RCBF0260
      WRITE(L,215)N                                                RCBF0270
      WRITE(L,220)PCO2                                             RCBF0280
      WRITE(L,225)BGND                                             RCBF0290
      WRITE(L,230)DT                                               RCBF0300

C     CHOOSE GAS THAT IS TO BE INJECTED,85 KR OR 133 XE            RCBF0320

      CALL DATSW(3,JD)                                             RCBF0340
      IF (JD - 1) 40,35,40                                         RCBF0350
   35 WRITE(L,235)                                                 RCBF0360
      GOTO 45                                                      RCBF0370
   40 WRITE(L,240)                                                 RCBF0380
   45 IF (INJ - 2) 50,55,60                                        RCBF0390

C     CHOOSE INJECTION SITE                                        RCBF0410

   50 WRITE(L,245)                                                 RCBF0430
      GOTO 65                                                      RCBF0440
   55 WRITE(L,250)                                                 RCBF0450
      GOTO 65                                                      RCBF0460
   60 WRITE(L,255)                                                 RCBF0470

C     GRAPHICAL ANALYSIS,LEAST SQUARES BEST FIT                    RCBF0490

   65 SOMXY = 0.                                                   RCBF0510
      SOMY = 0.                                                    RCBF0520
```

PAGE    7

```
      SOMXX = 0.                                                      RCBF0530
      SOMX = 0.                                                       RCBF0540
      DO 70 I=K,N                                                     RCBF0550
C     LOGARITHMIC CONVERSION                                          RCBF0570

      Y(I) = ALOG(A(I))                                               RCBF0590
      X = I                                                           RCBF0600
      SOMX = SOMX + X                                                 RCBF0610
      SOMY = SOMY + Y(I)                                              RCBF0620
      SOMXX = SOMXX + X * X                                           RCBF0630
      SOMXY = SOMXY + X * Y(I)                                        RCBF0640
   70 CONTINUE                                                        RCBF0650
      AN = (N - K) + 1                                                RCBF0660
      BETA = - (AN * SOMXY - SOMX * SOMY) / (AN * SOMXX - SOMX * SOMX) RCBF0670
      C2 = (SOMXX * SOMY - SOMX * SOMXY) / (AN * SOMXX - SOMX * SOMX)  RCBF0680
      B = 2.718282 * * C2                                             RCBF0690
      SOMX = 0.                                                       RCBF0700
      SOMY = 0.                                                       RCBF0710
      SOMXX = 0.                                                      RCBF0720
      SOMXY = 0.                                                      RCBF0730
      DO 80 I=1,20                                                    RCBF0740
      X = I                                                           RCBF0750
C     PROCEDURE TO PREVENT NEGATIVE LOGARITHMIC ARGUMENTS             RCBF0770

      IF ( (A(I) - B * 2.718282 * * ( - BETA * X)) - 0.1) 85,85,75    RCBF0790
   75 R = A(I) - B * 2.718282 * * ( - BETA * X)                       RCBF0800
      Y(I) = ALOG(R)                                                  RCBF0810
      SOMX = SOMX + X                                                 RCBF0820
      SOMXX = SOMXX + X * X                                           RCBF0830
      SOMY = SOMY + Y(I)                                              RCBF0840
      SOMXY = SOMXY + X * Y(I)                                        RCBF0850
   80 CONTINUE                                                        RCBF0860
   85 IF (X - 20.) 90,95,95                                           RCBF0870
   90 X = X - 1.                                                      RCBF0880
   95 ALPHA = - (X * SOMXY - SOMX * SOMY) / (X * SOMXX - SOMX * SOMX)  RCBF0890
      C1 = (SOMXX * SOMY - SOMX * SOMXY) / (X * SOMXX - SOMX * SOMX)   RCBF0900
      AA = 2.718282 * * C1                                            RCBF0910
      WRITE(L,260)                                                    RCBF0920
C     INITIAL GUESS VALUES                                            RCBF0940

      WRITE(L,265)                                                    RCBF0960
      WRITE(L,270)AA,ALPHA,B,BETA                                     RCBF0970

      ITERATIVE PROCEDURE FOR ESTIMATION OF A,ALPHA,B AND BETA        RCBF0990

      M = 0                                                           RCBF1010
  100 V = 0.                                                          RCBF1020
      DO 105 I=1,4                                                    RCBF1030
      HULP(I)=0.                                                      RCBF1040
      SOMV(I) = 0.                                                    RCBF1050
  105 CONTINUE                                                        RCBF1060
      DO 110 I=1,4                                                    RCBF1070
      DO 110 J=1,4                                                    RCBF1080
      SOM(I,J) = 0.                                                   RCBF1090
  110 CONTINUE                                                        RCBF1100
```

*References p. 241*

PAGE    8

```
C      MATRIX FORMATION                                              RCBF1120

       DO 115 I=1,N                                                  RCBF1140
       T = I - 1                                                     RCBF1150
       EXPA = 2.718282 * * ( - ALPHA * T)                           RCBF1160
       EXPB = 2.718282 * * ( - BETA * T)                            RCBF1170
       CA = AA * T                                                   RCBF1180
       CB = B * T                                                    RCBF1190
       SOM(1,1) = SOM(1,1) + EXPA * * 2.                            RCBF1200
       SOM(2,2) = SOM(2,2) + (CA * * 2.) * (EXPA * * 2.)           RCBF1210
       SOM(3,3) = SOM(3,3) + EXPB * * 2.                            RCBF1220
       SOM(4,4) = SOM(4,4) + (CB * * 2.) * (EXPB * * 2.)           RCBF1230
       SOM(2,1) = SOM(2,1) - CA * EXPA * * 2.                       RCBF1240
       SOM(3,1) = SOM(3,1) + EXPA * EXPB                            RCBF1250
       SOM(4,1) = SOM(4,1) - CB * (EXPA * EXPB)                     RCBF1260
       SOM(3,2) = SOM(3,2) - CA * (EXPA * EXPB)                     RCBF1270
       SOM(4,2) = SOM(4,2) + ( (T * * 2.) * (AA * B)) * (EXPA * EXPB)  RCBF1280
       SOM(4,3) = SOM(4,3) - CB * (EXPB * * 2.)                     RCBF1290
       V = A(I) - AA * EXPA - B * EXPB                              RCBF1300
       SOMV(1) = SOMV(1) + EXPA * V                                 RCBF1310
       SOMV(2) = SOMV(2) - CA * EXPA * V                           RCBF1320
       SOMV(3) = SOMV(3) + EXPB * V                                 RCBF1330
       SOMV(4) = SOMV(4) - CB * EXPB * V                           RCBF1340
   115 CONTINUE                                                     RCBF1350
       DO 120 J=1,4                                                 RCBF1360
       DO 120 I=1,4                                                 RCBF1370
       SOM(J,I) = SOM(I,J)                                          RCBF1380
   120 CONTINUE                                                     RCBF1390

C      DETERMINANT SOLUTION SUBPROGRAM                              RCBF1410

       CALL DETR4(SOM,DD1)                                          RCBF1430
       DO 125 I=1,4                                                 RCBF1440
       HULP(I)=SOM(I,1)                                             RCBF1450
       SOM(I,1) = SOMV(I)                                          RCBF1460
   125 CONTINUE                                                     RCBF1470
       CALL DETR4(SOM,DD2)                                          RCBF1480
       DA = DD2 / DD1                                               RCBF1490
       DO 130 I=1,4                                                 RCBF1500
       SOMV(I) = SOM(I,1)                                          RCBF1510
       SOM(I,1) = HULP(I)                                          RCBF1520
       HULP(I)=SOM(I,2)                                             RCBF1530
       SOM(I,2) = SOMV(I)                                          RCBF1540
   130 CONTINUE                                                     RCBF1550
       CALL DETR4(SOM,DD3)                                          RCBF1560
       DALPH = DD3 / DD1                                            RCBF1570
       DO 135 I=1,4                                                 RCBF1580
       SOMV(I) = SOM(I,2)                                          RCBF1590
       SOM(I,2) = HULP(I)                                          RCBF1600
       HULP(I)=SOM(I,3)                                             RCBF1610
       SOM(I,3) = SOMV(I)                                          RCBF1620
   135 CONTINUE                                                     RCBF1630
       CALL DETR4(SOM,DD4)                                          RCBF1640
       DB = DD4 / DD1                                               RCBF1650
       DO 140 I=1,4                                                 RCBF1660
       SOMV(I) = SOM(I,3)                                          RCBF1670
       SOM(I,3) = HULP(I)                                          RCBF1680
```

PAGE 9

```
      HULP(I)=SOM(I,4)                                              RCBF1690
      SOM(I,4) = SOMV(I)                                            RCBF1700
 140 CONTINUE                                                       RCBF1710
      CALL DETR4(SOM,DD5)                                           RCBF1720
      DBETA = DD5 / DD1                                             RCBF1730
      M = M + 1                                                     RCBF1740
      REST = ABS(DA / AA) + ABS(DALPH) + ABS(DB / B) + ABS(DBETA)   RCBF1750

C     PRECISION STATEMENT                                          RCBF1770

      IF (REST - 0.0001) 150,150,145                               RCBF1790
 145 AA = AA + DA                                                   RCBF1800
      ALPHA = ALPHA + DALPH                                         RCBF1810
      B = B + DB                                                    RCBF1820
      BETA = BETA + DBETA                                           RCBF1830
      GOTO 100                                                      RCBF1840

C     FINAL VALUES OF A,ALPHA,B AND BETA                           RCBF1860

 150 WRITE(L,275)AA,ALPHA,B,BETA                                    RCBF1880
      WRITE(L,280)M                                                 RCBF1890
      DO 155 I=1,N                                                  RCBF1900
      T = I - 1                                                     RCBF1910
      CUR(I)=(AA*2.718282**(-ALPHA*T))+(B*2.718282**(-BETA*T))      RCBF1920
      D(I) = DT * T                                                 RCBF1930
 155 CONTINUE                                                       RCBF1940

C     PARTITION COEFFICIENTS                                       RCBF1960

      CALL DATSW(3,JD)                                              RCBF1980
      IF (JD - 1) 165,160,165                                       RCBF1990
 160 PAR1 = 84.                                                     RCBF2000
      PAR2 = 157.                                                   RCBF2010
      GOTO 170                                                      RCBF2020
 165 PAR1 = 97.                                                     RCBF2030
      PAR2 = 132.                                                   RCBF2040
 170 FLOW1 = ALPHA * 1. / DT * PAR1                                 RCBF2050

C     CORRECTION FOR CO2 TENSION                                   RCBF2070

      CFL11 = FLOW1 / (1. + 0.025 * (PCO2 - PCORR))                RCBF2090
      FLOW2 = BETA * 1. / DT * PAR2                                 RCBF2100
      CFL22 = FLOW2 / (1. + 0.025 * (PCO2 - PCORR))                RCBF2110

C     DETERMINATION OF RELATIVE WEIGHTS                            RCBF2130

      WS = (B * FLOW1 / FLOW2) / (B * FLOW1 / FLOW2 + AA)          RCBF2150
      WF = 1. - WS                                                  RCBF2160
      FLOW3 = WF * FLOW1 + WS * FLOW2                               RCBF2170
      CFL33 = FLOW3 / (1. + 0.025 * (PCO2 - PCORR))                RCBF2180
      WRITE(L,285)(CUR(I),I=1,N)                                    RCBF2190
      WRITE(L,290)WF                                                RCBF2200
      WRITE(L,295)WS                                                RCBF2210
      WRITE(L,300)PCORR                                             RCBF2220
      WRITE(L,305)FLOW1,CFL11                                       RCBF2230
      WRITE(L,310)FLOW2,CFL22                                       RCBF2240
      WRITE(L,315)FLOW3,CFL33                                       RCBF2250
      WRITE(L,320)                                                  RCBF2260
```

*References p. 241*

```
C       HEIGHT OVER AREA METHOD (INTEGRAL)                              RCBF2280

        PAR3 =  WF * PAR1 + WS * PAR2                                   RCBF2300
        FLOW4 = ( (A(1) - A(N)) * PAR3 * (1. / DT)) / AREA             RCBF2310
        CFL44 = FLOW4 / (1. + 0.025 * (PCO2 - PCORR))                  RCBF2320
        WRITE(L,315)FLOW4,CFL44                                         RCBF2330
        CALL DATSW(15,IPP)                                              RCBF2340
        GOTO(185,175),IPP                                               RCBF2350

C       DUMMY STATEMENT TO PREVENT MISPUNCHING                          RCBF2370

    175 READ(2,195)                                                     RCBF2390
        WRITE(2,180)(D(I),A(I),CUR(I),I=1,N)                            RCBF2400
    180 FORMAT(3(F7.3,1H,,F8.1,1H,,F8.1,1H,))                           RCBF2410
    185 CALL DATSW(7,LLL)                                               RCBF2420
        GOTO(190,5),LLL                                                 RCBF2430
    190 CALL EXIT                                                       RCBF2440
    195 FORMAT(4F8.3,I5)                                                RCBF2450
    200 FORMAT( 2X,37HCBF PROGRAM DE VALOIS-SMITH      DATE, ///)       RCBF2460
    205 FORMAT (F5.0)                                                   RCBF2470
    210 FORMAT( 2X,28HINPUT DATA MINUS BACKGROUND, /)                   RCBF2480
    215 FORMAT( 2X,16HDATA ANALYSED,   I5 /)                            RCBF2490
    220 FORMAT( 2X,17HPCO2,            F8.3 /)                          RCBF2500
    225 FORMAT( 2X,17HBACKGROUND,      F8.3 /)                          RCBF2510
    230 FORMAT( 2X,17HTIME INTERVAL,   F8.3 /)                          RCBF2520
    235 FORMAT( 2X,30HGAS,                  XENON-133 /)                RCBF2530
    240 FORMAT( 2X,31HGAS,                  KRYPTON-85 /)               RCBF2540
    245 FORMAT( 2X,37HINJECTION SITE,       INTERNAL CAROTID //)        RCBF2550
    250 FORMAT( 2X,35HINJECTION SITE,       COMMON CAROTID //)          RCBF2560
    255 FORMAT( 2X,30HINJECTION SITE,       VERTEBRAL //)               RCBF2570
    260 FORMAT( 2X,26HTWO COMPARTMENTAL ANALYSIS /)                     RCBF2580
    265 FORMAT( 23X,1HA,6X,5HALPHA,6X,1HB,7X,4HBETA /)                  RCBF2590
    270 FORMAT( 2X,17HITERATION VALUES,F8.0,1X,F8.3,1X,F8.0,1X,F8.3 /)  RCBF2600
    275 FORMAT( 2X,17HDEFINITE VALUES, F8.0,1X,F8.3,1X,F8.0,1X,F8.3 ///) RCBF2610
    280 FORMAT( 2X,23HNUMBER OF ITERATIONS = I5 ///)                    RCBF2620
    285 FORMAT(10(F8.1,3X)/)                                            RCBF2630
    290 FORMAT( 2X,22HREL. WEIGHT FAST COMP.F8.3 /)                     RCBF2640
    295 FORMAT( 2X,22HREL. WEIGHT SLOW COMP.F8.3 ///)                   RCBF2650
    300 FORMAT( 28X,20HCORRECTED FOR PCO2= F7.3/)                       RCBF2660
    305 FORMAT( 2X,17HFLOW FAST COMP.  ,F8.3,15X,F8.3,8X,11HML/100G/MIN/) RCBF2670
    310 FORMAT( 2X,17HFLOW SLOW COMP.  ,F8.3,15X,F8.3,8X,11HML/100G/MIN/) RCBF2680
    315 FORMAT( 2X,17HFLOW MEAN        ,F8.3,15X,F8.3,8X,11HML/100G/MIN/) RCBF2690
    320 FORMAT( 2X,19HSTOCHASTIC ANALYSIS /)                            RCBF2700
        END                                                            RCBF2710

// FOR
*LIST SOURCE PROGRAM
*ONE WORD INTEGERS
*EXTENDED PRECISION
        SUBROUTINE DETR4(A,DET)
        DIMENSION A(4,4)                                               002
        X11=A(2,2)*(A(3,3)*A(4,4)-A(4,3)*A(3,4))                       003
        X12=A(3,2)*(A(2,3)*A(4,4)-A(4,3)*A(2,4))                       004
        X13=A(4,2)*(A(2,3)*A(3,4)-A(3,3)*A(2,4))                       005
        D1=X11-X12+X13                                                 006
        X21=A(1,2)*(A(3,3)*A(4,4)-A(4,3)*A(3,4))                       007
        X22=A(3,2)*(A(1,3)*A(4,4)-A(4,3)*A(1,4))                       008
        X23=A(4,2)*(A(1,3)*A(3,4)-A(3,3)*A(1,4))                       009
        D2=X21-X22+X23                                                 010
        X31=A(1,2)*(A(2,3)*A(4,4)-A(4,3)*A(2,4))                       011
        X32=A(2,2)*(A(1,3)*A(4,4)-A(4,3)*A(1,4))                       012
        X33=A(4,2)*(A(1,3)*A(2,4)-A(2,3)*A(1,4))                       013
        D3=X31-X32+X33                                                 014
        X41=A(1,2)*(A(2,3)*A(3,4)-A(3,3)*A(2,4))                       015
        X42=A(2,2)*(A(1,3)*A(3,4)-A(3,3)*A(1,4))                       016
        X43=A(3,2)*(A(1,3)*A(2,4)-A(2,3)*A(1,4))                       017
        D4=X41-X42+X43                                                 018
        DET=A(1,1)*D1-A(2,1)*D2+A(3,1)*D3-A(4,1)*D4                    019
        RETURN                                                        020
        END                                                           022
```

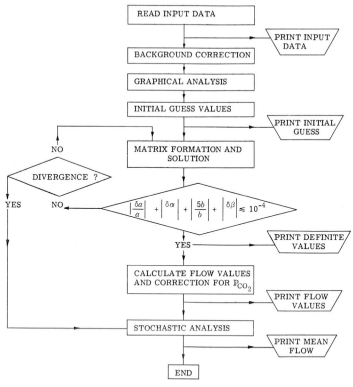

Fig. 3. Flow chart.

# REFERENCES

HOEDT-RASMUSSEN, K. (1967) Regional cerebral blood flow. The intra-arterial injection method. *Acta Neurol. Scand.*, **43**, Suppl. 27.

LASSEN, N. A. AND MUNCK, O. (1955) The cerebral blood flow in man determined by the use of radioactive Krypton. *Acta Physiol. Scand.*, **33**, 30.

SVEINSDOTTIR, E. (1965) Clearance curves of $Kr^{85}$ and $Xe^{133}$ considered as a sum of monoexponential outwash functions. *Acta Neurol. Scand.*, Suppl. **14**, 69.

# Quantitative Computer Analysis of Intracellularly Recorded Action Potentials

H. VAN WILGENBURG AND J. SMITH

*Central Institute for Brain Research, Amsterdam (The Netherlands)*

### INTRODUCTION

Descriptions in quantitative terms of action potentials may elucidate the mechanisms of generation and transmission of neuronal signals (Perkel *et al.*, 1967). The systematic statistical descriptions of spontaneous neural activity will enable the investigator to identify patterns of activity belonging to particular cells or neuronal networks. They also furnish the background for theoretical models and are necessary to any quantitative theory of information processing in the nervous system. Several neuronal models have already been proposed based on assumptions about synaptic input, threshold values, refractory periods and other intrinsic factors. Simple neural systems are being studied by many authors (Moore *et al.*, 1966). Most of these investigations deal with extracellular neuronal recordings. Present techniques make it possible to measure experimental parameters underlying neural variability with intracellular electrodes. Invertebrate nervous systems are especially suitable for this aim, because under appropriate conditions one can work with isolated neurons for many hours. In this paper an analysis is presented of intracellular recorded spike trains from the nervous system of the snail, *Helix pomatia*. Many cells show spontaneous firing patterns. The variability of the interspike intervals of the so-called pacemaker neurons is due to noise phenomena and molecular processes in the membrane (Junge and Moore, 1966). Other cells receive synaptic input even if the preparation is kept under constant conditions.

Special attention will be paid to the role of the synaptic noise on the neuronal variability.

### RESULTS

A few hundred intracellular recordings were made of different neurons in the snail nervous system (*Helix pomatia*). After impalement of the tissue 30% of the cells did not show action potentials, the other showed spontaneous spike potentials. Ten percent of these neurons (so-called pacemaker elements) exhibited the appearance of action potentials without detectable synaptic input. Systematic analysis of this activity may shed some light on the mechanisms underlying the neural variability in the absence of synaptic input. In other cells the pacemaker activity is influenced by exci-

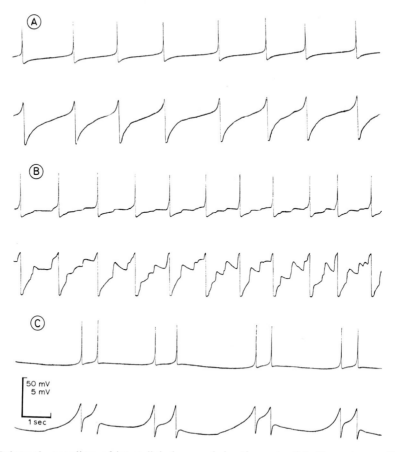

Fig. 1. Polygraph recordings of intracellularly recorded action potentials Upper traces after DC amplification. Lower traces AC amplifications. Time constant 0.3 sec. A. An autoactive neuron, B. As A with EPSPs, C. A phasic cell exhibiting serial dependency.

tatory or inhibitory postsynaptic input (Tauc, 1966) (Fig. 1). Some cells exhibited action potentials after sufficient excitatory input or after antidromic invasion (v. Wilgenburg, 1969). In order to obtain some insight in the role of synaptic noise on the probability density function (pdf) of the interspike interval distributions, the data were classified on the basis of the postsynaptic potentials. From polygraph recordings five categories of neuronal patterns were selected:

  I pacemaker neurons
 II auto-active neurons with postsynaptic potentials smaller than 1 mV
III neurons with excitatory postsynaptic potentials larger than 1 mV
IV neurons with excitatory and inhibitory postsynaptic potentials larger than 1 mV
 V neurons with inhibition of long duration.

   After classification the spike trains were considered as stochastic point processes. A process is stochastic owing to the random variation in the interspike intervals, and it is a point process owing to the instantaneity and indistinguishability of the individual spike events. Unit impulses were obtained with a pulse-shaping circuit

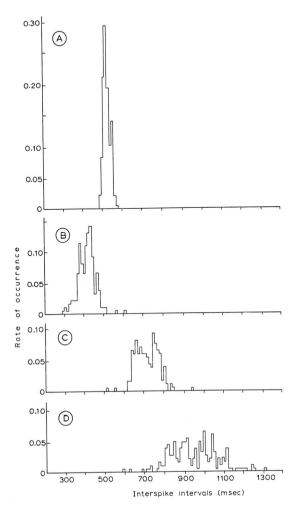

Fig. 2. Distributions of interspike intervals. A. Typical pacemaker neuron, B–D. Autoactive neurons
with synaptic input. Number of intervals 200.

ignoring all other characteristics of the action potentials, as duration, amplitude,
overshoot etc. A data retrieval computer (Nuclear Chicago), used in the interval
histogram mode, generated first order interval histograms (Fig. 2). Under certain
conditions this histogram may be considered as an approximation of the probability
density function of an interspike interval distribution. These conditions are the following: (a) the segment of the spike train to be analyzed should be reasonably stationary
and (b) the successive intervals should be independently distributed. In general each
stochastic process may be stationary or non-stationary. In a stationary process the
underlying probability distribution, of which the observed intervals constitute a
sample, do not themselves depend on the time of observation. A non-stationary process
is one in which a sustained trend exists in the mean firing rate. Stationarity means that
the statistical properties of the data are independent of the choice of the sample within

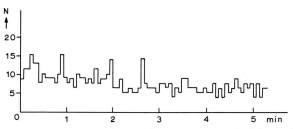

Fig. 3. Firing frequency (4-sec epochs) of a phasic neuron. A trend of decreasing activity is noted. Between 3 and 5 min after the onset the signal can be considered as reasonably stationary. N is the number of spikes.

a long run. The data thus obtained early in an experimental run are indistinguishable statistically from the data taken at a later time.

A definition of a stationary stochastic process is given by Parzen (1962): A stochastic process $X(t)$, $t$ $E$ $T$, whose index set $T$ is linear, is said to be:

1. *Strictly stationary of order k*, where $k$ is a given positive integer, if for any $k$ points, $t_1, \ldots \ldots t_k$ in $T$ and any $h$ in $T$, the $k$-dimensional *random vectors* $X(t_1), \ldots \ldots$ $X(t_k)$ and $X(t_1 + h), \ldots \ldots X(t_k + h)$ are identically distributed.

2. *Strictly stationary* if for any integer $k$ it is strictly stationary of order $k$.

To prove that a stochastic process is stationary, requires that $X(t)$, $t \geqslant 0$ is strictly stationary of order 1.

*Ensemble, sample of data*

Each random sample of data is a sample from an ensemble of theoretically possible samples. A sample is the set of times of spike occurrences, $X(t_0)$, $X(t_1)$, $X(t_2)$, $X(t_3)$, $\ldots \ldots \ldots \ldots$, $X(t_n)$ of the spike train. Most of the statistical measures of spike train activity assume a stationary process among intervals. The analysis should be applied either to the entire record (long run), or to segments of the record (samples), each of which has been found to be sufficiently stationary. A fully satisfactory test for stationarity in a finite spike train does not exist. A simple test of stationarity is to show that the chosen computation does not give widely different results for various samples of data that may be selected from a long run. Werner and Mountcastle (1963) have applied techniques of analysis of variance and random shuffling of intervals to detect non-stationarity. The situation regarding stationarity is mitigated by the fact that the statistical measurements for typical sample sizes are on the one hand not very sensitive to small departures and on the other hand large non-stationarities are fairly obvious.

In our experiments we used several qualitative judgements for stationarity. With a digital integrator (Nuclear, Chicago) the number of action potentials per four seconds was counted. The frequency distribution so obtained was written out with a pen recorder (Fig. 3). If the results were equally divided around a mean, the pattern was considered to be stationary. In another test 400 consecutive interspike interval discharges were measured with a precision of 1.25 msec. The results were written out as a

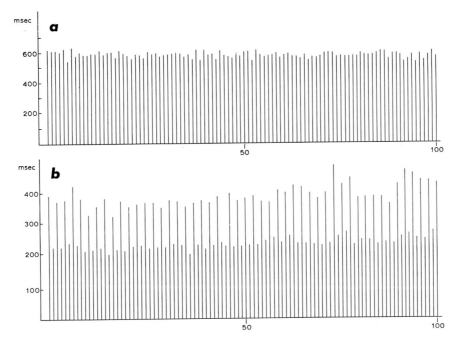

Fig. 4. Tachogram. The duration of 100 consecutive intervals is represented as vertical lines. A. Regular firing neuron, B. phasic firing neuron showing slight drifting.

tachogram (Fig. 4) and punched out on paper tape. Any drift, increase or decrease of interval length can easily be observed from the tachogram. A final test was performed by calculating the serial coefficients of these data between the intervals $j_{i+1}$ and $j_i$ up to $j_i + 20$ and $j_i$, with an IBM 1130 computer. This test is also a control on independency between the intervals (Fig. 5).

Several authors have published methods to analyse the statistical dependency of interspike intervals. Rodieck *et al.* (1962) introduced the joint interval density, in which the data are displayed in a scatter-diagram. The length of the *j*-th interval is presented on the abscissa and the length of the $(j + 1)$ th interval on the ordinate. An alternate form is the matrix equivalent of Smith and Smith (1965), which has been used in practice as a reliable test of independency.

Successive intervals are independently distributed when the normalized frequency distribution along the ordinate is the same for each abscissa value and *vice versa*. Constancy of the means of row and column is the necessary condition for independency of adjacent intervals in the record.

A comparative examination of dependency tests has been published by Poggio and Viernstein (1964). They tabulated the computated results of the linear regression analysis, the serial correlation coefficient and the expectation density for periodicities in neuronal impulse sequences. The main conclusion is that little difference exists for the indication of dependency in the tests.

We used the serial correlogram to describe serial dependence among interspike

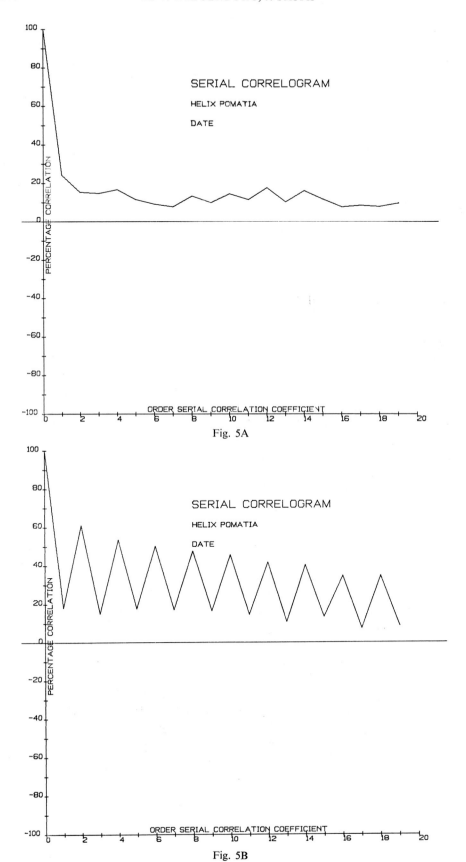

Fig. 5A

Fig. 5B

intervals. The serial correlation coefficient is then a quantitative measure. The first-order serial correlation coefficient compares each interval with the next interval, giving a single scalar quantity. This parameter summarizes the entire diagram of the joint interval distribution of lag 1. The second-order coefficient gives the same information, comparing each interval with the interval that follows one after the next. The $k$-th order coefficient compares each interval with the $k$-th interval following it.

The serial correlation coefficients have a range from $-1$ to $+1$, besides the zero-order coefficient which by definition equals $+1$. When the intervals are derived from a stationary renewal process (*e.g.*, the intervals are drawn independently from a common distribution) then the expected values of all orders of the serial correlation coefficient are approximately zero, indicating independency.

A long trend in the data is the source of a positive contribution to the serial correlation coefficients. Local trends in firing rate give rise to a positive contribution to the serial correlation coefficients. Alternation between long and short intervals gives a strongly negative first order coefficient followed by an alternation in sign of the higher order serial correlation coefficients. Thus a negative first order coefficient indicates that long intervals tend to be followed by short intervals and *vice versa*. A positive first order serial correlation coefficient indicates that long intervals tend to be followed by long ones and short intervals by short ones.

Cyclic variations in firing rate produce a damped oscillation in the serial correlogram (Fig. 5B).

When the coefficients stay positive for several orders it means that the data contain runs of high frequency. The length of the run equals the number of coefficients in a positive row. If, *e.g.*, the first 10 orders of coefficients are positive followed by an 11th order coefficient which is negative, then the runs of the intervals all stay above or below the mean interval. Irregular bursts of spikes produce negative low order serial correlation coefficients followed by slightly positive and 0 coefficients.

A gap in the record introduces a long interval, and affects the interval variance and thus distorts the serial correlogram. This effect is of primary importance in pacemaker neurons, where the interval variance is small.

For large interval variance coefficients the effect of trends and gaps on the serial correlogram is small. It is important to reveal this distorting effect, since significant information about the physiology of the neuron, such as refractory and synaptic effects, may be uncovered by correlational analysis of successive intervals (Junge and Moore, 1966). The use of the estimated spectrum of intervals (Cox and Lewis, 1966) overcomes these trends and effects.

Cells that showed obvious serial dependency were rejected for further analysis. It turned out that several registrations were not sufficiently stationary for long periods; therefore we used a sequence of 30–50 consecutive intervals. In some cases two or more series were taken from the same cell at different mean rates. From the first-order

---

Fig. 5. Serial correlogram. The serial coefficients between the intervals $j_{i+1}$ and $j_i$ up to $j_{i+20}$ and $j_i$ for: A. stationary firing neuron without serial dependency, B. drifting neuron with strong serial dependency due to phasic activity.

## TABLE I

STANDARD VARIATION *vs.* MEAN INTERVAL FOR THE FIVE CATEGORIES

$N$ is the number of single cells.

| Category | $N$ | Range of means (msec) | Range of CV | Standard deviation as function of mean |
|----------|-----|------------------------|-------------|----------------------------------------|
| I | 21 | 240–1940 | 0.02–0.10 | $0.005\,(T)^{1.60}$ |
| II | 29 | 320–3070 | 0.04–0.20 | $0.012\,(T)^{1.51}$ |
| III | 35 | 280–8100 | 0.03–0.38 | $0.021\,(T)^{1.47}$ |
| IV | 31 | 280–2720 | 0.03–0.89 | $0.068\,(T)^{1.33}$ |
| V | 19 | 590–3640 | 0.20–1.40 | $0.112\,(T)^{1.33}$ |

interval histograms the mean, standard deviation (SD), mean frequency (1/mean), and coefficient of variation (CV = SD/mean) were obtained with an IBM 1620 computer. The variation of SD with mean could also be described by the power function. The fitting procedure consisted of plotting log SD *vs.* log $X$ and finding the straight line of best fitting by the least square method for the five categories with the IBM 1130 computer. The findings are summarized in Fig. 6 and Table I.

// XEQ PLAN

```
 1   PAR, DDV 3
 2   SCA,SN1,ROTO,LOS10,SMO,SD2,ST1
 3   GRA,XGS12,GIDO
 4   SCA,SN2,SM-100,SD20,ST1,SLP-360
 5   CUR,CDA 120102F
 6   CFILE,NOV2,FDA I+0+1  C0101
 7   REF,RSN9,0,RAC5.5
 8   LAB,LCX18,18,LXC5,9,LTX SERIAL CORRELOGRAM
 9   LAB,LXC5,8.5,LTX   HELIX POMATIA
10   LAB,LXC5,8.0,LTX   DATE
11   TIT,TIN 1,TTX ORDER SERIAL CORRELATION COEFFICIENT
12   TIT,TIN2,TTX PERCENTAGE CORRELATION
13   FINISH
```

```
*ONE WORD INTEGERS
*IOCS(PAPER TAPE)
*IOCS(CARD)
*IOCS(1132PRINTER)
C         SERIAL CORRELATION COEFFICIENT COMPUTING PROGRAM      J.SMITH
C         IBM 1130, 8K SYSTEM, MAX.1600 VAR. AND 40 SERIAL ORDER COEFF.
C         1620 PAPER TAPE INPUT, BCD-CODE, FORMAT(F6.0), EOF SEPARATOR
C         A(1600) IS AN ARRAY OF MAX. 1600 REAL VARIABLES
C         R(1)=R(0) ALWAYS EQUAL TO 1
C         EQUATIONS USED FOR THE K-TH ORDER SERIAL CORR. COEFF.
C         R(K)=(SUM(I=1,M-K)(X(I)-MU(S))/SIGM(S)*(X(I+K)-MU(K))/SIGM(K))/
C         (M-K) IN WHICH, MU(S)=(SUM(I=1,M-K)X(I))/(M-K)   SIGM(S)**2=
C         (SUM(I=1,M-K)(X(I)-MU(S))**2)/(M-K)   MU(K)=(SUM(I=K+1,M)X(I))/
C         (M-K)   SIGM(K)**2=(SUM(I=K+1,M)(X(I)-MU(K))**2)/(M-K)
      DIMENSIONA(1600) ,R(40) ,ARRAY(40,5)
    5 FORMAT (A4,A2,I4,I3)
   10 FORMAT(F6.0)
   15 FORMAT (/////26H SERIAL-CORRELATION         ,A4,A2,// 21H TOTAL NR.OF
     1 DATA     ,I4//26H COMPUTED NR.SERIAL COEFF.,I3)
   20 FORMAT (///11H INPUT DATA///10(F7.0,4X))
   25 FORMAT (12H OUTPUT DATA///46H   COMPUTED VALUES OF   , 1.THE MEAN,
     1MU.      /57H                          2.THE STANDARD DEVIATION,SI
     1GMA./62H                          3.AND THE SERIAL CORR.COEFFICIEN
     1T,R./)
   30 FORMAT (///86H  MU(S)        SIGMA(S)       MU(L))
     1SIGMA(L))    SERIAL CORR.COEFF.  /)
   35 FORMAT (/5(F8.2,8X))
   40 FORMAT (10(F7.2,1H,))
   45 FORMAT(2I2)
   50 FORMAT (1H1)
C         READING THE PARAMETER CARDS, AND THE INPUT DATA, MX=OUTPUT UNIT
C         NUMBER, MY=INPUT UNIT NUMBER, PR=KIND OF ANIMAL, PR1=EXPERIMENT
C         NUMBER,NO=COMPUTED NR.OF SERIAL COEFF.,N=NR.OF INPUT DATA
      READ(2,45)MX,MY
      READ(2,5)PR,PR1,N,NO
C         READING 1620 PAPER-TAPE INPUT DATA
      NA = 0
      DO 55 J=1,N
      READ(4,10)A(J)
      IF (A(J) - 999999.) 55,60,60
   55 NA = NA + 1
C         COMPUTING THE MEAN AND STAND.DEVIATION BY CALLING THE SUBROUTI-
C         NE'MUSIG'
   60 N = NA
      DO 70 K=1,NO
      L = K - 1
      KK = 1
      LL = N - L
      CALL MUSIG(A,KK,LL,NO,AMU,SIGM)
      AMUS = AMU
      SIGMS = SIGM
      KK = L + 1
      LL = N
      CALL MUSIG(A,KK,LL,NO,AMU,SIGM)
      AMUL = AMU
      SIGML = SIGM
C         COMPUTING THE SERIAL ORDER CORRELATION COEFFICIENTS
      M = N - K + 1
```

```
      AM = M                                                    P B R   0 0 0 0
      ANORM = 0.0
      DO 65 I=1,M
      J = I + L
      ANORM = ANORM + ( (A(I) - AMUS) / SIGMS) * ( (A(J) - AMUL) / SIGML
     1)
   65 CONTINUE
      R(K) = (ANORM / AM) * 100.0
C         TABELLING OF THE MEAN, THE STAND.DEV., AND THE SERIAL ORDER COR
C         RELATION COEFFICIENTS
      ARRAY(K,1) = AMUS
      ARRAY(K,2) = SIGMS
      ARRAY(K,3) = AMUL
      ARRAY(K,4) = SIGML
      ARRAY(K,5) = R(K)
   70 CONTINUE
C     OUTPUT
      WRITE(MX,50)
      WRITE(MX,15)PR,PR1,N,NO
      WRITE(MX,20)(A(I),I=1,N)
      WRITE(MX,50)
      WRITE(MX,25)
      WRITE(MX,30)
      WRITE(MX,35)((ARRAY(K,L),L=1,5),K=1,NO)
      READ(2,45)
      WRITE(2,40)(R(K),K=1,NO)
      STOP
      END
*ONE WORD INTEGERS
C         SUBROUTINE COMPUTING THE MEAN(MU) AND STAND.DEV.(SIGM)
C         CALLING SEQUENCE CALL MUSIG(A,KK,LL,NO,AMU,SIGM)
C         KK=FIRST REAL VARIABLE, LL=LAST REAL VARIABLE, NO=NUMBER OF
C         SERIAL ORDER COEFFICIENTS, AMU=MEAN OF THE VARIABLES, SIGM=STAN
C         DEV.OF THE VARIABLES
      SUBROUTINEMUSIG(A,KK,LL,NO,AMU,SIGM)
      DIMENSIONA(1600)
      SOM = 0.0
      ANORM = 0.0
      AANT = LL - KK + 1
      DO 75 I=KK,LL
      SOM = SOM + A(I)
   75 CONTINUE
      AMU = SOM / AANT
      DO 80 I=KK,LL
      ANORM = ANORM + (A(I) - AMU) * * 2
   80 CONTINUE
      SIGM = SQRT(ANORM / AANT)
      RETURN
      END
*STORE      WS  UA  MUSIG
```

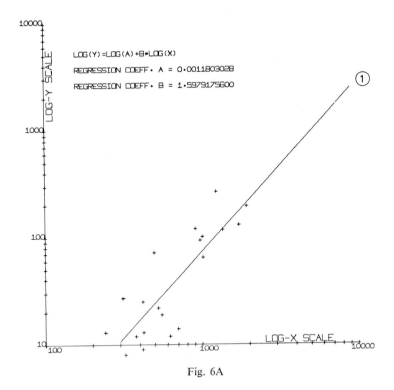

Fig. 6A

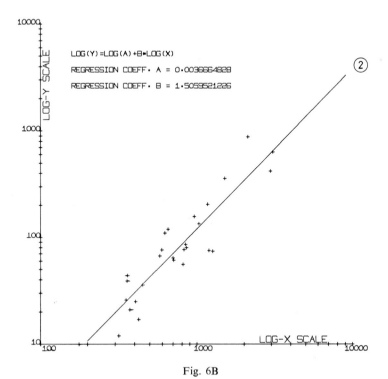

Fig. 6B

References p. 256

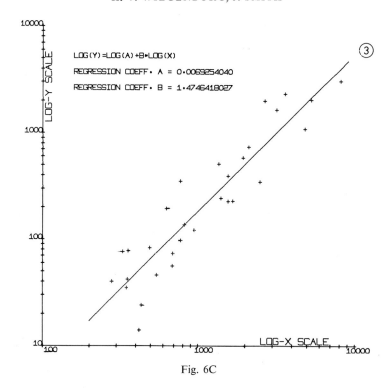

Fig. 6C

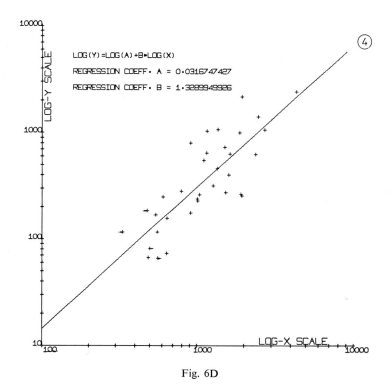

Fig. 6D

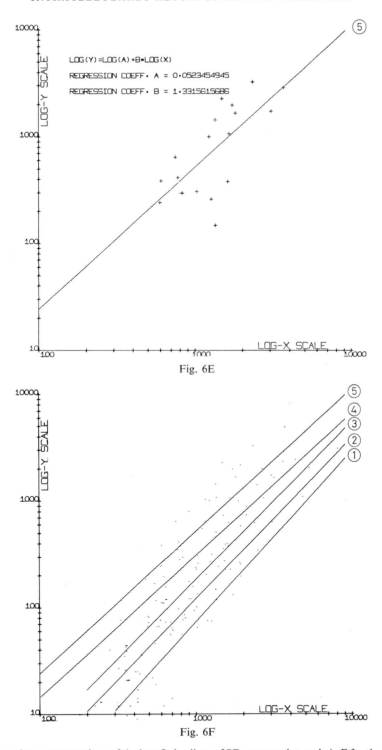

Fig. 6E

Fig. 6F

Fig. 6. Log–log representations of the best fitting lines of SD *vs.* mean interval. A–E for the individual categories. Dots represent single cells. F. the five regression lines of the above categories.

*References p. 256*

## DISCUSSION

The data from the snail neurons were divided into five categories. We must be careful in interpreting these data since the categories were based on the postsynaptic potentials We have tried to obtain the parameters from unimodel histograms with mean values close to the modes. This was not always the fact with cells that exhibited inhibition of long duration. At present it is difficult to understand the variation in the slope of the regression line from 1.60 for pacemaker neurons to 1.33 for cells with inhibition of long duration. Nevertheless we may safely assume that synaptic noise adds an extra source of neural variability to that of endogenous origin. As can be seen in Fig. 6, for the same mean value the standard deviation increases with more postsynaptic potentials for all firing rates. Synaptic noise as a source of randomness may be either of postsynaptic origin or of presynaptic origin, *e.g.*, spontaneous release of neurotransmitter or impulse activity arriving in the presynaptic terminals. The use of the power function to relate SD and mean of interval histograms has also been studied by Junge and Moore (1966) for *Aplysia* pacemaker neurons. They found a value of $0.00949 \cdot (T)^{1.21}$ for the standard deviation as a function of the mean. The difference in slope— 1.60 in our experiments for pacemaker neurons as compared to 1.21 for the *Aplysia* pacemaker neurons— might be due to differences in recording conditions.

## SUMMARY

An analysis of action potentials from spontaneous firing neurons in the central nervous system of the snail *Helix pomatia* was presented. On the basis of the postsynaptic potentials five categories of neurons have been selected. The interspike interval distributions were described by the interval histograms taking into account the phenomena of stationarity. The course of the firing frequency, the representation of consecutive intervals and the serial correlogram were used as tests of stationarity. The latter was also a test of independency between intervals. The standard deviation *vs.* mean interval was described by the coefficient of variation and the power function for the five categories.

## REFERENCES

Cox, D. R. and Lewis, P. A. W. (1966) *The Statistical Analysis of Series of Events*, Wiley, New York.

Junge, D. and Moore, G. P. (1966) Interspike interval fluctuations in *Aplysia* pacemaker neurons. *Biophys. J.,* 6, 411–434,

Moore, G. P., Perkel, D. H. and Segundo, J. S. (1966) Statistical analysis and functional interpretation of neuronal spike data. *Ann. Rev. Physiol.*, 28.

Parzen, E. (1962) Stochastic Processes, Holden-Day, San Francisco.

Perkel, D. H., Gerstein, G. L. and Moore, G. P. (1967) Neuronal spike trains and stochastic point-processes. *Biophys. J.*, 7, 391–440.

Poggio, G. F. and Viernstein, L. J. (1964) Time series analysis of impulse sequences of thalamic somatic sensory neurons. *J. Neurophysiol.*, 27, 517–545.

Rodieck, R. W., Kiang, N. Y. S. and Gerstein, G. L. (1962) Some quantitative methods for the study of spontaneous activity of single neurons. *Biophys. J.*, 2, 351.

Smith, D. R. and Smith, G. K. (1965) A statistical analysis of the continual activity of single cortical neurones in the cat unanaesthetized isolated forebrain. *Biophys. J.*, 5, 47–74.

Tauc, L. (1966) *Physiology of the Nervous System. Physiology of Mollusca II*, Academic Press, New York, pp. 387–411.

Werner, G. and Mountcastle, V. B. (1963) The variability of central neural activity in a sensory system and its implications for the central reflection of sensory events. *J. Neurophysiol.*, 26, 958–977.

Wilgenburg, H. van (1969) The axon reflex in *Helix pomatia*. *Curr. Mod. Biol.*, 3, 1–3.

# Author Index

# Subject Index

THE